Prenatal Screening and Diagnosis: An Update

Editors

ANTHONY O. ODIBO
DAVID A. KRANTZ

CLINICS IN LABORATORY MEDICINE

www.labmed.theclinics.com

Editorial Board
KENT B. LEWANDROWSKI
MATTHEW R. PINCUS

June 2016 • Volume 36 • Number 2

ELSEVIER

1600 John F. Kennedy Boulevard ● Suite 1800 ● Philadelphia, Pennsylvania, 19103-2899

http://www.theclinics.com

CLINICS IN LABORATORY MEDICINE Volume 36, Number 2
June 2016 ISSN 0272-2712, ISBN-13: 978-0-323-44620-4

Editor: Lauren Boyle
Developmental Editor: Colleen Viola

Reprints. For copies of 100 or more, of articles in this publication, please contact the Commercial Reprints Department, Elsevier Inc., 360 Park Avenue South, New York, New York 10010-1710. Tel. 212-633-3874, Fax: 212-633-3820, E-mail: reprints@elsevier.com.

Clinics in Laboratory Medicine (ISSN 0272-2712) is published quarterly by Elsevier Inc., 360 Park Avenue South, New York, NY 10010-1710. Months of issue are March, June, September, and December. Business and Editorial offices: 1600 John F. Kennedy Blvd., Suite 1800, Philadelphia, PA 19103-2899. Periodicals postage paid at NewYork, NY and additional mailing offices. Subscription prices are $250.00 per year (US individuals), $469.00 per year (US institutions), $100.00 per year (US students), $305.00 per year (Canadian individuals), $570.00 per year (Canadian institutions), $185.00 per year (Canadian students), $390.00 per year (international individuals), $570.00 per year (international institutions), $185.00 (international students). Foreign air speed delivery is included in all Clinics subscription prices. All prices are subject to change without notice. POSTMASTER: Send address changes to *Clinics in Laboratory Medicine*, Elsevier Health Sciences Division, Subscription Customer Service, 3251 Riverport Lane, Maryland Heights, MO 63043. **Customer Service: 1-800-654-2452 (US). From outside of the US and Canada, call 1-314-447-8871. Fax: 1-314-447-8029. E-mail: journalscustomerservice-usa@elsevier.com (for print support) or journalsonlinesuppor-t-usa@elsevier.com (for online support).**

Clinics in Laboratory Medicine is covered in *EMBASE/Exerpta Medica, MEDLINE/PubMed (Index Medicus), Cinahl, Current Contents/Clinical Medicine, BIOSIS and ISI/BIOMED*.

Contributors

EDITORS

ANTHONY O. ODIBO, MD, MSCE
Professor, Division of Maternal Fetal Medicine, Department of Obstetrics and Gynecology, University of South Florida Morsani College of Medicine, Tampa, Florida

DAVID A. KRANTZ, MA
Director of Biostatics, Eurofins/NTD, Melville, New York

AUTHORS

ALFRED Z. ABUHAMAD, MD
Professor and Chairman, Department of Obstetrics and Gynecology, Eastern Virginia Medical School, Norfolk, Virginia

STEPHANIE ANDRIOLE, MS, CGC
Comprehensive Genetics, PLLC, New York, New York

MATTHEW J. BLITZ, MD, MBA
Division of Maternal-Fetal Medicine, Department of Obstetrics and Gynecology, Hofstra North Shore-LIJ School of Medicine, North Shore University Hospital, Manhasset, New York

ADAM F. BORGIDA, MD
Associate Professor of Obstetrics and Gynecology, Division of Maternal Fetal Medicine, Prenatal Testing Center, Hartford Hospital, University of Connecticut School of Medicine, Farmington, Connecticut

EMMANUEL BUJOLD, MD, MSc
Department of Social and Preventive Medicine; Professor, Department of Obstetrics and Gynecology, Faculty of Medicine, Jeanne et Jean-Louis Lévesque Perinatal Research Chair, Université Laval, Quebec City, Quebec, Canada

MARY ASHLEY CAIN, MD
Assistant Professor, Division of Maternal Fetal Medicine, Department of Obstetrics and Gynecology, University of South Florida Morsani College of Medicine, Tampa, Florida

JONATHAN B. CARMICHAEL, PhD
Director of BioAssay Development, Eurofins/NTD, Melville, New York

ANGELINA CARTIN
Division of Maternal-Fetal Medicine, Department of Obstetrics and Gynecology, Maine Medical Partners Women's Health, Maine Medical Center, Portland, Maine

RENÉE L. CHARD, MSc, CGC
Division of Maternal-Fetal Medicine, Maine Medical Partners Women's Health, Portland, Maine

HOWARD CUCKLE, BA, MSc, DPhil
Adjunct Professor, Department of Obstetrics and Gynecology, Columbia University Medical Center, New York, New York

PE'ER DAR, MD, FACOG, FACMG
Associate Professor of Obstetrics and Gynecology; Division Director Fetal Medicine, Department of Obstetrics and Gynecology and Women's Health, Montefiore Medical Center, Albert Einstein College of Medicine, Bronx, New York

MARK I. EVANS, MD
Professor, Department of Obstetrics and Gynecology, Mt. Sinai School of Medicine; Director, Comprehensive Genetics and President, Fetal Medicine Foundation of America, New York, New York

SHARA M. EVANS, MSc, MPH
Comprehensive Genetics, PLLC, New York, New York; Senior Research Assistant, Department of Obstetrics and Gynecology, University of Colorado, Aurora, Colorado

DEBORAH M. FELDMAN, MD
Associate Professor of Obstetrics and Gynecology, Division of Maternal Fetal Medicine, Prenatal Testing Center, Hartford Hospital, University of Connecticut School of Medicine, Farmington, Connecticut

KATHERINE R. GOETZINGER, MD, MSCI
Assistant Professor, Department of Obstetrics, Gynecology and Reproductive Medicine, University of Maryland School of Medicine, Baltimore, Maryland

TERRENCE W. HALLAHAN, PhD
Laboratory Director, Eurofins/NTD, Melville, New York

ANTHONY N. IMUDIA, MD
Assistant Professor, Division of Reproductive Endocrinology and Infertility, University of South Florida Morsani College of Medicine, Tampa, Florida

KARL OLIVER KAGAN, MD, PhD
Professor, University of Tübingen, Tübingen, Germany

REBECCA KELLER, MD
Instructor in Obstetrics and Gynecology, Maternal Fetal Medicine, UConn Health Center, University of Connecticut School of Medicine, Farmington, Connecticut

DAVID A. KRANTZ, MA
Director of Biostatics, Eurofins/NTD, Melville, New York

BRYNN LEVY, MSc (Med), PhD, FACMG
Professor of Pathology and Cell Biology, Columbia University Medical Center, New York, New York

A. ASHLEIGH LONG, MD, PhD
Department of Obstetrics and Gynecology, Eastern Virginia Medical School, Norfolk, Virginia

JUDETTE M. LOUIS, MD, MPH
Assistant Professor, Division of Maternal Fetal Medicine, Department of Obstetrics and Gynecology, University of South Florida Morsani College of Medicine; Department of Community and Family Health, College of Public Health, University of South Florida, Tampa, Florida

ADETOLA F. LOUIS-JACQUES, MD
Fellow, Division of Maternal Fetal Medicine, Department of Obstetrics and Gynecology, University of South Florida Morsani College of Medicine, Tampa, Florida

LINDSAY MAGGIO, MD, MPH
Assistant Professor, Division of Maternal Fetal Medicine, Department of Obstetrics and Gynecology, University of South Florida Morsani College of Medicine, Tampa, Florida

KYPROS H. NICOLAIDES, MD
Professor, Harris Birthright Research Centre for Fetal Medicine, King's College Hospital, London, United Kingdom

MARY E. NORTON, MD
Department of Obstetrics, Gynecology, and Reproductive Sciences, University of California, San Francisco, San Francisco, California

ANTHONY O. ODIBO, MD, MSCE
Professor, Division of Maternal Fetal Medicine, Department of Obstetrics and Gynecology, University of South Florida Morsani College of Medicine, Tampa, Florida

MICHAEL G. PINETTE, MD
Division of Maternal-Fetal Medicine, Department of Obstetrics and Gynecology, Maine Medical Partners Women's Health, Maine Medical Center, Portland, Maine

SHAYNE PLOSKER, MD
Professor, Division of Reproductive Endocrinology and Infertility, University of South Florida Morsani College of Medicine, Tampa, Florida

STEPHANIE ROBERGE, MSc
Department of Social and Preventive Medicine, Faculty of Medicine, Université Laval, Quebec City, Quebec, Canada

BURTON ROCHELSON, MD
Chief of Maternal-Fetal Medicine; Director of Obstetrics and Gynecology; Professor, Hofstra North Shore-LIJ School of Medicine, North Shore University Hospital, Manhasset, New York

ALEJANDRO RODRIGUEZ, MD
Clinical Fellow, Division of Maternal-Fetal Medicine, Department of Obstetrics and Gynecology, University of South Florida Morsani College of Medicine, Tampa, Florida

STEPHANIE T. ROMERO, MD
Assistant Professor, Division of Maternal Fetal Medicine, Department of Obstetrics and Gynecology, University of South Florida Morsani College of Medicine, Tampa, Florida

HAGIT SHANI, MD
Fellow Clinical Genetics, Department of Obstetrics and Gynecology and Women's Health, Montefiore Medical Center, Albert Einstein College of Medicine, Bronx, New York

RACHEL G. SINKEY, MD
Division of Maternal-Fetal Medicine, Department of Obstetrics and Gynecology, University of South Florida, Tampa, Florida

JIRI D. SONEK, MD, RDMS
Center for Maternal-Fetal Medicine, Ultrasound, and Genetics, Fetal Medicine Foundation of USA, Clinical Professor, Wright State University, Dayton, Ohio

METHODIUS G. TUULI, MD, MPH
Assistant Professor, Division of Maternal-Fetal Medicine, Department of Obstetrics and Gynecology, Washington University School of Medicine, St Louis, Missouri

NIDHI VOHRA, MD
Director of Maternal-Fetal Medicine; Chief of Prenatal Diagnosis; Assistant Professor, Department of Obstetrics and Gynecology, Hofstra North Shore-LIJ School of Medicine, North Shore University Hospital, Manhasset, New York

RONALD J. WAPNER, MD
Professor of Obstetrics and Gynecology, Division of Maternal-Fetal Medicine, Department of Obstetrics and Gynecology, Columbia University Medical Center, New York, New York

STEVEN L. WARSOF, MD
Professor, Director of Genetics and Prenatal Diagnosis, Department of Obstetrics and Gynecology, Eastern Virginia Medical School, Norfolk, Virginia

JOSEPH R. WAX, MD
Division of Maternal-Fetal Medicine, Department of Obstetrics and Gynecology, Maine Medical Partners Women's Health, Maine Medical Center, Portland, Maine

KAREN WOU, MD
Clinical Genetics Fellow, Division of Clinical Genetics, Department of Pediatrics, Columbia University Medical Center, New York, New York

RUOFAN YAO, MD, MPH
Fellow, Maternal Fetal Medicine, Department of Obstetrics, Gynecology and Reproductive Medicine, University of Maryland School of Medicine, Baltimore, Maryland

Contents

> Cell-free fetal DNA screening for Down syndrome has gained rapid accep-
> tance over the past few years with increasing market penetration. Three
> main laboratory methodologies are currently used: a massive parallel
> shotgun sequencing (MPSS), a targeted massive parallel sequencing
> (t-MPS) and a single nucleotide polymorphism (SNP) based approach.
> Although each of these technologies has its own advantages and
> disadvantages, the performance of all was shown to be comparable and
> superior to that of traditional first-trimester screening for the detection of
> trisomy 21 in a routine prenatal population. Differences in performance
> were predominantly shown for chromosomal anomalies other than trisomy
> 21. Understanding the limitations and benefits of each technology is
> essential for proper counseling to patients. These technologies, as well
> as few investigational technologies described in this review, carry a great
> potential beyond screening for the common aneuploidies.

> Maternal plasma cell-free (cf) DNA testing has higher discriminatory power
> for aneuploidy than any conventional multi-marker screening test. Several
> strategies have been suggested for introducing it into clinical practice.
> Secondary cfDNA, restricted only to women with positive conventional
> screening test, is generally cost saving and minimizes the need for invasive
> prenatal diagnosis but leads to a small loss in detection. Primary cfDNA,
> replacing conventional screening or retaining the nuchal translucency
> scan, is not currently cost-effective for third-party payers. Contingent
> cfDNA, testing about 20% of women with the highest risks based on a con-
> ventional test, is the preferred approach.

> With the introduction of cell-free DNA screening for fetal aneuploidy and
> chromosomal microarray for prenatal diagnostic testing, options for preg-
> nant women have become increasingly complex. Discussions regarding
> options for prenatal testing for aneuploidy should occur prior to any testing
> and should include pertinent risks and benefits of each alternative test.
> There is no single screening or diagnostic test option that is the right

choice for all patients; patient decisions should be based on each individual woman's values and preferences after a discussion of all options.

Cost-effectiveness analyses allow assessment of whether marginal gains from new technology are worth increased costs. Several studies have examined cost-effectiveness of Down syndrome (DS) screening and found it to be cost-effective. Noninvasive prenatal screening also appears to be cost-effective among high-risk women with respect to DS screening, but not for the general population. Chromosomal microarray (CMA) is a genetic sequencing method superior to but more expensive than karyotype. In light of CMAs greater ability to detect genetic abnormalities, it is cost-effective when used for prenatal diagnosis of an anomalous fetus. This article covers methodology and salient issues of cost-effectiveness.

Noninvasive genomic assessments of the fetus while in utero have been made possible by the analysis of cell-free fetal DNA fragments from the serum of pregnant women, as part of a noninvasive prenatal testing screening strategy. Between 7% and 10% of total cell-free DNA in the maternal blood comes from placental trophoblasts, allowing for identification of the DNA associated with the fetal component of the placenta. Using simple venipuncture in the outpatient setting, this cell-free, extracellular fetal DNA can be isolated in the maternal serum from a single blood draw as early as the seventh week of gestation.

Chromosomal microarray analysis has replaced conventional G-banded karyotype in prenatal diagnosis as the first-tier test for the cytogenetic detection of copy number imbalances in fetuses with/without major structural abnormalities. This article reviews the basic technology of microarray; the value and clinical significance of the detection of microdeletions, microduplications, and other copy number variants; as well as the importance of genetic counseling for prenatal diagnosis. It also discusses the current status of noninvasive screening for some of these microdeletion and microduplication syndromes.

Historically, carrier screening for a small number of autosomal recessive disorders has been offered to targeted populations based on ethnicity and family history. These chosen disorders are associated with severe morbidity or mortality, have a well-established carrier frequency in the targeted population, and have an acceptably high detection rate to make screening efficient. With advancing genetic technology, expanded panels rapidly are being designed and offered to the panethnic general population. This article reviews current recommendations for ethnicity-specific carrier screening for common disorders as well as the limitations and counseling complexities associated with expanded panels.

The choice of screening or invasive procedure in twin pregnancies is a personal choice of whether the patient wishes to take a small risk of having a baby with a serious disorder versus a small risk of having a complication because she wishes to avoid that. How to interpret such risks has profound effects on the perceived value of techniques, either leading to a decision to screen or going directly to chorionic villus sampling. There are profound issues surrounding the data and the interpretation of the data. No single short review can exhaustively examine all of the issues.

First-trimester pregnancy evaluation using fetal and maternal parameters not only allows for diagnoses to be made early in gestation but can also assess the risk of complications that become clinically evident later in pregnancy. This evaluation makes it possible for pregnancy care to be individualized. In select cases, treatment that reduces the risk of complications can be started early in pregnancy. Even though cell-free DNA is a significant advance in diagnosing fetal aneuploidy, the combination of first-trimester ultrasound and maternal serum biochemistries casts a much wider diagnostic net; therefore, the two technologies are best used in combination.

Low-dose aspirin (LDA) has been used for several years for the prevention of preeclampsia (PE). LDA started in early pregnancy is associated with improvement of placental implantation. The best evidence suggests that LDA can prevent more than half of PE cases in high-risk women when started before 16 weeks of gestation. Moreover, LDA started in early pregnancy reduces the risk of other placenta-mediated complications such as intrauterine growth restriction (IUGR) and perinatal death. The efficacy of LDA has been demonstrated in women with abnormal first-trimester uterine artery Doppler or with prior history of chronic hypertension or preeclampsia.

Preeclampsia and intrauterine growth restriction are major contributors
to perinatal mortality and morbidity. Accurate prediction is important
for identifying those who require more intensive monitoring, permitting
earlier recognition and intervention and targeting of potential preventive
measures. Although measures of placental dysfunction have been associated with increased risk adverse pregnancy outcomes, the ability of
any single measure to predict these outcomes is poor. Predictive models
combining analytes and measurements of placental structure and blood
flow have produced mixed results. Biochemical markers plus uterine artery Doppler screening throughout gestation show promise as screening
tools. Published studies, however, suggest limited clinical applicability.

Abnormal levels of maternal serum analytes have been associated with
fetal growth restriction (FGR) and preeclampsia secondary to placental
vascular dysfunction. Accurately identifying the FGR fetuses at highest
risk for adverse outcomes remains challenging. Placental function can
be assessed by Doppler analysis of the maternal and fetal circulation.
Although the combination of multiple abnormal maternal serum analytes
and abnormal Doppler findings is strongly associated with adverse outcomes, the predictive value remains too low to be used as a screening
test in a low-risk population. Stratification of cases based on the severity
of Doppler abnormalities may improve predictive models.

The heterogeneous causes of spontaneous preterm birth make prediction
and prevention difficult. Recently developed biochemical and biophysical
tests add significantly to clinicians' ability to evaluate and treat women at
risk for spontaneous preterm birth. The primary importance of transvaginal
cervical sonography and cervicovaginal fetal fibronectin lies in the high
negative predictive values of the tests for preterm delivery risk. Cervical
length may be useful in identifying women who are candidates for cervical
cerclage or progesterone therapy for preterm birth prevention. Together,
cervical length and fibronectin can be used in the triaging of women symptomatic for preterm labor.

Preimplantation genetic testing (PGT) of oocytes and embryos is the
earliest form of prenatal testing. PGT requires in vitro fertilization for

embryo creation. In the past 25 years, the use of PGT has increased dramatically. The indications of PGT include identification of embryos harboring single-gene disorders, chromosomal structural abnormalities, chromosomal numeric abnormalities, and mitochondrial disorders; gender selection; and identifying unaffected, HLA-matched embryos to permit the creation of a savior sibling. PGT is not without risks, limitations, or ethical controversies. This review discusses the techniques and clinical applications of different forms of PGT and the debate surrounding its associated uncertainty and expanded use.

David A. Krantz, Terrence W. Hallahan, and Jonathan B. Carmichael

Biochemical prenatal screening was initiated with the use of maternal serum alpha fetoprotein to screen for open neural tube defects. Screening now includes multiple marker and sequential screening protocols involving serum and ultrasound markers to screen for aneuploidy. Recently cell-free DNA screening for aneuploidy has been initiated but does not screen for neural tube defects. Although ultrasound is highly effective in identifying neural tube defects in high-risk populations, in decentralized health systems maternal serum screening still plays a significant role. Abnormal maternal serum alpha fetoprotein alone, or in combination with other markers, may indicate adverse pregnancy outcome in the absence of open neural tube defects.

Deborah M. Feldman, Rebecca Keller, and Adam F. Borgida

There are several infections in adults that warrant special consideration in pregnant women given the potential fetal consequences. Among these are toxoplasmosis, parvovirus B19, and cytomegalovirus. These infections have an important impact on the developing fetus, depending on the timing of infection. This article reviews the modes of transmission as well as maternal and neonatal effects of each of these infections. In addition, the article outlines recommended testing, fetal surveillance, and treatment where indicated.

Adetola F. Louis-Jacques, Lindsay Maggio, and Stephanie T. Romero

Pregnancy is associated with increased clotting potential and decreased fibrinolysis. Women with thrombophilias have an increased risk of venous thromboembolism during pregnancy. At least 50% of cases of venous thromboembolism in pregnant women are associated with an inherited or acquired thrombophilia. Acquired thrombophilias have also been linked with adverse pregnancy outcomes, such as recurrent pregnancy loss, intrauterine fetal demise, early onset severe preeclampsia, placental abruption, and fetal growth restriction. This article addresses indications for thrombophilia testing, the appropriate laboratory tests, and timing of testing to ensure reliability of results.

Sleep disordered breathing (SDB) occurs in 0.6% to 15% of reproductive-aged women. Because of an overlap in symptoms of SDB and normal pregnancy findings, the diagnosis of SDB in pregnancy is challenging. The repetitive arousals, sleep fragmentation, and hypoxias experienced by patients with SDB lead to an increase in oxidative stress and inflammation. In the nonpregnant population, SDB is associated with an increased risk of diabetes mellitus, heart disease, and stroke. Increasing evidence identifies an association between SDB in pregnancy and gestational diabetes, preeclampsia, and fetal growth abnormalities.

CLINICS IN LABORATORY MEDICINE

Preface

Prenatal Screening: The Birth of a New Era

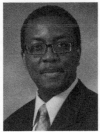
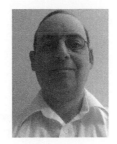

Anthony O. Odibo, MD, MSCE   David A. Krantz, MA
Editors

We cannot believe that it is just over 5 years ago that we were invited as guest editors for a *Clinics in Laboratory Medicine* issue dedicated to Prenatal Screening. Yet, these last 5 years have witnessed a tremendous paradigm shift in aneuploidy screening, mostly resulting from the breakthrough in research and introduction of cell-free fetal DNA technology. Although this new technology has been rapidly adopted for high-risk pregnancies, the application of such technology to the general population remains the focus of debate, with several authors commenting on this subject in this issue. Also in the last 5 years, we have seen the introduction into clinical practice of genetic carrier screening as well as greater use of chromosome microarray analysis to identify micro-duplications and microdeletions. Recent reports have evaluated the possibility of iden-tifying a limited number of microdeletions and duplications using cell-free fetal DNA technology as well.

While these advances in genetic analysis were taking place, new applications for serum and ultrasound markers were being developed. The most promising of these are screening tools for pre-eclampsia and intrauterine growth restriction, especially the early-onset and more clinically significant form of these conditions. Coincident with the development of these new tools has been a re-evaluation of the ability of low-dose aspirin to prevent pre-eclampsia, thus providing a potential clinical pathway following high-risk screening results for these disorders.

With the obesity epidemic occurring in the United States and globally, a major complication, sleep apnea, and its contribution to adverse pregnancy outcome, is becoming recognized. A new article dedicated to this has been added. In addition, previous articles that were retained have been updated. Previous articles addressing screening for preterm birth risk and viral and parasitic infections have been updated.

We are deeply honored that the authors of the following articles, representing the leading experts in prenatal screening and diagnosis, participated in this issue. We also acknowledge the contributions of the authors of the previous issue; some of

Clin Lab Med 36 (2016) xv–xvi
http://dx.doi.org/10.1016/j.cll.2016.01.014   **labmed.theclinics.com**
0272-2712/16/$ – see front matter © 2016 Published by Elsevier Inc.

whom could not help with the current issue. Their prior work, however, was updated for inclusion.

Anthony O. Odibo, MD, MSCE
University of South Florida–
Morsani College of Medicine
2 Tampa General Circle
Tampa, FL 33606, USA

David A. Krantz, MA
Eurofins/NTD
80 Ruland Road, Suite 1
Melville, NY 11747, USA

E-mail addresses:
aodibo@health.usf.edu (A.O. Odibo)
david.krantz@perkinelmer.com (D.A. Krantz)

Cell-free DNA
Comparison of Technologies

Pe'er Dar, MD[a], Hagit Shani, MD[a], Mark I. Evans, MD[b,c],*

KEYWORDS

- Cell-free fetal DNA • Noninvasive prenatal screening • Next-generation sequencing
- Multiple parallel shotgun sequencing • Selected probes • Selective sequencing
- Single nucleotide polymorphisms • DNA methylation

KEY POINTS

- Use of cell-free fetal DNA has increased dramatically over the past few years.
- There are 2 main methods currently in use: next-generation sequencing and selected probes or selected sequencing.
- Expansion to microdeletion and duplication analysis is emerging. Statistical performance is variable among chromosomes.
- There is confusion among patients and physicians as to the capabilities and limitations of such screening.

INTRODUCTION

For more than half a century, definitive prenatal diagnosis of chromosome and mendelian disorders has been possible and widely available, but it has been done only by obtaining fetal cells through invasive diagnostic procedures.[1,2] Because such procedures carry associated risks of miscarriage, are expensive, and require labor intensive care and sophisticated technology, they cannot be realistically offered to all patients.[3] Screening tests, using maternal serum screening and ultrasonography, made significant advancements in the last 4 decades but can alter odds and are not diagnostic.[3]

Looking for fetal cells has been the goal of prenatal diagnosis for more than a century.[4] Therefore, the first approach to obtain fetal DNA noninvasively centered on the search for fetal cells in the maternal circulation.[5–7] Following Lo and colleagues'[8] patent and publication in 1997 on the presence of paternally derived fetal cell-free DNA (cfDNA) in maternal serum, a second line of investigation has focused first on cfDNA, then free fetal RNA, and back to cfDNA in the mother's circulation.[9,10]

[a] Department of Obstetrics & Gynecology and Women's Health, Montefiore Medical Center, Albert Einstein College of Medicine, 1695 Eastchester Road, Bronx, New York 10461, USA; [b] Department of Obstetrics and Gynecology, Mt. Sinai School of Medicine, New York, NY, USA; [c] Comprehensive Genetics and Fetal Medicine Foundation of America, 131 East 65th Street, New York, NY 10065, USA
* Corresponding author. Comprehensive Genetics, 131 East 65th Street, New York, NY 10065.
E-mail address: evans@compregen.com

Clin Lab Med 36 (2016) 199–211
http://dx.doi.org/10.1016/j.cll.2016.01.015
0272-2712/16/$ – see front matter © 2016 Elsevier Inc. All rights reserved.

labmed.theclinics.com

Since it became commercially available in late 2011, cfDNA-based noninvasive prenatal screening (NIPS) for fetal aneuploidy has seen an unprecedentedly rapid increase in clinical implementation.[11,12] Although most cfDNA screens initially targeted trisomy 21, screening quickly expanded to include detection of trisomy 18, trisomy 13, and some sex chromosome aneuploidies, and now also selected microdeletions and microduplications for numerous other conditions.[11–23]

The initial investigation of noninvasive fetal DNA evaluation focused on NIH-funded studies of fetal cells in maternal blood but were unsuccessful. After these failed attempts, research and funding shifted from government funding in the academic domain to the private sector and the focus shifted from fetal cell DNA to cfDNA. This approach also experienced difficulties as companies attempted to rush to commercialization before tests were appropriately validated. Nevertheless, cfDNA screening was eventually validated by several clinical studies, and each showed considerable improvements in sensitivities and specificities compared with conventional serum screening approaches.[12–14,16,19,20,24–28]

The use of noninvasive diagnostics has potential far beyond aneuploidy, including screening for microdeletions, microduplications, and even single gene mutations; more than 1 company now offers screening for microdeletions and microduplications syndromes through cfDNA. This topic is discussed in more detail, elsewhere in this issue (See Wou K, Levy B, Wapner RJ: Chromosomal Microarrays for the Prenatal Detection of Microdeletions and Microduplications, in this issue).

CELL-FREE DNA

Lo and colleagues[9] suggested that most cfDNA in maternal serum is of maternal origin. In their report from 1998, the fraction of cfDNA of fetal origin was between 3% and 6% depending on gestational age. More recent studies show a much higher variability and larger range of cfDNA in maternal plasma (closer to 10%). Dar and colleagues[29] reported on an average fetal fraction of 10.2% and a wide range from 0.6% to 50% in a large clinical data set. Fetal fraction is associated with several factors, the most significant being the gestational age. By 9 weeks, fetal fraction averages 8% to 10%. There is a modest increase of 0.1% per week from 9 to 20 weeks' gestation. A more significant increase of 0.6% per week is seen from 21 weeks onwards. There is also a significant inverse correlation between maternal weight and fetal fraction. For every 4.5-kg (10 pound) increase in maternal weight there is roughly a 0.5% decrease in fetal fraction for maternal weights between 36.5 and 91 kg (80 and 200 pounds), and a 0.3% decrease for maternal weights more than 91 g. The decrease in fetal fraction with increased maternal weight could be attributed to a dilutional effect caused by increased maternal blood volume or increased maternal adipocyte cfDNA release.[30] Fetal fractions were also lower in women of Afro-Caribbean origin than in white people.[30]

Fetal fraction have been observed to vary based on presence of aneuploidy. Fetal fractions were decreased for trisomy 13 (0.741 Multiple of Medians [MoM]), trisomy 18 (0.919 MoM) and monosomy X (0.84 MoM). In contrast, fetal fractions for trisomy 21 samples were increased (1.045 MoM). Palomaki and colleagues[31] showed similar results for trisomy 21 and for trisomy 18. The median fetal fraction in Down syndrome pregnancies is, on average, 17% higher than in euploid pregnancies and the median level in trisomy 18 pregnancies is 29% lower. Digynic triploidy also has a median fetal fraction that is 81% lower than euploid pregnancies. In contrast, in trisomy 13, monosomy X, sex trisomies, and mosaic fetuses fetal fraction medians were similar to those found in euploid pregnancies.[31]

The second aspect of cfDNA of fetal origin is the size. Fetal cfDNA fragments tend to be shorter than maternal fragments, averaging only about 300 versus greater than 500 base pairs for maternal fragments.[32,33] The difference has been attributed to differential mechanisms of apoptosis between syncytiotrophoblasts and maternal cell apoptosis and serves as the basis for attempts to discriminate fetal and maternal DNA for evaluation.

In addition, although it is commonly referred to as cfDNA of fetal origin, the origin of the so-called fetal cfDNA is placental, and more specifically the syncytiotrophoblast. Although, in most cases, the placenta and the fetus share the same genetics, 1% to 2% of placentae have confined placental mosaicism,[34,35] most commonly involving chromosomal trisomy.

ISOLATION OF FETAL CELL-FREE DNA

Circulating cfDNA is a challenging analyte for extraction owing to its low concentration in plasma. Fetal cfDNA represents only a small portion of the total cfDNA in maternal plasma, and added to the fact that half of fetal DNA originates from the mother, this makes its isolation even more complicated. Several approaches have been suggested that allow enrichment of the fetal component. The most obvious approach was trying to separate the DNA fragments by size.[36]

A few laboratories showed some success in sample enrichment by using gel size fractionation with or without whole-genome amplification of the smaller fragments. An alternative strategy, developed by the laboratory of Dennis Lo in Hong Kong, was the use of matrix-assisted laser desorption ionization time-of-flight mass spectrometry for the detection of fetal point mutations.[37] Dhallan and colleagues[38] tried to lower the maternal DNA fraction by suppressing maternal DNA release from the cells, adding formaldehyde to stabilize the cells.

Another approach was trying to take advantage of the different methylation pattern of fetal DNA. Papageorgiou and colleagues[39] tried to use the different immunoprecipitation pattern of the fetal hypermethylated DNA. Chim and colleagues[40] investigated markers on chromosome 21 that might be amenable to epigenetic differences and found 19 markers that are differentially methylated between maternal and fetal tissues. However, at this time, these approaches have not been accepted into clinical practice to identify chromosome abnormalities. However, differentiating fetal DNA from maternal DNA based on methylation markers[12,21] or by comparing relative representation of fetal and maternal haplotypes[23] is currently being used for the calculation of fetal fraction.

SCREENING FOR ANEUPLOIDY

Three main NIPS approaches have been developed and commercialized: the massively parallel shotgun sequencing (MPSS), a counting-based, approach; the targeted massively parallel sequencing (t-MPS), a progeny of the MPSS approach; and the single nucleotide polymorphism (SNP)–based approach (**Box 1**).

THE MASSIVE PARALLEL SHOTGUN SEQUENCING APPROACH

MPSS uses a universal amplification and sequencing of all cfDNA, fetal and maternal, isolated from maternal plasma. Fetal chromosome copy number is then determined by comparing the absolute number of sequence reads from the chromosomes of interest (eg, chromosome 21) with the number of reads from reference chromosomes.[12,13,24,41]

Box 1
Methods for prenatal screening for fetal aneuploidy

Methods for prenatal screening

Maternal serum biochemistry (triple and quadruple test)

Combined biochemistry and nuchal translucency

Cell-free fetal DNA
  MPSS
  t-MPS
  SNP

Free fetal RNA[a]

Methylation differences[a]

Fetal cells in maternal serum[a]

Endocervical trophoblasts[a]

[a]Investigational.

The reads are processed to exclude poor-quality data and then mapped (tagged) to their chromosome of origin according to the known human genome build. The fraction of reads is proportionate to chromosome size. Thus, typically 8.5% of all reads are from chromosome 1, whereas only about 1.2% are from chromosome 22.[42] The fraction of reads is also proportionate to the repeat sequences and to the guanine-cytosine (GC) content of each chromosome.[23] The higher the GC content, the higher the mean tag sequence. As a result, counts of the chromosome of interest must be normalized against referenced chromosomes that are expected to be disomic.[21,42] The ratio of the number of reads that belong to chromosome 21 to the total number of reads is calculated for each sample and compared with the mean and standard deviation of this ratio in control samples. This standardized fractional genomic representation expresses the reads result as a Z-score, which represents the degree to which the normalized counts for the chromosome of interest differ from the expected normalized counts when there is normal diploid status. The patient-specific trisomy risk can be calculated based on the Z-score and the patient's a priori risk. Nevertheless, major commercial providers of this test either currently choose to present their results only in terms of positive or negative based on Z-scores exceeding a predefined threshold.[43] Benn and colleagues[43] showed that the expected counts in a fetus with trisomy 21 depend on the fetal fraction and that the difference between a trisomic and disomic fetus is small. For example, when the fetal fraction is 20%, the relative excess in chromosome 21 DNA fragments is $(0.8 \times 2) + (0.2 \times 3) = 2.2$ compared with the situation for a euploid fetus $(0.8 \times 2) + (0.2 \times 2) = 2$, which is an increase in the number of chromosome 21 counts of only 10%. As a result, a large number of reads are required to detect trisomy.

If the ratio of reads originating from the test chromosome to 1 or more reference chromosomes that are presumed to be disomic is greater than or less than a predetermined threshold, fetal trisomy or monosomy, respectively, is inferred. Although cfDNA methods that rely on this counting approach for detecting trisomy 21 and trisomy 18 show improved sensitivity compared with traditional serum and ultrasonography screening,[13,21,24] sensitivity for trisomy 13 and chromosome X aneuploidies is reduced compared with that for trisomies 21 and 18,[12,17,24] mostly because of amplification variation. Chromosome 13 has lower GC content than chromosome

21. As a result, the measurement of the genomic representations of chromosome 13 is less precise than that for chromosome 21.[42] The detection of trisomy 13 therefore necessitates quantitative correction of its GC content and in part explains the poorer performance for trisomy 13 than for trisomy 21.[44]

Additional algorithms were proposed to detect the excess counts of reads. Senhert and colleagues[18] suggested the normalized chromosome value (NCV) method. Yeang and colleagues[45] developed an algorithm using read counts from all 22 autosomes. Comparison of the different algorithms (Z-score, NCV, and using counts of all 22 chromosomes) was equally efficient. The performance of cfDNA screening using the MPSS approach in a commercial setting has been reported.[11,13,41,46–48] Although follow-up information was incomplete and reports on false-negative cases were voluntary by providers, the detection rate (DR) on confirmed cases was 96.2% for trisomy 21 (with DR in the best possible scenario, assuming all miscarriages and unconfirmed cases are eventually confirmed as trisomy 21, to be 98.5%) and 94% for combination of trisomy 21, 18, 13, and monosomy X.

The main advantage of the MPSS approach is that it does not necessitate the separation of fetal DNA from maternal DNA, or the enrichment of fetal fraction. The method was shown to correctly identify ploidy status with excellent positive predictive values, especially for trisomy 21. Furthermore, MPSS enables analyzing several different samples together using barcodes attached to all DNA fragments (short synthetic oligonucleotide sequence), hence multiplexing. High-level multiplexing limits the depth of sequencing. Multiplexing is highly dependent on the fetal fraction, therefore a minimum fetal fraction of 4% is currently required. Other limitations of MPSS are the cost of the assay and the need to compare reads count with a reference chromosome.

THE TARGETED MASSIVELY PARALLEL SEQUENCING APPROACH

Because of the high cost and complexity of data analysis of the MPSS method, Sparks and colleagues[20] developed a targeted assay for cfDNA, referred to as t-MPS, by sequencing and counting only selected regions on the chromosomes of interest. Using this chromosome-selective sequencing method, called digital analysis of selected regions (DANSR) only 420,000 reads per sample were required to achieve performance similar to MPSS. In comparison, 10.8 million sequencing reads per sample are required, on average, in MPSS. In addition, DANSR mapping efficiency was estimated to be more than 96%, whereas MPSS mapping rates are up to 50%, showing very high specificity of the selected regions. Using this new technology decreased costs significantly. The addition of a new risk calculation algorithm, the Fetal Fraction Optimized Risk of Trisomy Evaluation (FORTE), which takes into account both age-related risk and fetal fraction, was validated in several clinical trials, including the multicenter Non-invasive Chromosomal Evaluation (NICE) study.[11] Using the DANSR/FORTE on a microarray-based quantitation platform had similar performance to the original new-generation sequencing DANSR/FORTE approach.[49]

THE SINGLE NUCLEOTIDE POLYMORPHISM APPROACH

The second approach entails specific amplification and sequencing of SNPs.[15,16,22,50] SNPs are the most common type of genetic variation in humans, serving as a genetic fingerprint and accounting for 1.6% of the human genome. Each SNP represents a difference in a single nucleotide. For example, an SNP may replace the nucleotide cytosine (C) with the nucleotide thymine (T) in AAGCCTA to AAGCTTA. Most commonly, these variations are found in the DNA between genes. The method uses comparison of SNPs with high levels of heterozygosity, from parental genome to the SNPs on the cfDNA. Thousands of SNP sequences are designed for each chromosome of interest. Only SNP sequences for which at least 1 of the parents is heterozygous are informative in determining fetal fraction and copy number count.

The feasibility of a noninvasive aneuploidy test that takes advantage of SNPs was first shown by Dhallan and colleagues.[51] After centrifugation, the maternal DNA is present in the buffy coat and a blend of maternal and fetal DNA is present in maternal plasma. Using paternal blood, the investigators could identify the intensities of the uniquely inherited paternal SNPs in the plasma, allowing an estimation of the fetal fraction. Comparison of the maternal plus fetal bands with the unique fetal band intensity also allowed estimation of the fetal chromosome 21 dosage.

Zimmermann and colleagues[22] developed a novel method named parental support, which abandoned the need for a reference chromosome. His approach involved a multiplex amplification of 11,000 SNP sequences in a single polymerase chain reaction (PCR) performed on the plasma DNA followed by sequencing. Each product was evaluated based on the hypothesis that the fetus is monosomic, disomic, or trisomic. After considering the positions of the SNPs on the chromosomes and the possibility that they may have been recombined, a maximum likelihood is calculated that the fetus is either normal, aneuploid (chromosome 21, 18, 13, or sex chromosome) or triploid, or that uniparental disomy is present. If the measured data resemble more than 1 hypothesis (ie, both euploid and trisomy) then a no-call result is issued. Prior age-related risk could be included in the calculated accuracy as well. Because, realistically, in most cases the father is not available for the test, the algorithm uses the human genome SNP map data as the paternal representation.

Clearly, the SNP approach requires a sophisticated informatics-based method to compute aneuploidy risk through SNP distribution. The main advantage of the SNP approach is being less prone to amplification variation and therefore expected to return equally accurate copy number calls across chromosomes.[13,23,52] In addition, it carries a theoretic advantage in detecting triploidy, the ploidy state of dizygotic twins, origin of dichorionic twins, maternal mosaicism (maternal cancer), and a parental origin of a chromosome, including detection of uniparental disomy. The main disadvantages include its inability to provide a read when there is high genetics homology between the parents (consanguinity) and it cannot be offered in pregnancies from egg donation or following bone marrow transplantation.

Validation of this SNP-based noninvasive prenatal testing method at 11 to 13 weeks' gestation was reported in a prospective blinded study, showing 100% sensitivity for detection of trisomy 21, trisomy 18, trisomy 13, Turner syndrome, and triploidy cases.[16] Recently, the SNP-based approach, using about 20,000 SNP sequences, was evaluated in clinical setting in more than 31,000 pregnancies. Results showed that performance in clinical settings was consistent with validation studies.[29] Using only cases confirmed through chromosome analysis or clinical evaluation at birth, the positive predictive value in this mixed low-risk and high-risk population was 90.9% for trisomy 21. However, complete genetic or clinical confirmation of all cases was not feasible, precluding accurate assessment of negative screens.

SCREENING FOR ANEUPLOIDY: INVESTIGATIONAL APPROACHES

In addition to the commercially available screening methods, several other approaches are currently under investigation and are briefly described here.

METHYLATED DNA–BASED ASSAY

The fetal genome differs from maternal in areas of hypermethylation and hypomethylation. Tong and colleagues[53] first showed the correct detection of fetal trisomy 18 by calculating the allelic ratio of maternal methylated and fetal-specific unmethylated SERPINB5 allele located on chromosome 18. Investigating specific and single loci mandates the use of specific restriction enzymes and narrows the number of loci suitable for testing.[54] Tong and colleagues[55] later published their experience with detecting markers on chromosome 21 that are differently methylated among fetal and maternal DNA. They correctly assigned 23 of 24 euploid pregnancies and all 5 trisomy 21 pregnancies. Papageorgiou and colleagues[56] presented a strategy of immunoprecipitation of fetal hypermethylated DNA combined with reverse transcription PCR for fetal fraction enrichment. They analyzed fetal-specific differentially methylated regions on chromosome 21 and calculated the ratio of the methylated regions in trisomy 21 to normal pregnancies. The method enabled the correct determination of 34 of 34 trisomy 21 pregnancies and 46 of 46 euploid pregnancies. A recent advancement that may enhance the evolution of this approach is the development of maternal and fetal methylomic profiles using genomewide bisulfite sequencing.[57]

Clinical trials were not done for methylated fetal DNA–based detection of fetal aneuploidy in maternal blood. However, if this approach is fully developed, it could be substantially cheaper than sequencing-based methods.

FREE FETAL RNA IN MATERNAL PLASMA

Cell-free fetal RNA is present in maternal plasma[58] and is fairly stable.[59] It represents the entire fetal transcriptome, the set of all RNA molecules, including messenger RNA (mRNA), ribosomal RNA, transfer RNA, and other noncoding RNA,[60] and the expression levels of placenta-specific transcripts in the plasma positively correlate with expression levels in the placenta.[61] The use of placental-expressed mRNA and microRNA in maternal plasma for the noninvasive detection of fetal aneuploidy has been an area of research in recent years. Calculating deviation in RNA-SNPs from expected maternal/fetal ratio, using mass spectrometry, allowed detection of T21 affected pregnancies by targeting the PLAC4 gene mRNA, which is transcribed from chromosome 21.[62] A major limitation of this approach is that it is informative only when the fetus is heterozygotic for the studied SNPs. Tsui and colleagues[63] further optimized the method in fetuses homozygous for the PLAC4 SNPs. They showed that mRNA quantification by digital PCR direct counting of the alleles in maternal plasma correctly detected the increased PLAC4 mRNA concentration in maternal plasma in T21 pregnancies. Although showing some success in the initial proof-of-principle studies, data from follow up studies were disappointing.[64] A major practical problem was that cell processing had to begin within 12 hours of the plasma being obtained. Thus, standard overnight shipment to commercial laboratories is insufficient for routine use, which severely limits its potential.

REINTRODUCTION OF FETAL CELLS

The presence of fetal cells in maternal circulation was initially described more than a century ago, but attempts to use fetal cells as a diagnostic or screening test to date have been frustrating.[4,7] The number of fetal cells in maternal blood is extremely low, speculated at perhaps 1 part per 10 million.[65] In 20 mL of maternal blood there may be no more than 20 fetal cells, so isolation, purification, and enhancement methods need to be nearly perfect to find and reliably analyze these cells. Even slight handling losses can render the technique nearly or completely useless, and conversely imperfections in techniques can produce high proportions of false-positive results by reading maternal cells as fetal. It is well appreciated in the screening literature that in situations in which rare event detection is required, even an excellent screening test will have a high proportion of false-positive results.[66]

The considerable difficulty in separating the signal to noise of fetal cells from maternal cells has been a function of many factors, including ignorance of the total number and type of fetal cells, the timing of their appearance, the possibility of detecting them in all pregnancies, and the best approach for their enrichment and analysis.[7] For example, in 2002 the NICHD (National Institute for Child health and Human Development)-sponsored NIFTY (NICHD Fetal cell isolaTion studY) trial was only able to detect the correct fetal gender or aneuploidy in less than 50% of cases.[4] There were many important contributions from NIFTY, and many lessons were learned that will be important to the ultimate success of the concept, but the overall conclusion from NIFTY was that the technology was not yet ready for a clinical trial. There were too many variables that needed to be standardized within and across the centers involved before a clinical trial could have been feasible. Furthermore, it the available fluorescence in situ hybridization probes could not easily penetrate and stain the fetal cells that were isolated.[67]

Development has taken a step back and encouraged the private sector to develop the technology. Several companies have taken up the challenge. There have been several recent publications with the differing groups focusing on slightly different areas of expertise. The rarity of the cells being sought suggests an automated approach to sample analysis.[68] One such approach, automated fluorescence microscopy, has been taken to the detection and analysis of fetal cells based on both immunohistochemical and molecular markers. Seppo and colleagues[69] used this system to show rapid and reliable detection of apparently fetal cells on slides of maternal blood. Huang and colleagues[70] used a microfluidic filtration device to separate erythrocytes from other nucleated cells in maternal blood samples. The next step still needs to be optimized; namely, the definitive identification of fetal cells. There have been suggestions that laser capture microdissection methodologies might be useful, but so far there are too few data to reach any conclusions.[71] Recent research suggests the use of the marker set CD105 and CD141 for fetal cell enrichment.[72] Using this set, these investigators were able to identify fetal cells in 90% of samples.

ENDOCERVICAL FETAL TROPHOBLASTS

Although most approaches to noninvasive prenatal diagnosis have centered on maternal peripheral blood as a source of fetal material, other potential sources of cells have been suggested. An attractive alternative to peripheral blood is isolation and analysis of transcervical trophoblasts. Unlike maternal blood, in which the fetal cells consist of multiple circulating fetal cell types, fetal cells in the cervix are all of placental origin and probably overwhelmingly trophoblasts. Thus, fetal cell recovery has the potential to be more amenable to unique markers that distinguish fetal from surrounding maternal cells. Noninvasive recovery of endocervical fetal trophoblasts during early pregnancy could permit definitive prenatal genetic testing. Several studies support the potential of this approach.[73,74] Sampling methods include lavage, cytobrush, and aspiration of cervical specimens. Although the optimal endocervical sampling procedure has yet to be determined, fetal cell DRs from 60% to more than 80% of cases have been reported.[75,76] Millions of pregnant women have undergone some type of cervical sampling while pregnant and several studies have shown no increase in adverse pregnancy events following endocervical sampling.[76–79] Fetal cells obtained by such an approach are amenable to analysis by both immunohistochemical and molecular techniques, making the approach suitable for the various analytical methods described in this article. The study of fetal cells is ongoing.

ROLE OF CELL-FREE DNA IN PRENATAL SCREENING

As discussed in several other articles in this issue, there are many issues to be considered when evaluating the proper role for this new technology, which is a better screen for Down syndrome, per se, but is also very expensive for what it does. From a public health perspective, Cuckle and colleagues[80] and Evans and colleagues[81] showed that the cost to find an additional case not detected by combined screening in low-risk populations is more than $3 million. Furthermore, the developments in array comparative genomic hybridization (CGH) technologies have vastly increased the detection capabilities from direct fetal tissue (ie, from chorionic villus sampling and amniocentesis) such that the objectives have changed considerably. cfDNA cannot be considered a replacement for diagnostic procedures until its capabilities can match the advanced performance of the direct tissue methods.

REFERENCES

1. Evans MI, Wapner RJ. Invasive prenatal diagnostic procedures 2005. Semin Perinatol 2005;29(4):215–8.
2. Evans MI, Johnson MP, Yaron Y, et al. Prenatal diagnosis: genetics, reproductive risks, testing and management. , New York: McGraw-Hill; 2006.
3. Evans MI, Krivchenia EL, Wapner RJ, et al. Principles of screening. Clin Obstet Gynecol 2002;45(3):657–60 [discussion: 730–2].
4. Bianchi DW, Simpson JL, Jackson LG, et al. Fetal gender and aneuploidy detection using fetal cells in maternal blood: analysis of NIFTY I data. National Institute of Child Health and Development Fetal Cell Isolation Study. Prenat Diagn 2002; 22(7):609–15.
5. Herzenberg LA, Bianchi DW, Schroder J, et al. Fetal cells in the blood of pregnant women: detection and enrichment by fluorescence-activated cell sorting. Proc Natl Acad Sci U S A 1979;76(3):1453–5.
6. Hahn S, Holzgreve W. Fetal cells and fetal DNA in maternal blood: new developments for a new millennium. Basel (Switzerland): Karger; 2001.
7. Holzgreve W, Zhong XY, Troeger C, et al. Fetal cells and fetal DNA in maternal blood: an overview of the Basel experience. In: Holzgreve W, Hahn S, editors. Fetal cells and fetal DNA in maternal blood: new developments for a new millennium. Basel (Switzerland): Karger; 2001.
8. Lo YM, Corbetta N, Chamberlain PF, et al. Presence of fetal DNA in maternal plasma and serum. Lancet 1997;350(9076):485–7.
9. Lo YM, Tein MS, Lau TK, et al. Quantitative analysis of fetal DNA in maternal plasma and serum: implications for noninvasive prenatal diagnosis. Am J Hum Genet 1998;62(4):768–75.
10. Heung MM, Tsui NB, Leung TY, et al. Development of extraction protocols to improve the yield for fetal RNA in maternal plasma. Prenat Diagn 2009;29(3): 277–9.
11. Norton ME, Brar H, Weiss J, et al. Non-invasive Chromosomal Evaluation (NICE) study: results of a multicenter prospective cohort study for detection of fetal trisomy 21 and trisomy 18. Am J Obstet Gynecol 2012;207(2):137.e1–8.

12. Palomaki GE, Deciu C, Kloza EM, et al. DNA sequencing of maternal plasma reliably identifies trisomy 18 and trisomy 13 as well as Down syndrome: an international collaborative study. Genet Med 2012;14(3):296–305.

13. Palomaki GE, Kloza EM, Lambert-Messerlian GM, et al. DNA sequencing of maternal plasma to detect Down syndrome: an international clinical validation study. Genet Med 2011;13(11):913–20.

14. Verweij EJ, Jacobsson B, van Scheltema PA, et al. European Non-invasive Trisomy Evaluation (EU-NITE) study: a multicenter prospective cohort study for non-invasive fetal trisomy 21 testing. Prenat Diagn 2013;33(10):996–1001.

15. Samango-Sprouse C, Banjevic M, Ryan A, et al. SNP-based non-invasive prenatal testing detects sex chromosome aneuploidies with high accuracy. Prenat Diagn 2013;33(7):643–9.

16. Nicolaides KH, Syngelaki A, Gil M, et al. Validation of targeted sequencing of single-nucleotide polymorphisms for non-invasive prenatal detection of aneuploidy of chromosomes 13, 18, 21, X, and Y. Prenat Diagn 2013;33(6):575–9.

17. Mazloom AR, Dzakula Z, Oeth P, et al. Noninvasive prenatal detection of sex chromosomal aneuploidies by sequencing circulating cell-free DNA from maternal plasma. Prenat Diagn 2013;33(6):591–7.

18. Sehnert AJ, Rhees B, Comstock D, et al. Optimal detection of fetal chromosomal abnormalities by massively parallel DNA sequencing of cell-free fetal DNA from maternal blood. Clin Chem 2011;57(7):1042–9.

19. Sparks AB, Struble CA, Wang ET, et al. Noninvasive prenatal detection and selective analysis of cell-free DNA obtained from maternal blood: evaluation for trisomy 21 and trisomy 18. Am J Obstet Gynecol 2012;206(4):319.e1–9.

20. Sparks AB, Wang ET, Struble CA, et al. Selective analysis of cell-free DNA in maternal blood for evaluation of fetal trisomy. Prenat Diagn 2012;32(1):3–9.

21. Ehrich M, Deciu C, Zwiefelhofer T, et al. Noninvasive detection of fetal trisomy 21 by sequencing of DNA in maternal blood: a study in a clinical setting. Am J Obstet Gynecol 2011;204(3):205.e1–11.

22. Zimmermann B, Hill M, Gemelos G, et al. Noninvasive prenatal aneuploidy testing of chromosomes 13, 18, 21, X, and Y, using targeted sequencing of polymorphic loci. Prenat Diagn 2012;32(13):1233–41.

23. Fan HC, Blumenfeld YJ, Chitkara U, et al. Noninvasive diagnosis of fetal aneuploidy by shotgun sequencing DNA from maternal blood. Proc Natl Acad Sci U S A 2008;105(42):16266–71.

24. Bianchi DW, Platt LD, Goldberg JD, et al, MatErnal BLood IS Source to Accurately diagnose fetal aneuploidy (MELISSA) Study Group. Genome-wide fetal aneuploidy detection by maternal plasma DNA sequencing. Obstet Gynecol 2012; 119(5):890–901.

25. Ashoor G, Syngelaki A, Wagner M, et al. Chromosome-selective sequencing of maternal plasma cell-free DNA for first-trimester detection of trisomy 21 and trisomy 18. Am J Obstet Gynecol 2012;206(4):322.e1–5.

26. Ashoor G, Syngelaki A, Wang E, et al. Trisomy 13 detection in the first trimester of pregnancy using a chromosome-selective cell-free DNA analysis method. Ultrasound Obstet Gynecol 2013;41(1):21–5.

27. Nicolaides KH, Wright D, Poon LC, et al. First-trimester contingent screening for trisomy 21 by biomarkers and maternal blood cell-free DNA testing. Ultrasound Obstet Gynecol 2013;42(1):41–50.

28. Zhang H, Gao Y, Jiang F, et al. Non-invasive prenatal testing for trisomies 21, 18 and 13: clinical experience from 146,958 pregnancies. Ultrasound Obstet Gynecol 2015;45(5):530–8.

29. Dar P, Curnow KJ, Gross SJ, et al. Clinical experience and follow-up with large scale single-nucleotide polymorphism-based noninvasive prenatal aneuploidy testing. Am J Obstet Gynecol 2014;211(5):527.e1–17.

30. Ashoor G, Syngelaki A, Poon LC, et al. Fetal fraction in maternal plasma cell-free DNA at 11-13 weeks' gestation: relation to maternal and fetal characteristics. Ultrasound Obstet Gynecol 2013;41(1):26–32.

31. Palomaki GE, Kloza EM, Lambert-Messerlian GM, et al. Circulating cell free DNA testing: are some test failures informative? Prenat Diagn 2015;35(3):289–93.

32. Chan KC, Zhang J, Hui AB, et al. Size distributions of maternal and fetal DNA in maternal plasma. Clin Chem 2004;50(1):88–92.

33. Li Y, Di Naro E, Vitucci A, et al. Detection of paternally inherited fetal point mutations for beta-thalassemia using size-fractionated cell-free DNA in maternal plasma. JAMA 2005;293(7):843–9.

34. Choi H, Lau TK, Jiang FM, et al. Fetal aneuploidy screening by maternal plasma DNA sequencing: 'false positive' due to confined placental mosaicism. Prenat Diagn 2013;33(2):198–200.

35. Harrison KJ, Barrett IJ, Lomax BL, et al. Detection of confined placental mosaicism in trisomy 18 conceptions using interphase cytogenetic analysis. Hum Genet 1993;92(4):353–8.

36. Li Y, Zimmermann B, Rusterholz C, et al. Size separation of circulatory DNA in maternal plasma permits ready detection of fetal DNA polymorphisms. Clin Chem 2004;50(6):1002–11.

37. Lun FM, Tsui NB, Chan KC, et al. Noninvasive prenatal diagnosis of monogenic diseases by digital size selection and relative mutation dosage on DNA in maternal plasma. Proc Natl Acad Sci U S A 2008;105(50):19920–5.

38. Dhallan R, Au WC, Mattagajasingh S, et al. Methods to increase the percentage of free fetal DNA recovered from the maternal circulation. JAMA 2004;291(9):1114–9.

39. Papageorgiou EA, Fiegler H, Rakyan V, et al. Sites of differential DNA methylation between placenta and peripheral blood: molecular markers for noninvasive prenatal diagnosis of aneuploidies. Am J Pathol 2009;174(5):1609–18.

40. Chim SS, Jin S, Lee TY, et al. Systematic search for placental DNA-methylation markers on chromosome 21: toward a maternal plasma-based epigenetic test for fetal trisomy 21. Clin Chem 2008;54(3):500–11.

41. Futch T, Spinosa J, Bhatt S, et al. Initial clinical laboratory experience in noninvasive prenatal testing for fetal aneuploidy from maternal plasma DNA samples. Prenat Diagn 2013;33(6):569–74.

42. Chiu RW, Chan KC, Gao Y, et al. Noninvasive prenatal diagnosis of fetal chromosomal aneuploidy by massively parallel genomic sequencing of DNA in maternal plasma. Proc Natl Acad Sci U S A 2008;105(51):20458–63.

43. Benn P, Cuckle H, Pergament E. Non-invasive prenatal testing for aneuploidy: current status and future prospects. Ultrasound Obstet Gynecol 2013;42(1):15–33.

44. Chen EZ, Chiu RW, Sun H, et al. Noninvasive prenatal diagnosis of fetal trisomy 18 and trisomy 13 by maternal plasma DNA sequencing. PLoS One 2011;6(7): e21791.

45. Yeang CH, Ma GC, Hsu HW, et al. Genome-wide normalized score: a novel algorithm to detect fetal trisomy 21 during non-invasive prenatal testing. Ultrasound Obstet Gynecol 2014;44(1):25–30.

46. Dan S, Wang W, Ren J, et al. Clinical application of massively parallel sequencing-based prenatal noninvasive fetal trisomy test for trisomies 21 and 18 in 11,105 pregnancies with mixed risk factors. Prenat Diagn 2012;32(13):1225–32.

47. Song Y, Liu C, Qi H, et al. Noninvasive prenatal testing of fetal aneuploidies by massively parallel sequencing in a prospective Chinese population. Prenat Diagn 2013;33(7):700–6.

48. Lau TK, Chen F, Pan X, et al. Noninvasive prenatal diagnosis of common fetal chromosomal aneuploidies by maternal plasma DNA sequencing. J Matern Fetal Neonatal Med 2012;25(8):1370–4.

49. Stokowski R, Wang E, White K, et al. Clinical performance of non-invasive prenatal testing (NIPT) using targeted cell-free DNA analysis in maternal plasma with microarrays or next generation sequencing (NGS) is consistent across multiple controlled clinical studies. Prenat Diagn 2015;35(12):1243–6.

50. Liao GJ, Chan KC, Jiang P, et al. Noninvasive prenatal diagnosis of fetal trisomy 21 by allelic ratio analysis using targeted massively parallel sequencing of maternal plasma DNA. PLoS One 2012;7(5):e38154.

51. Dhallan R, Guo X, Emche S, et al. A non-invasive test for prenatal diagnosis based on fetal DNA present in maternal blood: a preliminary study. Lancet 2007;369(9560):474–81.

52. Fan HC, Gu W, Wang J, et al. Non-invasive prenatal measurement of the fetal genome. Nature 2012;487(7407):320–4.

53. Tong YK, Ding C, Chiu RW, et al. Noninvasive prenatal detection of fetal trisomy 18 by epigenetic allelic ratio analysis in maternal plasma: theoretical and empirical considerations. Clin Chem 2006;52(12):2194–202.

54. Old RW, Crea F, Puszyk W, et al. Candidate epigenetic biomarkers for noninvasive prenatal diagnosis of Down syndrome. Reprod Biomed Online 2007; 15(2):227–35.

55. Tong YK, Jin S, Chiu RW, et al. Noninvasive prenatal detection of trisomy 21 by an epigenetic-genetic chromosome-dosage approach. Clin Chem 2010;56(1):90–8.

56. Papageorgiou EA, Karagrigoriou A, Tsaliki E, et al. Fetal-specific DNA methylation ratio permits noninvasive prenatal diagnosis of trisomy 21. Nat Med 2011;17(4): 510–3.

57. Lun FM, Chiu RW, Sun K, et al. Noninvasive prenatal methylomic analysis by genomewide bisulfite sequencing of maternal plasma DNA. Clin Chem 2013; 59(11):1583–94.

58. Poon LL, Leung TN, Lau TK, et al. Presence of fetal RNA in maternal plasma. Clin Chem 2000;46(11):1832–4.

59. Tsui NB, Ng EK, Lo YM. Stability of endogenous and added RNA in blood specimens, serum, and plasma. Clin Chem 2002;48(10):1647–53.

60. Tsui NB, Jiang P, Wong YF, et al. Maternal plasma RNA sequencing for genomewide transcriptomic profiling and identification of pregnancy-associated transcripts. Clin Chem 2014;60(7):954–62.

61. Go AT, Visser A, Mulders MA, et al. Detection of placental transcription factor mRNA in maternal plasma. Clin Chem 2004;50(8):1413–4.

62. Lo YM, Tsui NB, Chiu RW, et al. Plasma placental RNA allelic ratio permits noninvasive prenatal chromosomal aneuploidy detection. Nat Med 2007;13(2): 218–23.

63. Tsui NB, Akolekar R, Chiu RW, et al. Synergy of total PLAC4 RNA concentration and measurement of the RNA single-nucleotide polymorphism allelic ratio for the noninvasive prenatal detection of trisomy 21. Clin Chem 2010;56(1):73–81.

64. Yang L, Sun HY, Chen DZ, et al. Explore the dynamic alternation of gene PLAC4 mRNA expression levels in maternal plasma in second trimester for nonivasive detection of trisomy 21. Obstet Gynecol Sci 2015;58(4):261–7.

65. Bianchi DW, Klinger KW, Vadnais TJ, et al. Development of a model system to compare cell separation methods for the isolation of fetal cells from maternal blood. Prenat Diagn 1996;16(4):289–98.
66. Evans MI, Hyett J, Nicolaides KH. Genetic screening and clinical testing. In: Funai E, Evans MI, Lockwood J, editors. High risk obstetrics in the requisites in obstetrics and gynecology. Philadelphia: Elsevier Science; 2008. p. 33–60.
67. Bischoff FZ, Hahn S, Johnson KL, et al. Intact fetal cells in maternal plasma: are they really there? Lancet 2003;361(9352):139–40.
68. Kilpatrick MW, Tafas T, Evans MI, et al. Automated detection of rare fetal cells in maternal blood: eliminating the false-positive XY signals in XX pregnancies. Am J Obstet Gynecol 2004;190(6):1571–8 [discussion: 1578–81].
69. Seppo A, Frisova V, Ichetovkin I, et al. Detection of circulating fetal cells utilizing automated microscopy: potential for noninvasive prenatal diagnosis of chromosomal aneuploidies. Prenat Diagn 2008;28(9):815–21.
70. Huang R, Barber TA, Schmidt MA, et al. A microfluidics approach for the isolation of nucleated red blood cells (NRBCs) from the peripheral blood of pregnant women. Prenat Diagn 2008;28(10):892–9.
71. Burgemeister R. New aspects of laser microdissection in research and routine. J Histochem Cytochem 2005;53(3):409–12.
72. Hatt L, Brinch M, Singh R, et al. A new marker set that identifies fetal cells in maternal circulation with high specificity. Prenat Diagn 2014;34(11):1066–72.
73. Adinolfi M, Sherlock J. First trimester prenatal diagnosis using transcervical cells: an evaluation. Hum Reprod Update 1997;3(4):383–92.
74. Fejgin MD, Diukman R, Cotton Y, et al. Fetal cells in the uterine cervix: a source for early non-invasive prenatal diagnosis. Prenat Diagn 2001;21(8):619–21.
75. Bussani C, Cioni R, Scarselli B, et al. Strategies for the isolation and detection of fetal cells in transcervical samples. Prenat Diagn 2002;22(12):1098–101.
76. Cioni R, Bussani C, Scarselli B, et al. Comparison of two techniques for transcervical cell sampling performed in the same study population. Prenat Diagn 2005; 25(3):198–202.
77. Rodeck C, Tutschek B, Sherlock J, et al. Methods for the transcervical collection of fetal cells during the first trimester of pregnancy. Prenat Diagn 1995;15(10): 933–42.
78. Massari A, Novelli G, Colosimo A, et al. Non-invasive early prenatal molecular diagnosis using retrieved transcervical trophoblast cells. Hum Genet 1996; 97(2):150–5.
79. Katz-Jaffe MG, Mantzaris D, Cram DS. DNA identification of fetal cells isolated from cervical mucus: potential for early non-invasive prenatal diagnosis. BJOG 2005;112(5):595–600.
80. Cuckle H, Benn P, Pergament E. Maternal cfDNA screening for Down syndrome– a cost sensitivity analysis. Prenat Diagn 2013;33(7):636–42.
81. Evans MI, Sonek JD, Hallahan TW, et al. Cell-free fetal DNA screening in the USA: a cost analysis of screening strategies. Ultrasound Obstet Gynecol 2015;45(1): 74–83.

Strategies for Implementing Cell-Free DNA Testing

Howard Cuckle, BA, MSc, DPhil

KEYWORDS

- cfDNA • Aneuploidy • Screening • Prenatal • Maternal plasma

KEY POINTS

- Maternal plasma cell-free (cf) DNA is much more discriminatory for Down syndrome than conventional screening.
- Secondary cfDNA is generally cost saving and prevents iatrogenic fetal loss but reduces detection, and primary cfDNA is currently too expensive. Contingent cfDNA has a detection rate closer to primary than secondary cfDNA and is affordable.
- Noncalls present less of a practical problem for contingent than primary cfDNA.
- Extending testing to include other common aneuploidies and subchromosome abnormalities vastly increases the false-positive rate to that approaching conventional screening.
- The continuing utility of the nuchal translucency scan may be in detecting structural abnormalities, particularly severe cardiac defects and biochemical markers in detecting adverse pregnancy outcomes, such as preeclampsia and growth restriction.

INTRODUCTION

Until recently antenatal screening for Down syndrome and other common aneuploidies was based on the determination of markers in maternal serum and by ultrasound examination. Tests based on the combination of markers have been used to estimate the individual's risk of an affected pregnancy. Those with a high enough risk (designated positive) are offered invasive prenatal diagnosis using either first-trimester chorionic villus sampling (CVS) or second-trimester amniocentesis, both being associated with fetal loss. The choice of cutoff risk varies according to local or national guidelines. In most health care systems, invasive testing is not offered to those with negative results, although in some localities such testing is a matter of individual choice.

Consultant: PerkinElmer Inc, Venadis Diagnostics AB, Hy-Laboratories Ltd; director: Genome Ltd.
Department of Obstetrics & Gynecology, Columbia University Medical Center, 622 West 168th Street, New York, NY 10032, USA
E-mail address: h.s.cuckle@leeds.ac.uk

Clin Lab Med 36 (2016) 213–226
http://dx.doi.org/10.1016/j.cll.2016.01.010
labmed.theclinics.com

This approach, which had developed over decades, is about to change radically with the discovery that a single marker, maternal plasma cell-free (cf) DNA, has a vastly superior performance than any of the conventional screening tests. However, the new marker has several limitations; the conventional tests have roles beyond aneuploidy. These complications mean that there is no single strategy that can be recommended when implementing cfDNA testing in clinical practice. For the near future it is likely that different strategies will be used worldwide.

Screening Tests

The performance of antenatal screening tests for aneuploidy are evaluated by 2 factors: the detection rate (DR), the proportion of affected pregnancies with positive screening results, and the false-positive rate (FPR), the proportion of euploid pregnancies with positive results. Two further factors might be evaluated, which are a function of both test performance and the population being tested: the positive predictive value (PPV), the risk of aneuploidy among the positives, and negative predictive value (NPV), the risk among the negatives. These factors can be calculated at the time of screening or at birth; because the common aneuploidies have a high intrauterine fatality, the rate at birth will be much lower.

Conventional Down Syndrome Screening

The most widely used markers are maternal serum pregnancy-associated plasma protein (PAPP)-A, human chorionic gonadotrophin (hCG), free-β subunit of hCG, α-fetoprotein (AFP), unconjugated estriol (uE$_3$) and inhibin-A, and ultrasound nuchal translucency (NT). The discriminatory power of each varies according to gestational age, limiting the possible concurrent combination of markers. Additionally there is now increasing experience with further first-trimester ultrasound markers: absence of the fetal nasal bone (NB), abnormal blood flow in the ductus venosus, tricuspid regurgitation, and the frontal-maxillary facial angle. A further first-trimester maternal serum marker, placental growth factor (PlGF), is also being considered as is the second-trimester ultrasound facial profile markers, nuchal skinfold (NF), nasal bone length (NBL) and prenasal thickness (PT).

The performance of conventional screening tests is best evaluated using statistical modeling because prospective screening studies are subject to viability bias, which necessarily overestimates aneuploidy detection rates. Modeling shows that performance is higher for tests that combined first-trimester markers than for second-trimester tests and highest for those using markers from both trimesters.

Table 1 shows model-predicted performance for 5 of the best protocols: NT, PAPP-A and free β-hCG at 12 weeks (combined test); second-trimester free β-hCG, AFP, uE$_3$, and inhibin A (Quad test); combined test markers, but restricting invasive testing to the 1% with the highest risks and for 19% with an initial borderline risk, second-trimester Quad markers followed by risk revision (contingent test); NT and PAPP-A at 12 weeks together with second-trimester Quad markers for all women (integrated test); same but without NT (serum integrated test). **Table 1** also shows some variants with additional markers. Tests that include ultrasound markers perform best.

Types of Cell-Free DNA Test

Currently there are 3 broad methods available from large laboratories in the United States and China. These methods are shotgun (genome-wide) massively parallel sequencing (s-MPS), targeted MPS (t-MPS), and a single nucleotide polymorphism (SNP) method. Outside of these countries the tests can either be obtained through

Table 1
Conventional tests: model-predicted Down syndrome screening performance

Test	FPR 5%		FPR 3%		FPR 1%	
	DR (%)	PPV (%)	DR (%)	PPV (%)	DR (%)	PPV (%)
Standard						
Combined	84.5	2.2	80.5	3.4	71.7	8.3
Quad	70.8	1.8	64.0	2.8	49.9	6.2
Contingent (1% very high, 19% borderline risks)	91.7	2.4	89.4	3.8	80.2	10
Integrated	91.6	2.4	89.0	3.8	82.9	10
Serum integrated test	75.7	2.0	70.1	3.3	52.2	7.1
Variants						
Combined with NB	92.9	2.4	90.7	3.8	84.9	10
Combined with PIGF & AFP	87.6	2.3	83.8	3.6	75.2	9.1
Quad test with NF, NBL, & PT	93.4	2.4	90.6	3.8	83.4	10

Based on standardized maternal age distribution,[1] serum, and ultrasound parameters at 12 weeks from a published meta-analysis,[2] a meta-analysis of first-trimester PIGF, and AFP studies (cited in Refs.[2,3]).
PPV calculated at term rather than the time of the test.
Data from Refs.[1–3]

distributers representing the United States and China laboratories or in some case through local laboratories under license. In the near future it is expected that newer cfDNA methods will become available that are simpler, cheaper, and capable of high throughput.

Table 2 summarizes the technical differences between s-MPS, t-MPS, and SNPs. With the 2 counting methods, millions of genome-wide fetal and maternal fragments are sequenced and informative sequences are mapped to discrete chromosome-specific loci; for t-MPS there is enrichment for the chromosomes of interest. In aneuploidy the distribution of chromosomes will be skewed by the excess or deficit of one

Table 2
Methods of cell-free DNA testing for aneuploidy in a specific chromosome

Method	Chromosomes Sequenced	Measurement	Detection	Result
s-MPS	All	Fragment count	Proportion compared with expected for euploidy	Z-score, likelihood ratio, adjusted for GC content or not
t-MPS	Few	Fragment count	Proportion compared with expected for euploidy	Risk, adjusted for FF, maternal age, and gestation
SNP	All	SNP array	Pattern compared with expected for aneuploidy and euploidy	Maximum likelihood Z-score

Abbreviations: FF, fetal fraction; GC, guanine-cytosine.

chromosome. The other approach does not use counting but amplifies about 20,000 SNPs both in the buffy coat (maternal) and plasma (maternal and fetoplacental), which are then sequenced. In aneuploidy the pattern of products will differ between the 2 sources. All 3 methods are sensitive to the proportion of cfDNA arising from the feto-placental unit, the fetal fraction (FF).

Lately, commercial providers are considering the introduction of methods that do not require sequencing of large numbers of fragments, which is a costly and time-consuming step in the procedure.

Discriminatory Power of Cell-Free DNA Testing for Down Syndrome

There have been 13 published studies carried out in plasma samples drawn before invasive prenatal diagnosis (so-called high-risk studies).[4–16] In addition, there are 7 published studies whereby samples were drawn as part of existing screening programs[17–23] and an additional one with a mixture of both study designs.[24] Meta-analysis of the high-risk studies yields a DR of 99.3% and FPR of 0.11%. Performance is even better for the other studies, but these are less reliable because of both incomplete follow-up and viability bias.

Cell-Free DNA Screening Strategies

At present, 3 types of strategies are being discussed, with cfDNA testing offered only to women with positive conventional screening results (secondary cfDNA test); to all women, replacing conventional screening (primary cfDNA test); and to 10% to 30% of women selected according to their conventional screening result (contingent cfDNA test). There are 4 variants of the last strategy: the selected group has the highest conventional test risks; a very small group with the highest risk is offered invasive prenatal diagnosis and the rest have cfDNA; using additional conventional test markers; and women of advanced maternal age (AMA) are automatically offered cfDNA, and younger women are selected according to their conventional test risk. In all strategies those with a positive cfDNA result are offered invasive prenatal diagnosis.

Table 3 shows the model-predicted performance of each strategy. Secondary cfDNA will substantially reduce the number of amniocenteses or CVS procedures performed by conventional screening, thereby reducing iatrogenic fetal losses; but it will also lead to a small reduction in detection. Primary cfDNA maximizes detection while ensuring that relatively few women have invasive prenatal diagnosis. Contingent cfDNA vastly reduces the number of women requiring a costly (see later discussion) cfDNA test while maintaining a detection rate much closer to primary cfDNA than the combined test. The version whereby those with very high risks are offered invasive testing has a slightly higher detection rate and, despite a much higher false-positive rate, is considered worthwhile because about two-thirds of affected pregnancies are in the very-high-risk group and waiting for cfDNA results is avoided. All other strategies have a much higher PPV than conventional tests, and all strategies have an extremely low NPV.

Cost-Effectiveness

In public health aneuploidy screening programs, the most useful measure of cost-effectiveness is the marginal cost or the incremental cost ratio (ICR). This ICR is the cost of each additional affected birth avoided by the new test over and above those avoided by the existing test. This cost can be compared with the lifetime cost of an affected individual, restricted to the direct medical, educational, and social services costs or including indirect societal costs, such as loss of income. In some

Table 3
Cell-free DNA strategies: model-predicted Down syndrome screening performance

Selected for cfDNA	DR (%)	FPR (%)	PPV (%)
Secondary cfDNA (after combined test)			
5% positives	83.9	0.006	95
3% positives	79.9	0.003	97
1% positives	71.2	0.001	99
Primary cfDNA			
100%	99.3	0.11	54
Contingent cfDNA (using combined test)			
20% with highest risk	93.6	0.02	85
Except 0.5% with very high risk have IPND	94.1	0.52	19
20% with highest risk using additionally PlGF & AFP	95.6	0.02	85
AMA and 20% highest risk in remainder	94.8	0.03	81

Based on standardized maternal age distribution,[1] serum, and ultrasound parameters at 12 weeks from a published meta-analysis,[2] a meta-analysis of first-trimester PlGF and AFP studies (cited in Refs.[2,3]) and a meta-analysis of cfDNA studies.[4–16]
   PPV and NPV calculated at term rather than the time of the test.
   Abbreviations: AMA, advanced maternal age older than 35 years; IPND, invasive prenatal diagnosis.
   Data from Refs.[1–16]

cost-effectiveness studies, the lifetime cost is included in the ICR, which is then compared with some general measure of affordability, a function of the amount of resources available in a country, such as the gross domestic product (GDP) per capita. For example, according to World Health Organization's guidelines,[25] a new intervention is very cost-effective if the cost per disability adjusted life-years averted is less than the GDP per capita. In addition to the marginal cost, public health planners need to consider the total cost of changing to the new strategy or the average cost per woman screened.

Secondary cfDNA strategies are generally cost-neutral or lead to cost savings because the unit cost of the cfDNA test is of the same order of magnitude or cheaper than the unit cost of invasive prenatal diagnosis. A more detailed cost-effectiveness analysis is required to draw conclusions about the primary cfDNA and contingent cfDNA strategies. In its most simple form the inputs are the unit costs of the conventional screening test, of cfDNA, and of invasive prenatal diagnosis as well as uptake rates. These costs will vary considerably between countries as will lifetime costs, but the costs are probably in the same relative proportion everywhere. **Table 4** is an illustration assigning unit costs appropriate for a country, such as the United States, where the direct lifetime costs of a Down syndrome birth are about $0.9 million.[26] This illustration shows that the marginal cost of switching to primary cfDNA only becomes less than the lifetime cost of a Down syndrome birth avoided when the unit cost of cfDNA testing decreases to less than 1.5 to 2.5 times the unit cost of the combined test. The higher end of this range will apply if the NT scan is retained (see later discussion). Contingent cfDNA is much cheaper than primary cfDNA and is affordable at a unit cost of cfDNA testing 4 to 5 times that of the combined test. It should be understood that the unit cost of these tests is not just the price of reagents but includes laboratory overheads, technician time, and, outside a public health setting, profit.

Table 4 makes the simplistic assumption that cfDNA and conventional strategies will have a similar uptake. If uptake depends on perceptions about the eventual

Table 4
Marginal cost ($ million) per additional Down syndrome birth avoided compared with the combined test, according to the unit cost of cell-free DNA

Selected for cfDNA	Unit Cost of cfDNA					
	$1200	$1000	$800	$600	$400	$200
Primary cfDNA						
100%	4.72	3.71	2.69	1.67	0.65	[b]
100%, assuming that NT is retained	5.49	4.47	3.45	2.43	1.41	0.39
Contingent cfDNA						
20% with highest risk	1.39	1.06	0.72	0.39	0.05	[b]
Except 0.5% with very high risk[a]	1.32	1.01	0.70	0.40	0.09	[b]
20% with highest risk using additionally PlGF & AFP	1.51	1.23	0.95	0.67	0.39	0.11
AMA and 20% highest risk in rest	1.71	1.31	0.92	0.52	0.12	[b]
Assuming NT retained in AMA	1.81	1.41	1.01	0.62	0.22	[b]

Based on the following: unit cost of NT $150, serum markers $25 each, and invasive prenatal diagnosis $1500; assuming uptake same for cfDNA and the combined test, 100% for invasive prenatal diagnosis and that once diagnosed all Down syndrome pregnancies will be terminated; standardized maternal age distribution,[1] serum, and ultrasound parameters at 12 weeks from a published meta-analysis,[2] a meta-analysis of first-trimester PlGF and AFP studies (cited in Refs.[2,3]), and a meta-analysis of cfDNA studies.[4-16]
PPV and NPV calculated at term rather than the time of the test.
Abbreviation: AMA, maternal age more than 35 years.
[a] Offered invasive prenatal diagnosis.
[b] Cost saving.
Data from Refs.[1-16]

need for invasive prenatal diagnosis, the former may have higher uptake and the marginal cost will be lower. Preliminary results in one study indicate that this may be the case, but this is compensated by the reduced uptake of invasive prenatal diagnosis when the cfDNA result is positive.

Test No-Calls

Table 5 shows that a large proportion of cfDNA tests carried out by the large United States and China laboratories do not yield a positive or negative result. These figures

Table 5
No-call rate and time to report: clinical experience in large commercial laboratories

Laboratory	Number of Screens	Initial No-Call (%)	Repeat No-Call (%)	Time to Report (d)
United States				
Ariosa[a]	—	2.2	32	5
Natera[27]	30,725	6.4	36	7–9
Sequenome[28]	100,000	1.9	27	7
Verinata[29]	6123	2.4	—	5[b]
China				
BGI[30]	146,958	2.2	4.5	—

[a] Thomas Musci, personal communication, 2015.
[b] Business days.
Data from Refs.[27-30]

have been reported from their routine clinical experience rather than the published high-risk or general population screening studies whereby criteria for calling may have been more stringent. There are 3 circumstances when a no-call can happen: a poor sample or quality assessment failure, a low FF, or an uninterpretable result regarded by the laboratory as too close to the cutoff. The last circumstance occurs only in one laboratory, and they do not measure FF.

Those laboratories that do measure FF have set a lower limit of 4%. This limit was chosen to take account of both the measurement error of FF and the necessary association between the average copies of chromosome 21 per genome in Down syndrome according to FF given by the formula $3*FF+2*(1-FF)$. As FF decreases, the number of copies approaches 2 and the discriminatory power of cfDNA diminishes. However, it can be argued that if the precision of cfDNA measurement is high (eg, using deeper sequencing), discrimination can be sufficient at even very low levels, accepting that cfDNA is a screening test and does not purport to be diagnostic.

The FF will be largely determined by the size of the placenta, and samples tested earlier in pregnancy when the placenta is smaller have a higher noncall rate. Another important factor is maternal body mass because a given amount of fetal DNA will be diluted by a greater blood volume in a larger woman resulting in a lower FF. **Table 5** shows that the chance of a second no-call on a fresh sample is even higher than the first. This chance will be partly due to the placental size not changing sufficiently between tests and the body mass being stable.

Table 5 also shows that the turnaround time is extensive for all the laboratories. Consequently for no-call samples, there is a major practical problem, especially for samples being sent from abroad. Some would consider not repeating the test, thus, reducing the detection rate or having invasive prenatal diagnosis (because of the increased risk of non-Down syndrome aneuploidy in no-calls; see later discussion) and, thus, increasing the false-positive rate. This issue is more of a problem for primary cfDNA because with contingent cfDNA the combined test risk can be used by itself to inform choice.

Cell-Free DNA Performance for Other Aneuploidies

Conventional screening protocols detect a large number of aneuploidies other than Down syndrome. Some laboratories have separate algorithms to calculate the risk for Edwards and Patau syndromes, but the combined test using only a cutoff for Down syndrome risk has a high incidental diagnosis of these trisomies. Modeling predicts that for a Down syndrome false-positive rate of 5%, the detection rates for Edwards and Patau syndromes will be 85.0% and 96.2%, respectively (parameters in Ref.[2]). Conventional screening also leads to the incidental diagnosis of other aneuploidies. In one meta-analysis, Down syndrome represented only 58% of aneuploidies detected and even all 3 common trisomies together only 76%.[31]

Table 6 shows the discriminatory power of cfDNA for Edwards and Patau syndromes based on a meta-analysis of the high-risk studies cited earlier for Down syndrome and Palomaki and colleagues.[32] Rates are comparable with conventional screening, but the inclusion of these aneuploidies in the cfDNA test by all commercial providers will substantially increase the false-positive rate compared with Down syndrome alone. **Table 6** also shows the discriminatory power of cfDNA for the detection of Turner syndrome based on meta-analysis of all types of published studies.[34] These rates are less secure than for Edwards and Patau syndromes because they largely include only monosomy X cases, whereas mosaic cases of Turner syndrome are much more common than monosomy X at birth. Consequently, it is likely that a large proportion of the cases studied were pregnancies destined to spontaneously abort

Table 6
Discriminatory power of cell-free DNA test for all common aneuploidies

Aneuploidy	DR (%)	FPR (%)
Down syndrome	99.3	0.11
Edwards syndrome	96.9	0.09
Patau syndrome	87.3	0.23
Turner syndrome	90.3	0.23
Other SCAs	93.0	0.14
All autosomal trisomies	98.3	0.43
Plus Turner syndrome	97.5	0.66
Plus all SCAs	95.2	0.80

Based on meta-analyses of cfDNA studies[4–16,32] and prevalence at birth for Edwards and Patau syndromes, 1 of 8 and 1 of 14 Down syndrome, respectively, and SCAs from Ref.[33]
Data from Refs.[4–16,32,33]

and do not reflect the more clinically important surviving cases of Turner syndrome.[35] Other sex chromosome abnormalities (SCAs) are also detectable by cfDNA; **Table 6** shows the discriminatory power of 47,XXX, 47,XXY, and 47,XYY from a meta-analysis of all types of published studies.[34]

Table 7 shows the model-predicted performance in the detection of all 3 common autosomal trisomies. The same general conclusions can be drawn about the relative efficiency of the secondary, primary, and contingent cfDNA strategies. For primary and secondary cfDNA, the higher false-positive rate is reflected in reduced PPV apart from the version of contingent cfDNA whereby 0.5% with very high risk have invasive

Table 7
Model-predicted autosomal trisomy screening performance for cell-free DNA strategies

Selected for cfDNA	DR (%)	FPR (%)	PPV (%)
Secondary cfDNA (after combined test positive for Down syndrome)			
5% positives	84.8	0.02	86
3% positives	80.0	0.01	91
1% positives	71.7	0.004	96
Primary cfDNA			
100%	98.3	0.43	27
Contingent cfDNA (using combined test Down syndrome risks to select)			
20% with highest risk	92.8	0.09	63
Except 0.5% with very high risk have IPND	94.1	0.58	18
20% with highest risk using additionally PlGF & AFP	94.7	0.09	64
AMA and 20% highest risk in remainder	94.0	0.12	56

Based on standardized maternal age distribution,[1] serum, and ultrasound parameters at 12 weeks from a published meta-analysis,[2] a meta-analysis of first-trimester PlGF & AFP studies (cited in Refs.[2,3]), a meta-analysis of cfDNA sudies[4–16,32] and prevalence at birth for Edwards and Patau syndromes, 1 of 8 and 1 of 14 Down syndrome, respectively, from Ref.[33]
PPV and NPV calculated at term rather than the time of the test.
Abbreviations: AMA, advanced maternal age older than 35 years; IPND, invasive prenatal diagnosis.
Data from Refs.[1–16,32,33]

prenatal diagnosis. Because in the absence of screening the birth prevalence of all 3 trisomies is only about one-fifth higher than Down syndrome alone and infant mortality is extremely high, the inclusion of the additional trisomies has little effect on cost-benefit analyses.

Reasons for False-Positive and False-Negative Results

Conventional aneuploidy screening tests generate a high rate of false positives, in the range of 1% to 5% depending on the cutoff chosen. The rate of false negatives is even higher with a minimum of about 7% for the best combination of markers. This rate is to be expected for screening tests, which are by their nature simply designed to identify a subgroup of the population to have a definitive diagnostic test. Because the discriminatory power of cfDNA testing is vastly superior to the conventional tests some regard it as almost diagnostic. From this perspective the small number of false positives and false negatives are considered discordant. Although this is misleading, it is worth documenting the known reasons for such results, which are summarized in **Table 8**.

There are 2 *test-related* causes. Like biochemical and ultrasound markers, there is overlap in the distribution of cfDNA results between affected and unaffected pregnancies due to imprecision of measurement. Generally, the more steps in the assay process, the greater the accumulated imprecision. For cfDNA, methods based on counting, precision can be improved by increasing the depth of sequencing the number of DNA fragments counted. Another test-related factor is the FF. As discussed earlier in samples with low FF, albeit greater than the acceptable limit for laboratories that do have one, the distribution of results in affected pregnancies will be closer to that of euploid pregnancies, which leads to false-negative results. For an individual case, considering possible *biological* causes of discordancy may determine the appropriate clinical management.

Biological causes of false-positive cell-free DNA results

It is relatively common for an undiscovered twin pregnancy to spontaneously reduce to a singleton in early pregnancy. When such a vanishing twin occurs, the additional placental tissue can persist and be detected by the cfDNA test. Because a large proportion of aneuploidies are nonviable, there is an increased chance that the persisting tissue is affected, leading to a false-positive result. The SNP-based cfDNA method can identify additional haplotypes that may indicate a vanishing twin.

Some phenotypically normal women have an abnormal karyotype. The most common will be SCAs, such as 47,XXX or mosaic cases with cell lines with loss of an X

Table 8
Reasons for cell-free DNA false-positive and false-negative results

Reason	False Positive	False Negative
Test related		
Precision	✔	✔
Low FF	✗	✔
Biological		
Vanishing twin	✔	✗
Maternal karyotype	✔	✗
Maternal malignancy	✔	✗
CPM	✔	✔
True mosaicism	✗	✔

chromosome. Low-level mosaicism for trisomy 21, 18, or 13 is also possible as well as a small copy number variant (CNV) on one of those chromosomes. In all such cases a positive cfDNA result may be produced. A related problem, but a much greater challenge for counseling, is occult maternal malignancy. In such cases, there can be a positive cfDNA result for more than one type of aneuploidy, which in itself might alert the laboratory to possible malignancy.

Confined placental mosaicism (CPM), whereby there are karyotypic differences between the placenta and the fetus, is a well-known phenomenon in cytogenetics. Because fetal cfDNA is substantially derived from the placenta, a cfDNA result can be discordant with the fetal karyotype obtained by amniocentesis. When the placenta is affected and the fetus is normal, this will yield a false-positive cfDNA result.[36]

Biological causes of false-negative cell-free DNA results

Similarly to the position with false positives, CPM can also cause false negatives, which occurs when the placenta is karyotypically normal and the fetus is affected. Edwards, Patau, and Turner syndromes have high intrauterine fatality; the more viable cases have mosaic placentae. Hence, there will be a tendency for false-negative cfDNA results caused by CPM to be more viable. In principle, true mosaicism whereby the fetus is a clone of different cell lines is more likely to have false-negative cfDNA results than nonmosaic cases.

Twins

In monochorionic twins, conventional screening can be carried out using the protocol as for singletons, albeit using a risk algorithm that takes account of the increased (about double) biochemical marker concentrations. In dichorionic twins, the discriminatory power of the biochemical markers is reduced because if one fetus has Down syndrome and the other is unaffected, the abnormal concentration from the affected fetus can be masked by that of the unaffected co-twin. To avoid this, many centers rely on ultrasound markers alone; even with the most optimal algorithms, which take account of correlations between the fetuses, detection is relatively low. For example, in one study the model-predicted Down syndrome detection rate was 77% for a 5% false-positive rate.[37]

A similar problem arises with cfDNA screening. For a given FF, if one twin is affected and the other normal, the expected number of chromosome 21 counts per genome will be reduced to $2.5*FF+2*(1-FF)$. This number will be offset to some extent by the general increase in the total FF for twin pregnancies, estimated to be one-third in one study,[38] presumably because of greater placental volume. Another problem is that in twins FF is an aggregate of cfDNA from both fetuses, so it can happen that the affected twin contributes a low FF limit but the aggregate is greater than the limit for the method, so the test result is acceptable.

At total of 957 cfDNA results in twins have been reported in the literature.[38–45] The overall detection rates in cases whereby one fetus is affected were as follows: Down syndrome 95.3% (41 of 43), Edwards syndrome 88.9% (8 of 9), and Patau syndrome 100% (2 of 2). The rates when both were affected were as follows: Down syndrome 100% (5 of 5) and Edwards syndrome 100% (2 of 2). The false-positive rate was 0.0% (0 of 897).

Although the detection rate in twins is lower than estimated for singletons, it can still be argued that primary cfDNA testing is indicated in such pregnancies. Firstly, the conventional screening detection rate is also lower than in singletons. More importantly, a large proportion of twins are in women who have had assisted reproductive technologies. Such women, especially those who have had an extended period of infertility, are less likely to undergo the hazards of invasive prenatal diagnosis.

Subchromosomal Abnormalities

Commercial providers of cfDNA tests are beginning to include in the panel a limited number of relatively common serious abnormalities related to CNVs. These abnormalities include the following: DiGeorge syndrome (22q11.2 deletion), 1p36 deletion syndrome, Prader-Willi, and Angelman and Cri-du-Chat syndromes. By far the most frequent is DiGeorge syndrome, which some have estimated to be as frequent as Down syndrome.[46] The discriminatory power of cfDNA tests for these abnormalities has been estimated from a study using both plasma samples from pregnant women and artificial plasma mixtures.[47] The estimated detection rate for DiGeorge syndrome was 83.3% with a false-positive rate of 0.71% and for the other syndromes combined 45.5% and 0.06%, respectively. Hence, inclusion of such abnormalities in the panel is expected to almost double the false-positive rate. Including all the common aneuploidies and these subchromosomal abnormalities would lead to a 1.6% rate of invasive prenatal diagnosis, approaching that of conventional screening. And in centers that routinely provide a microarray analysis on CVS and amniocentesis samples, patients would need to be counseled that a much larger number of subchromosomal abnormalities would be detected with invasive testing.[48]

Continuing Role for Nuchal Translucency and First-Trimester Markers

If the unit cost of a cfDNA test decreases substantially, primary cfDNA will be affordable by third-party payers, including public health systems. At that point health planners may consider abandonment of the first-trimester ultrasound NT scan, perhaps replacing it by a simpler dating scan. However, a large NT is associated with an increased risk of structural abnormalities and genetic syndromes even in the absence of aneuploidy. Among the former are major cardiac defects; this aspect alone may be sufficient to justify retaining the scan. A meta-analysis of 20 studies found a detection rate of 44% for a false-positive rate of 5.5%.[49]

A case may also be made for retaining some first-trimester biochemical markers, specifically for use in screening for adverse pregnancy outcomes, such as preeclampsia and growth restriction. These outcomes are much more common than all aneuploidies combined. A large proportion can be prevented through first-trimester screening using maternal serum PAPP-A and PlGF, together with ultrasound uterine artery Doppler and blood pressure measurement[50–52] followed by daily low-dose soluble aspirin in screen positives.[53] Cost-benefit analysis has indicated that this type of screening is affordable.[54]

REFERENCES

1. Cuckle H, Aitken D, Goodburn S, et al. Age-standardisation for monitoring performance in Down's syndrome screening programmes. Prenat Diagn 2004;24(11): 851–6.
2. Cuckle HS, Pergament E, Benn P. Multianalyte maternal serum screening for chromosomal abnormalities and neural tube defects. In: Milunsky A, Milunsky JM, editors. Genetic disorders and the fetus: diagnosis, prevention and treatment - 7th edition. Hoboken (NJ): Wiley-Blackwell; 2016. p. 483–540.
3. Huang T, Dennis A, Meschino WS, et al. First trimester screening for Down syndrome using nuchal translucency, maternal serum pregnancy-associated plasma protein A, free-β human chorionic gonadotrophin, placental growth factor and α-fetoprotein. Prenat Diagn 2015;35(7):709–16.
4. Chiu RW, Akolekar R, Zheng YW, et al. Non-invasive prenatal assessment of trisomy 21 by multiplexed maternal plasma DNA sequencing: large scale validation study. Br Med J 2011;342:c7401.

5. Ehrich M, Deciu C, Zweifellhofer T, et al. Noninvasive detection of fetal trisomy 21 by sequencing of DNA in maternal blood: a study in a clinical setting. Am J Obstet Gynecol 2011;204:205.e201–11.

6. Palomaki GE, Kloza EM, Lambert-Messerlian GM, et al. DNA sequencing of maternal plasma to detect Down syndrome: an international clinical validation study. Genet Med 2011;13:913–20.

7. Bianchi DW, Platt LD, Goldberg JD, et al, on behalf of the MatErnal Blood IS Source to Accurately diagnose fetal aneuploidy (MELISSA) Study Group. Genome-wide fetal aneuploidy detection by maternal plasma DNA sequencing. Obstet Gynecol 2012;119:890–901.

8. Sparks AB, Wang ET, Song K, et al. Noninvasive prenatal detection and selective analysis of cell-free DNA obtained from maternal blood: evaluation for trisomy 21 and trisomy 18. Am J Obstet Gynecol 2012;206:319.e1–9.

9. Ashoor G, Syngelaki A, Wagner M, et al. Chromosome-selective sequencing of maternal plasma cell-free DNA for first-trimester detection of trisomy 21 and trisomy 18. Am J Obstet Gynecol 2012;206:322.e1–5.

10. Norton ME, Brar H, Weiss J, et al. Non-invasive chromosomal evaluation (NICE) study: results of a multicenter prospective cohort study for detection of fetal trisomy 21 and trisomy 18. Am J Obstet Gynecol 2012;207:137.e1–8.

11. Verweij EJ, Jacobsson B, van Scheltema PA, et al. European non-invasive trisomy evaluation (EU-NITE) study: a multicenter prospective cohort study for non-invasive fetal trisomy 21 testing. Prenat Diagn 2013;33(10):996–1001.

12. Stumm M, Entezami M, Haug K, et al. Diagnostic accuracy of random massively parallel sequencing for non-invasive prenatal detection of common autosomal aneuploidies: a collaborative study in Europe. Prenat Diagn 2014;34(2):185–91.

13. Nicolaides KH, Syngelaki A, Gil M, et al. Validation of targeted sequencing of single-nucleotide polymorphisms for non-invasive prenatal detection of aneuploidy of chromosomes 13, 18, 21, X, and Y. Prenat Diagn 2013;33(6):575–9.

14. Zimmermann B, Hill M, Gemelos G, et al. Noninvasive prenatal aneuploidy testing of chromosomes 13, 18, 21, X, and Y, using targeted sequencing of polymorphic loci. Prenat Diagn 2012;32(13):1233–41.

15. Liang D, Lv W, Wang H, et al. Non-invasive prenatal testing of fetal whole chromosome aneuploidy by massively parallel sequencing. Prenat Diagn 2013;33(6):409–15.

16. Porreco RP, Garite TJ, Maurel K, et al. Noninvasive prenatal screening for fetal trisomies 21, 18, 13 and the common sex chromosome aneuploidies from maternal blood using massively parallel genomic sequencing of DNA. Am J Obstet Gynecol 2014;211(4):365.e1–12.

17. Dan S, Wang W, Ren J, et al. Clinical application of massively parallel sequencing-based prenatal noninvasive fetal trisomy test for trisomies 21 and 18 in 11,105 pregnancies with mixed risk factors. Prenat Diagn 2012;32:1225–32.

18. Nicolaides KH, Syngelaki A, Ashoor G, et al. Noninvasive prenatal testing for fetal trisomies in a routinely screened first-trimester population. Am J Obstet Gynecol 2012;207:374.e1–6.

19. Song Y, Liu C, Qi H, et al. Noninvasive prenatal testing of fetal aneuploidies by massively parallel sequencing in a prospective Chinese population. Prenat Diagn 2013;33(7):700–6.

20. Lau TK, Cheung SW, Lo PS, et al. Non-invasive prenatal testing for fetal chromosomal abnormalities by low-coverage whole-genome sequencing of maternal plasma DNA: review of 1982 consecutive cases in a single center. Ultrasound Obstet Gynecol 2014;43(3):254–64.

21. Gil MM, Quezada MS, Bregant B, et al. Implementation of maternal blood cell-free DNA testing in early screening for aneuploidies. Ultrasound Obstet Gynecol 2013;42(1):34–40.

22. Bianchi DW, Parker RL, Wentworth J, et al, CARE Study Group. DNA sequencing versus standard prenatal aneuploidy screening. N Engl J Med 2014;370(9): 799–808.

23. Norton ME, Jacobsson B, Swami G, et al. Non-invasive examination of trisomy using directed cell free DNA analysis: the NEXT study. J Med 2015;372(17): 1589–97.

24. Pergament E, Cuckle H, Zimmermann B, et al. Single-nucleotide polymorphism-based non-invasive prenatal testing in a high- and low-risk cohort. Obstet Gynecol 2014;124(2 Pt 1):210–8.

25. WHO Commission on MacroEconomics and Health. Macroeconomics and health: investing in health for economic development. Report of the commission on macroeconomics and health. Geneva, Switzerland: World Health Organization; 2001.

26. Cuckle H, Benn P, Pergament E. Maternal cfDNA screening for Down's syndrome – a cost sensitivity analysis. Prenat Diagn 2013;33(7):636–42.

27. Dar P, Curnow KJ, Gross SJ, et al. Clinical experience and follow-up with large scale single-nucleotide polymorphism-based noninvasive prenatal aneuploidy testing. Am J Obstet Gynecol 2014;211(5):527.e1–17.

28. McCullough RM, Almasri EA, Guan X, et al. Non-invasive prenatal chromosomal aneuploidy testing - clinical experience: 100,000 clinical samples. PLoS One 2014;9(10):e109173.

29. Futch T, Spinosa J, Bhatt S, et al. Initial clinical laboratory experience in noninvasive prenatal testing for fetal aneuploidy from maternal plasma DNA samples. Prenat Diagn 2013;33(6):569–74.

30. Zhang H, Gao Y, Jiang F, et al. Noninvasive prenatal testing for trisomy 21, 18 and 13-clinical experience from 146,958 pregnancies. Ultrasound Obstet Gynecol 2015;46(1):130.

31. Davis C, Cuckle H, Yaron Y. Screening for Down syndrome – incidental diagnosis of other aneuploidies. Prenat Diagn 2014;34(11):1044–8.

32. Palomaki GE, Deciu C, Kloza EM, et al. DNA sequencing of maternal plasma reliably identifies trisomy 18 and trisomy 13 as well as Down syndrome: an international collaborative study. Genet Med 2012;14:296–305.

33. Hook EBH. Chromosomal abnormalities: prevalence, risks and recurrence. In: Brock DJH, Rodeck CH, Ferguson-Smith MA, editors. Prenatal diagnosis and screening. London: Churchill Livingstone; 1992. p. 351–92.

34. Gil MM, Quezada MS, Revello R, et al. Analysis of cell-free DNA in maternal blood in screening for fetal aneuploidies: updated meta-analysis. Ultrasound Obstet Gynecol 2015;45(3):249–66.

35. Hook EB, Warburton D. Turner syndrome revisited: review of new data supports the hypothesis that all viable 45X cases are cryptic mosaics with a rescue cell line implying an origin by mitotic loss. Hum Genet 2014;133:417–24.

36. Grati FR, Malvestiti F, Ferreira JC, et al. Fetoplacental mosaicism: potential implications for false-positive and false-negative noninvasive prenatal screening results. Genet Med 2014;16(8):620–4.

37. Maymon R, Rozen H, Baruchin O, et al. Model predicted Down's syndrome detection rates for nuchal translucency screening in twin pregnancies. Prenat Diagn 2011;31(5):426–9.

38. Canick JA, Kloza EM, Lambert-Messerlian GM, et al. DNA sequencing of maternal plasma to identify Down syndrome and other trisomies in multiple gestations. Prenat Diagn 2012;32:1–5.
39. Grömminger S, Yagmur E, Erkan S, et al. Fetal aneuploidy detection by cell-free DNA sequencing for multiple pregnancies and quality issues with vanishing twins. Clin Med 2014;3:679–92.
40. Leung TY, Qu JZZ, Liao GJW, et al. Noninvasive twin zygosity assessment and aneuploidy detection by maternal plasma DNA sequencing. Prenat Diagn 2013;33(7):675–81.
41. Lau TK, Jiang F, Chan MK, et al. Non-invasive prenatal screening of fetal Down syndrome by maternal plasma DNA sequencing in twin pregnancies. J Matern Fetal Neonatal Med 2013;26:434–7.
42. Srinivasan A, Bianchi D, Liao W, et al. Maternal plasma DNA sequencing: effects of multiple gestation on aneuploidy detection and the relative cell-free fetal DNA (cffDNA) per fetus. Am J Obstet Gynecol 2013;208:S31.
43. Huang X, Zheng J, Chen M, et al. Noninvasive prenatal testing of trisomies 21 and 18 by massively parallel sequencing of maternal plasma DNA in twin pregnancies. Prenat Diagn 2014;34(4):335–40.
44. del Mar Gil M, Quezada MS, Bregant B, et al. Cell-free DNA analysis for trisomy risk assessment in first-trimester twin pregnancies. Fetal Diagn Ther 2014;35(3):204–11.
45. Bevilacqua E, Gil MM, Nicolaides KH, et al. Performance of screening for aneuploidies by cell-free DNA analysis of maternal blood in twin pregnancies. Ultrasound Obstet Gynecol 2015;45(1):61–6.
46. Grati FR, Molina Gomes D, Ferreira JC, et al. Prevalence of recurrent pathogenic microdeletions and microduplications in over 9500 pregnancies. Prenat Diagn 2015;35(8):801–9.
47. Wapner RJ, Babiarz JE, Levy B, et al. Expanding the scope of non-invasive prenatal testing: detection if fetal microdeletion syndromes. Am J Obstet Gynecol 2015;212(3):332.e1–9.
48. Wapner RJ, Martin CL, Levy B, et al. Chromosomal microarray versus karyotyping for prenatal diagnosis. N Engl J Med 2012;367(23):2175–84.
49. Sotiriadis A, Papatheodorou S, Eleftheriades M, et al. Nuchal translucency and major congenital heart defects in fetuses with normal karyotype: a meta-analysis. Ultrasound Obstet Gynecol 2013;42(4):383–9.
50. Akolekar R, Syngelaki A, Poon L, et al. Competing risks model in early screening for preeclampsia by biophysical and biochemical markers. Fetal Diagn Ther 2013;33(1):8–15 [Erratum appears in Fetal Diagn Ther 2013;34(1):43].
51. Park F, Russo K, Pellosi M, et al. The impact of aspirin on the prevalence of early onset pre-eclampsia after first trimester screening. Prenat Diagn 2014;34(Suppl 1):e4.
52. Poon L, Syngelaki A, Akolekar R, et al. Combined screening for preeclampsia and small for gestational age at 11-13 weeks. Fetal Diagn Ther 2013;33:16–27.
53. Roberge S, Nicolaides KH, Demers H, et al. Prevention of perinatal death and adverse perinatal outcome using: a meta-analysis. Ultrasound Obstet Gynecol 2013;41:491–9.
54. Shmueli A, Meiri H, Gonen R. Economic assessment of screening for pre-eclampsia. Prenat Diagn 2012;32(1):29–38.

Genetic Counseling for Patients Considering Screening and Diagnosis for Chromosomal Abnormalities

Renée L. Chard, MSc, CGC[a], Mary E. Norton, MD[b],*

KEYWORDS

- Genetic counseling • Chromosome abnormalities • Prenatal care
- Noninvasive prenatal screening • Maternal serum multiple marker screening
- Chorionic villi sampling • Amniocentesis

KEY POINTS

- With the introduction of cell-free DNA (cfDNA) screening for fetal aneuploidy, as well as chromosomal microarray for prenatal diagnostic testing, options for pregnant women have become increasingly complex.
- Discussions regarding options for prenatal testing for aneuploidy should occur prior to any testing and need not be lengthy or complex but should include pertinent risks and benefits of each alternative test.
- It is also important that the family history be assessed so that a focus on aneuploidy screening does not occur at the expense of missing a serious condition in a family that warrants evaluation and formal genetic counseling.
- There is no single screening or diagnostic test option that is the right choice for all patients; patient decisions should be based on each individual woman's values and preferences after a discussion of all options.

INTRODUCTION

With the advent of cfDNA screening for fetal aneuploidy, and the transition of chromosomal microarray from the pediatric clinic to the prenatal setting, testing options for pregnant women have entered a new era, and the number of testing options is overwhelming. Although the continued expansion of available tests offers expectant parents more options than ever before, it becomes paramount to equip prenatal care providers with the resources and support they need to assure their patients are

[a] Division of Maternal-Fetal Medicine, Maine Medical Partners Women's Health, 887 Congress Street, Suite 200, Portland, ME 04102, USA; [b] Department of Obstetrics, Gynecology, and Reproductive Sciences, University of California, San Francisco, 550 16th Street, 7th Floor, San Francisco, CA 94143, USA
* Correspondence:
E-mail address: mary.norton@ucsf.edu

Clin Lab Med 36 (2016) 227–236
http://dx.doi.org/10.1016/j.cll.2016.01.005
0272-2712/16/$ – see front matter © 2016 Elsevier Inc. All rights reserved.

labmed.theclinics.com

counseled adequately to make informed decisions about testing that best satisfies their needs. Ideally, as a result of genetic counseling, patients should not only be educated about the details of the testing protocols but also feel that their values and concerns have been heard and their provider understands and respects their decisions. To achieve this goal requires excellent pretest counseling that encompasses the components outlined in this article.

Professional societies, including the American College of Obstetricians and Gynecologists, agree that screening and invasive diagnostic testing for aneuploidy should be available to all women, regardless of maternal age.[1,2] The offer of prenatal testing requires a discussion of the risks and benefits of invasive testing compared with screening tests, including the potential for a false-positive result (the false-positive rate) as well as the possibility for a false-negative result and how many chromosomally abnormal fetuses will be detected (the detection rate). In addition, the detection rate for aneuploidies other than Down syndrome and the type and prognosis of the aneuploidies likely to be missed by different screening tests should be discussed. The practitioner providing this information should be familiar with these details and able to answer any questions that arise. The differences between screening and diagnostic testing should be discussed with all women; an individual's decision as to whether to have screening or diagnostic testing, or any testing at all, is based on many factors, including the risk that the fetus will have a chromosomal abnormality, the risk of pregnancy loss from an invasive procedure, and the consequences of having an affected child. Studies that have evaluated women's preferences have shown that women weigh these potential outcomes differently.[3] The decision to have invasive testing should take into account these preferences and the offer of an invasive test should not be based solely on age. It is generally agreed that maternal age of 35 years alone should no longer be used as a threshold to determine who is offered screening versus who is offered invasive testing.[1–4]

Since the introduction of amniocentesis, prenatal genetic testing guidelines have focused on identifying patients at increased risk of giving birth to an infant with Down syndrome or another chromosomal abnormality, for whom invasive diagnostic testing should be recommended. Although initially advanced maternal age was the only recognized risk factor, identification of serum and ultrasonographic markers that can better estimate the risk of an affected fetus has led to the incorporation of screening into routine prenatal care for women of all ages.[5–9] Introduction of cfDNA testing has intensified the complexity of prenatal testing decision making.

PRETEST COUNSELING

Discussions regarding options for prenatal testing for aneuploidy should occur prior to any screening or diagnostic testing and typically occur in the context of routine prenatal care. The conversation usually includes each woman's provider; this may be a midwife, nurse practitioner, family practitioner, generalist obstetrician, or perinatologist. A discussion of testing options should begin with the reminder that most babies are born healthy but that all fetuses have an estimated 3% to 4% chance of being born with a birth defect or intellectual disability.[10] Some women have risk factors, including maternal age, family history, underlying maternal medical conditions, and/or environmental exposures, that affect their a priori risks for specific conditions. Although there is no test that can identify all conditions, prenatal screening and diagnostic tests can shed light on some conditions. Some risk factors are not addressed by routine prenatal genetic testing, however, and patients with a family history of a genetic disorder should be referred for formal genetic counseling.

Pretest counseling need not be lengthy or complex, particularly for low-risk women without significant anxiety or concern.[11] It is important for a provider to explain a few basic concepts, however. These include the fact that tests for chromosome abnormalities in pregnancy generally fall into 1 of 2 categories: screening tests and diagnostic tests. Although the distinction between the 2 might be obvious to clinicians, many patients do not appreciate the differences, especially when results of some screening tests are reported as positive or negative, which imply presence or absence rather than increased or decreased risk.

USE OF EDUCATIONAL TOOLS

Although a pretest discussion of prenatal testing options need not be complex or time consuming, in many settings, educational pamphlets and videos are a useful means of providing information to educate patients and to help in decision making. Such tools are most appropriate for pretest counseling, generally of low-risk patients, and should be used to enhance, not replace, counseling by a provider. It is important that the family history be assessed if such tools are used so that a focus on aneuploidy screening does not occur at the expense of missing a serious condition in a family that warrants evaluation and formal genetic counseling.[12] Although pamphlets and videos can reinforce points made by a provider, each woman should still be provided with an opportunity to ask questions and discuss the testing options.

SCREENING VERSUS DIAGNOSTIC TESTING

Maternal age has historically been the most common screening test used to identify women at increased risk for fetal chromosome abnormalities and to determine who should be offered prenatal diagnostic testing. As maternal age increases, the chance of delivering a child with Down syndrome increases from approximately 1/1000 at 30 years of age to almost 1/400 at 35 years of age and 1/100 at 40 years of age.[13] Because of this association of advancing maternal age with aneuploidy, prenatal diagnosis has been offered to women 35 years of age or older for many years.[14]

In general, screening tests are noninvasive tests that provide risk estimates, whereas diagnostic tests are more commonly invasive tests that provide certainty about the presence of a given condition. Because screening tests provide only risk estimates, a result indicating increased risk is not considered incorrect or inaccurate if the disorder is not present. As an example, if a patient has a first-trimester combined screening test that indicates an increased chance for trisomy 18, and follow-up chorionic villi sampling (CVS) procedure yields normal chromosomes, it does not mean that the combined test was incorrect or inaccurate in identifying that increased risk. Likewise, a 40-year-old woman who has a normal CVS result is nevertheless accurately identified as at increased risk based on age prior to her diagnostic test.

It is also important that women appreciate the range of conditions that can be identified with screening tests, which typically screen for a few conditions, versus diagnostic testing, which can detect a large number of abnormalities, particularly if chromosomal microarray is chosen.[15,16] Although cfDNA tests have the highest detection rates with low false-positive rates for trisomy 21 and trisomy 18, making them the most accurate screening tests for these conditions, cfDNA does not test for other chromosome abnormalities, copy number variants, or structural birth defects, such as open neural tube defects. Trisomies 13, 18, and 21 account for approximately two-thirds of aneuploidy, and the proportion of fetuses with less common aneuploidies is higher in younger women. Norton and colleagues[17] found that approximately 71% of fetal karyotype abnormalities could be detected with cfDNA screening. In part for this reason, in a study of outcomes, including fetal abnormalities detected, quality of life, and cost, Kaimal and colleagues[18] found that for most women a screening strategy that begins with traditional maternal serum multiple marker screening followed by diagnostic testing, including chromosomal microarray, is the most effective and also the least costly.

For women who undergo primary cfDNA screening, the additional benefit of nuchal translucency (NT) ultrasound is the topic of debate. In general, NT is most beneficial for the detection of the common aneuploidies for which cfDNA screening has high sensitivity and adds little to the detection of rare, uncommon abnormalities. In 1 study, it was determined that only 19% of fetuses with a rare chromosomal abnormality, not detectable by cfDNA screening, had an NT measurement of greater than or equal to 3.5 mm.[19]

The addition of NT measurement to cfDNA screening also allows the opportunity for first-trimester anatomy examination. With increased ultrasound resolution, first-trimester assessment of fetal anatomy is feasible and some major anomalies are confidently detected between 11 weeks' and 14 weeks' gestation. Studies in experienced centers have reported detection rates of approximately 50% for major anomalies.[20] A complete examination, however, is only possible in 65% to 70% of cases[21]; there are more false-positive results, the expertise required to perform such an examination is limited, and a second-trimester anatomy scan is still required. Therefore, the benefit of an additional first-trimester ultrasound is uncertain. A further benefit of multiple marker screening, which incorporates NT measurement, is, therefore, the opportunity for a first-trimester anatomy ultrasound without the need for a separate examination that by itself is of uncertain benefit. Ultimately, for women who want comprehensive and definitive information, diagnostic testing may be preferable to the more limited information provided by screening.

Poor understanding of the purpose of screening can lead to distrust and avoidance of either screening or follow-up diagnostic testing and is best explained before any testing is undertaken. It is helpful for a woman to recognize that a screening test is an assessment of risk for a certain outcome, for example, that measurement of the maternal serum alpha fetoprotein level indicates if the pregnancy is at increased or reduced risk for an open neural tube defect, but that in the case of an abnormal screening result, additional testing is needed to determine whether or not the finding is present in the fetus. A screening test can be considered a starter test to help a woman decide if she wants to pursue diagnostic testing.

This point is especially important when the recommended follow-up test is an invasive diagnostic test. A pregnant woman should understand before undergoing maternal serum multiple marker or cfDNA screening that the recommended follow-up in the event of a positive result is a CVS procedure or amniocentesis. A woman who wishes to avoid the small risk of pregnancy loss associated with these invasive procedures, or who prefers not to receive diagnostic information regarding the chromosomal status of her fetus, may chose not to have a screening test that could end in a result that only increases her anxiety. So, although a screening test might be perceived as "just a blood test," the consequences of an abnormal result should be considered and discussed when the test is offered.

For a patient to make an informed decision regarding testing options, it is also important for her to understand the condition for which the testing is performed. In the authors' experience, when asked, many women admit that although they have heard of Down syndrome, they are not really familiar with the condition. The same is true for spina bifida, cystic fibrosis, and many other conditions for which obstetric care providers routinely offer screening or testing. At minimum, a brief description of the type of conditions for which screening is offered is an important component of pretest counseling. Again, this does not need to be lengthy or complex for typical, low-risk patients.

Each woman should also know that she may choose to undergo – or decline – testing for several personal reasons. For example, although some women have testing because they would consider pregnancy termination after certain diagnoses, other women have testing primarily to relieve anxiety or because they are not sure how they would manage an abnormal result and, therefore, prefer to gather more information and keep their options open. An offer of testing, and a decision to undergo testing, in no way implies that an abortion would or should be chosen in the event of an abnormal result.

Counseling should be a dialogue that occurs early in pregnancy to assure all options are available. The provider should evaluate the woman's understanding and elucidates her needs, fears, and preferences. It is important that assumptions regarding choices based on age, history of fertility treatment, prior pregnancy choices, or race/ethnicity be avoided. Each woman is a unique individual and best ethical practice requires that balanced information and options be offered to all women equally.[22]

COUNSELING AFTER POSITIVE ANEUPLOIDY SCREENING

Women who screen positive for Down syndrome, trisomy 18, open neural tube defects, or Smith-Lemli-Opitz syndrome based on traditional biochemical screening benefit from detailed genetic counseling regarding follow-up testing. Previously, testing options were limited to CVS or amniocentesis for fetal karyotyping. Now cfDNA screening is a follow-up option and might be especially useful for women who otherwise would not have any additional testing. It is important, however, that women are informed of what might be missed if cfDNA testing is used rather than diagnostic testing.[19]

Norton and colleagues[19] reviewed results of fetal karyotyping on specimens obtained from singleton pregnancies as a result of positive maternal serum multiple marker screening and found that 83% of the chromosomal abnormalities identified were common aneuploidies that would have been detected though cfDNA screening. The 17% that would have been missed included conditions, such as triploidy, mosaicism, rare trisomies, large duplications and deletions, and translocations. The number of findings undetectable by cfDNA was inversely proportional to maternal age, with 20% to 25% of abnormalities found in women under the age of 25 undetectable by cfDNA testing and only 8% undetectable by cfDNA testing in women over the age of 45.

RECOGNITION OF THE IMPORTANCE OF PATIENT VALUES AND PREFERENCES IN DECISION MAKING

At 35 years of age, the chance of identifying a fetus with Down syndrome approximates the chance of miscarriage due to an amniocentesis procedure. This is part of the reason that testing has traditionally been offered at this point.[4,13] For many women, however, the decision to undergo diagnostic testing is difficult, because not all women weigh the risks and advantages equally.[3,22] Every patient brings unique values, concerns, and needs, and each should be encouraged to consider what a positive test result would mean for her. For some, the possibility of miscarriage is more of a concern than the possibility of having a child with Down syndrome or another intellectual disability or birth defect. For others, concerns over caring for a child with disabilities may be more serious.[22] All patients considering invasive prenatal diagnosis should, therefore, undergo genetic counseling to discuss the options available and the risks, benefits, and limitations of each testing choice.

Studies have questioned the routinization of prenatal screening[23] and documented substantial variation in how women view the outcomes of decisions to undergo, or forego, testing.[3,22] Low uptake rates of invasive testing among women who receive positive screening results have also been reported,[24] raising concerns about the extent to which the purpose and potential outcomes of screening are understood, particularly among women of lower literacy and numeracy levels. The same may also apply to women who are non-English speakers. Nonetheless, clinicians continue to use standardized approaches to counseling, often simply recommending screening and deferring conversations about invasive diagnostic testing[25] or cfDNA screening until screen positive results are received. This practice is a disservice to patients who might be left with information they would rather not have or who feel pressured into having screening or invasive testing they feel ambivalent about because of increased anxiety they would have avoided if they had chosen not to have screening or any testing.

In a randomized controlled trial that assessed the prenatal testing choices women made in the context of being fully informed about testing options, it was found that, after receiving comprehensive prenatal testing information and having the opportunity to explicitly consider their values and preferences, women were less likely to opt for invasive diagnostic testing. They were also more likely to forego all testing for aneuploidy. In this study, women who received more comprehensive counseling had improved knowledge regarding prenatal testing, amniocentesis-related miscarriage, and age-adjusted Down-syndrome risk, suggesting that it resulted in more informed patient decision making. This study also demonstrated that offering diagnostic testing to women of all risk levels in the context of informed decision making did not result in increased use of these procedures,[26] a finding that has been demonstrated in other studies as well.[27]

The findings of these studies, that women who are offered all screening and diagnostic options after comprehensive counseling are less likely to undergo invasive testing and more likely to decline all forms of prenatal screening and diagnostic testing, add support to the contention that women may not be receiving adequate counseling about their options. This underscores the need for clinicians to provide comprehensive counseling, be clear that prenatal testing is not appropriate for everyone, and present foregoing testing as a reasonable choice. A patient should not have a test because she thinks the results are important to her provider or because she feels she will receive better care if she does so. In the era of cfDNA testing for aneuploidy, it is particularly important that women understand the purpose and potential consequences of undergoing testing, because cfDNA screening may easily be routinized as simply another blood test in the large panel of routine prenatal laboratory tests.[28]

INDICATIONS FOR GENETIC COUNSELING

Genetic counselors are health care professionals with advanced degrees who are uniquely trained to explain complex genetic information in an understandable format to patients and to facilitate the informed decision-making process. Providing comprehensive genetic counseling takes time but should be considered an investment, because thorough genetic counseling can enhance the patient-provider relationship and increase a woman's trust of and satisfaction with her provider.

Genetic counseling is appropriate for pregnant women for a variety of different indications. Traditionally, women aged 35 years and older were referred for genetic counseling to discuss the option of diagnostic testing, given their increased risk of aneuploidy. With improvements in screening options, more women are selecting screening and often make this choice without formal genetic counseling. This is reasonable, provided that each woman understand the tradeoffs of screening versus diagnostic testing and is comfortable with those risks and benefits. In some cases, this information can be effectively provided by alternative means, such as videos, on-line decision aids, and other tools. The provision of such information and patient education should be documented in the medical record.

Women should be referred for formal genetic counseling, however, if they have a positive screening result for aneuploidy (either multiple marker screening or cfDNA screening), have a positive family history of concern, if they or their partner carries a chromosomal rearrangement, if both parents are carriers of the same single gene disorder, if the woman carries an X-linked condition, or if the fetus is found to have a structural abnormality on an ultrasound that potentially has a genetic basis. All patients should have some form of history screening taken to assure these risk factors are not present.

GENETIC COUNSELING AFTER ABNORMAL DIAGNOSTIC TESTING

Reporting an abnormal diagnostic test result is never an easy task. Comprehensive pretest counseling, including a conversation about a patient's needs and understanding of the testing, however, lays the groundwork for effective post-test discussion. Disclosure of an abnormal diagnostic test should include a review of the accuracy of the test result, especially the very low false-positive rates associated with diagnostic testing. Results should be disclosed in a confident, judgement-neutral manner by a provider familiar enough with the diagnosed condition to provide some information to the patient, although referral for further counseling may be indicated. If results are initially provided by telephone, an appointment for a face-to-face meeting should be offered. The patient should be given time to react and to grieve.

It is also important that women be provided with accurate, up-to-date information about the condition that has been diagnosed. Sex chromosome abnormalities are among the mildest of the common aneuploidies and some individuals are phenotypically normal. There is an associated increased chance, however, for neurodevelopmental delay, mild dysmorphic features, and reduced fertility.[29,30] Trisomy 21 is the most common trisomy and the most common genetic cause of intellectual disability, usually in the mild to moderate range. Features of trisomy 21 include short stature, characteristic facies, and an increased chance for cardiac defects, hearing loss, and thyroid disease. Life expectancy is currently 50 to 60 years.[29,31]

Trisomy 18 and trisomy 13 are associated with severe medical problems and poor prognosis. Features of trisomy 18 include intrauterine growth restriction, micrognathia, clenched fists, cardiac defects, and severe intellectual disability. Approximately 50% of newborns with trisomy 18 die within the first week and fewer than 10% survive a year.[29] Prognosis is similar for newborns with trisomy 13, which is associated with holoprosencephaly, oral clefting, cardiac defects, and renal disease, among other findings.[29] Referral to a board-certified genetic counselor is recommended, and referral to other subspecialists also may be helpful as well as to support groups, such as the National Down Syndrome Society, or a Web site, such as perinatalhospice.org, if there is a diagnosis of an aneuploidy with poor prognosis, such as trisomy 13 or trisomy 18.

Many less common chromosomal disorders, in particular copy number variants detected by chromosomal microarray, have a less certain prognosis. The outcome for such variants of uncertain significance can range from essentially normal to poor with potential for significant birth defects and severe intellectual disability. Consultation with a geneticist and/or a genetic counselor is suggested when such disorders are diagnosed.

GENETIC NONDISCRIMINATION ACT

Individuals who undergo some types of genetic testing may be concerned about the possibility of discrimination based on their genetic testing results. The 2008 federal Genetic Information Nondiscrimination Act (GINA) was passed to protect against discrimination by employers and/or health insurance providers based on their genetic information. The act has 2 parts. Title I makes it illegal for health insurance providers to use or require genetic information to make decisions about an individual's health insurance eligibility or coverage. GINA protections do not extend to other forms of insurance, such as life, disability, or long-term care insurance. Title II makes it illegal for employers to use an individual's genetic information when making decisions about hiring, promotion, and several other terms of employment.

SUMMARY

The field of genetics and genomics has developed at a dizzying pace. These developments have had an impact on all areas of medicine, including obstetrics. All women should be offered prenatal testing for chromosomal disorders, but the broad array of options makes this a challenge for busy obstetric providers. Although optimal education likely is provided by 1-on-1 formal genetic counseling for every patient, this is not feasible or practical. Rather, all women should receive an adequate amount of balanced and nondirective information to allow making an individual and informed choice, based on preferences and values. For women identified as at increased risk for chromosomal or other genetic disorders, or those requesting invasive diagnostic testing, referral to a geneticist or genetic counselor is appropriate.

REFERENCES

1. American College of Obstetricians and Gynecologists. Practice bulletin No. 77: screening for fetal chromosomal abnormalities. Obstet Gynecol 2007;109: 217–27.
2. American College of Obstetricians and Gynecologists. ACOG Practice Bulletin No. 88: invasive prenatal testing for aneuploidy. Obstet Gynecol 2007;110(6): 1459–67.
3. Kuppermann M, Nease RF, Learman LA, et al. Procedure-related miscarriages and Down syndrome-affected births: implications for prenatal testing based on women's preferences. Obstet Gynecol 2000;96(4):511–6.
4. Kuppermann M, Goldberg JD, Nease RF Jr, et al. Who should be offered prenatal diagnosis? The 35-year-old question. Am J Public Health 1999;89(2):160–3.
5. Haddow JE, Palomaki GE, Knight GJ, et al. Reducing the need for amniocentesis in women 35 years of age or older with serum markers for screening. N Engl J Med 1994;330(16):1114–8.
6. Malone FD, Canick JA, Ball RH, et al. First-trimester or second-trimester screening, or both, for Down's syndrome. N Engl J Med 2005;353:2001–11.
7. Wald NJ, Rodeck C, Hackshaw AK, et al. First and second trimester antenatal screening for Down's syndrome: the results of the Serum, Urine and Ultrasound Screening Study (SURUSS). J Med Screen 2003;10:56–104.

8. Wapner RJ, Thom EA, Simpson JL, et al. First-trimester screening for trisomies 21 and 18. First trimester maternal serum biochemistry and fetal nuchal translucency screening (BUN) study group. N Engl J Med 2003;349:1405–13.

9. Baer R, Flessel MC, Jelliffe-Pawlowski LL, et al. Detection rates for aneuploidy by first-trimester and sequential screening. Obstet Gynecol 2015;126:753–9.

10. Hoyert DL, Mathews TJ, Menacker F, et al. Annual summary of vital statistics. Pediatrics 2004;2006(117):168–83.

11. "Podcast: Counseling an AMA Patient for Genetic Testing." Available at: https://www.perinatalquality.org. Accessed December 5, 2015.

12. Williams J 3rd, Rad S, Beauchamp S, et al. Utilization of noninvasive prenatal testing: impact on referrals for diagnostic testing. Am J Obstet Gynecol 2015; 213(1):102.e1–6.

13. Savva GM, Morris JK, Mutton DE, et al. Maternal age-specific fetal loss rates in Down syndrome pregnancies. Prenat Diagn 2006;26:499.

14. National Institute of Child Health and Human Development. Antenatal diagnosis. Natl Inst Health Consens Dev Conf Summ 1979;2:11–5.

15. American College of Obstetricians and Gynecologists Committee on Genetics. Committee Opinion No. 581: the use of chromosomal microarray analysis in prenatal diagnosis. Obstet Gynecol 2013;122(6):1374–7.

16. Wapner RJ, Martin CL, Levy B, et al. Chromosomal microarray versus karyotyping for prenatal diagnosis. N Engl J Med 2012;367:2175–84.

17. Norton ME, Baer RJ, Wapner RJ, et al. Cell free DNA versus sequential screening for the detection of fetal chromosomal abnormalities. Am J Obstet Gynecol 2015. [Epub ahead of print].

18. Kaimal AJ, Norton ME, Kuppermann M. Prenatal testing in the genomic age: clinical outcomes, quality of life, and costs. Obstet Gynecol 2015;126(4):737–46.

19. Norton ME, Jelliffe-Pawlowski LL, Currier RJ. Chromosome abnormalities detected by current prenatal screening and noninvasive prenatal testing. Obstet Gynecol 2014;124(5):979–86.

20. Rossi AC, Prefumo F. Accuracy of ultrasonography at 11-14 weeks of gestation for detection of fetal structural anomalies: a systematic review. Obstet Gynecol 2013;122:1160–7.

21. Lim J, Whittle WL, Lee YM, et al. Early anatomy ultrasound in women at increased risk of fetal anomalies. Prenat Diagn 2013;33:863–8.

22. Kuppermann M, Learman LA, Gates E, et al. Beyond race or ethnicity and socio-economic status: predictors of prenatal testing for Down syndrome. Obstet Gynecol 2006;107(5):1087–97.

23. Press N, Browner CH. Why women say yes to prenatal diagnosis. Soc Sci Med 1997;45(7):979–89.

24. Chetty S, Garabedian MJ, Norton ME. Uptake of noninvasive prenatal testing (NIPT) in women following positive aneuploidy screening. Prenat Diagn 2013; 33(6):542–6.

25. Driscoll DA, Morgan MA, Schulkin J. Screening for down syndrome: changing practice of obstetricians. Am J Obstet Gynecol 2009;200(4):459.e1–9.

26. Kuppermann M, Pena S, Bishop JT, et al. Effect of enhanced information, values clarification, and removal of financial barriers on use of prenatal genetic testing: a randomized clinical trial. JAMA 2014;312(12):1210–7.

27. Norton ME, Nakagawa S, Norem C, et al. Effects of changes in prenatal aneuploidy screening policies in an integrated health care system. Obstet Gynecol 2013;121(2 Pt 1):265–71.

28. van den Heuvel A, Chitty L, Dormandy E, et al. Will the introduction of non-invasive prenatal diagnostic testing erode informed choices? An experimental study of health care professionals. Patient Educ Couns 2010;78(1):24–8.
29. Hutaff-Lee C, Cordeiro L, Tartaglia N. Cognitive and medical features of chromosomal aneuploidy. Handb Clin Neurol 2013;111:273–9.
30. Linden MG, Bender BG, Robinson A. Intrauterine diagnosis of sex chromosome aneuploidy. Obstet Gynecol 1996;87(3):468–75.
31. Sheets KB, Crissman BG, Feist CD, et al. Practice guidelines for communicating a prenatal or postnatal diagnosis of Down syndrome: recommendations of the National Society of Genetic Counselors. J Genet Couns 2011;20(5):432–41.

Cost-Effectiveness of Old and New Technologies for Aneuploidy Screening

Rachel G. Sinkey, MD*, Anthony O. Odibo, MD, MSCE

KEYWORDS

- Cost-benefit analysis • Cost-effectiveness analysis • Down syndrome • Economics
- Prenatal diagnosis–economics • Noninvasive prenatal screening

KEY POINTS

- Cost-effectiveness analyses allow assessment of whether marginal gains from new technology are worth the increased costs.
- Several studies have examined cost-effectiveness of Down syndrome (DS) screening and found it to be cost-effective across most clinical scenarios.
- Noninvasive prenatal screening also appears to be cost-effective among high-risk women with respect to DS screening, but not for the general population as a first-line screening tool.
- Chromosomal microarray (CMA) is a genetic sequencing method superior to but more expensive than karyotype; it is cost-effective when used for prenatal diagnosis of an anomalous fetus.

INTRODUCTION

Increases in health care costs continue to outpace inflation.[1] In 2011, total expenditures on health care were greater than $2.7 trillion, or 17.9% of the gross domestic product.[2] In this setting, health care systems, health insurance providers, health care providers, the government, and patients themselves are increasingly aware of rising costs and interested in controlling them.

Efforts to balance health care quality with expenditures have led to a new emphasis on comparative effectiveness research, which examines both the differences in outcomes and the costs of health care interventions. To compare the marginal benefits to be gained from new procedures, medications, and screening tests to their often increased costs, economic evaluations of such innovations are now commonly

The authors have no disclosures.
Division of Maternal-Fetal Medicine, Department of Obstetrics and Gynecology, University of South Florida, 2 Tampa General Circle, Tampa, FL 33606, USA
* Corresponding author. Division of Maternal-Fetal Medicine, Department of Obstetrics and Gynecology, University of South Florida Morsani College of Medicine, 2 Tampa General Circle, STC, 6th Floor, Tampa, FL 33606.
E-mail address: rsinkey@health.usf.edu

Clin Lab Med 36 (2016) 237–248
http://dx.doi.org/10.1016/j.cll.2016.01.008
0272-2712/16/$ – see front matter © 2016 Elsevier Inc. All rights reserved.
labmed.theclinics.com

used.[3,4] These analyses may help guide health care providers, organizations, professional societies, and policymakers to determine how and to whom particular health care services are provided.[5]

Economic analyses have been used for decades to inform the development of prenatal screening and diagnosis guidelines. Prenatal diagnosis has several attributes that make such analyses challenging.[6,7] These features include tradeoffs of the risks and benefits to both the mother and the fetus, redundancy of screening and diagnostic tests both in the current pregnancy and in subsequent pregnancies, balancing short- and long-term outcomes, ethical issues regarding termination of pregnancy, and the incorporation of patient preferences, which can range widely for the possible outcomes. This review discusses the different types of economic analyses commonly used in health care with a particular focus on the diagnosis of Down syndrome (DS), the use of chromosomal microarray (CMA) among fetuses with sonographically detected anomalies, and the cost-effectiveness of noninvasive prenatal screening.

ECONOMIC ANALYSES IN HEALTH CARE

The simplest economic analysis in health care takes into account only the costs. Such a cost analysis or cost-only analysis may be limited to just the direct costs of the provision of health care or may be expanded to incorporate the indirect costs of patients' travel time and lost work productivity. A cost-benefit analysis (CBA) assumes that the health outcomes from 2 or more strategies are essentially equal and makes a comparison between multiple programs or strategies on a purely financial level. In a CBA, all direct and indirect costs of health care are included as well as economic valuations of the outcomes. In this purely financial analytical tool, only economic distinctions are made between the value to society or individuals of having particular health outcomes.

The term cost-effectiveness analysis (CEA) specifically refers to an analysis in which costs and outcomes between 2 or more health care programs or strategies are compared. A cost-effectiveness ratio is composed of a numerator, which is the difference between the costs of 2 programs, and a denominator, which is the difference between the outcomes of 2 programs. The denominator in a CEA can be any of a variety of outcomes, including the commonly used years of life saved (life-years), number of diagnoses made, and number of cases prevented. Within a particular clinical arena, these may all be reasonable outcomes to compare. However, attempts to compare the outcomes from disparate procedures such as routine dental care and cardiothoracic surgery are more difficult, suffering from the "apples-to-oranges" problem. Comparing the cost-effectiveness of different programs is not particularly important if the new program is both cheaper and leads to better outcomes (a dominant strategy), in which case the new program should be adopted. A careful comparison is also less important if the new program both costs more and leads to worse outcomes (a dominated strategy). However, for new strategies that cost more and lead to better outcomes or cost less but lead to worse outcomes, CEA is a useful tool to evaluate differences between programs.

It is relatively straightforward to make comparisons between programs in different clinical arenas using CBA. By converting all of the outcomes into financial ones, they become comparable. However, CBA is limited when considering outcomes that lead not to financial burdens but rather to burdensome morbidities. A way to compare such outcomes is by quality-adjusting the value of one's life using utilities. Utility is the unit of value that some product or outcome or, in this case, health state, brings to an individual's life. It is the common valuation given to consumption of goods and services in economics and is defined as ranging from 0 (no utility or death) to 1 (perfect happiness). In CEAs, these valuations are defined as 0 for death and 1 for perfect health, with all other health states falling between these 2. There is occasionally debate about whether there are certain health states that should be scored as worse than death, but most analyses use death as the bottom anchor of utilities, which is assigned the value 0.[8] Once utilities are assigned to particular health states, they can be multiplied by the time spent in that particular health state to generate quality-adjusted life-years (QALYs). When QALYs are used as the outcome measure in the denominator of a CEA, the analysis is considered a cost-utility analysis (CUA).

Estimation of utilities has been done in many ways, but the 2 most commonly used are the standard gamble and time tradeoff metrics.[9] In the standard gamble, patients are asked what probability of death they would be willing to take to avoid a particular health outcome and live in perfect health.[10] For example, if an individual is willing to take a 5% chance of death to avoid losing their sight, then the sightless state has a utility of 0.95 (1 − 0.05). In the time tradeoff, an individual is asked how many years of life they would give up to avoid a particular health outcome and live in perfect health.[11] Thus, if a 25-year-old individual has a life expectancy of 50 additional years and is willing to give up 5 years of life to avoid losing their sight, a valuation of 0.9 (1 − 5/50) would be the estimated utility. Methodologic concerns with these metrics include realism and avoidance of loss of life in standard gamble and different valuations for different times of life in time tradeoff. Despite these problems, their estimation allows comparison between different clinical outcomes.

Given the importance of estimating the benefits from different interventions in health care, these economic analytical techniques can be quite useful. The US Public Health Service convened a panel in 1996 to establish strict criteria for the effective application of CEA.[12] These criteria have been used to analyze the methodologic quality of published CEAs in health care,[13,14] specifically in obstetrics and gynecology.[15,16] These criteria should be carefully considered when either performing or evaluating a CEA.

COST-EFFECTIVENESS ANALYSIS OF THE PRENATAL DIAGNOSIS

CEAs of prenatal diagnosis have been performed for more than 3 decades and have informed the development of guidelines surrounding particular screening and diagnostic strategies. However, even the more recent analyses could be improved with careful consideration of several methodologic issues particular to prenatal diagnosis.

The benefits of prenatal screening and diagnosis include diagnosing a problem that can be treated prenatally (eg, fetal anemia in cases of alloimmunization or prenatal surgery for a subset of fetuses with a myelomeningocele), diagnosing a problem that can be treated postnatally (eg, cardiac anomalies),[17] diagnosing severe genetic disorders, anomalies, and syndromes so that termination of pregnancy can be performed (eg, cystic fibrosis, renal agenesis, or DS), and reassurance of women and their partners that their fetus has either a very low risk of or is without any of the more common diagnosable conditions (eg, reassuring nuchal translucency (NT) or normal karyotype). Unfortunately, how each of these benefits is accounted for in CEAs is inconsistent at best. For example, most studies in the literature examining the cost-effectiveness of screening for DS focus specifically on the benefits to the woman undergoing prenatal diagnosis rather than on the benefits to either her partner or her other children. When considering the benefits from screening for neural tube defects, the biggest financial gain is achieved by society when a diagnosed fetus is terminated.[18] With increased interest in fetal surgery programs, costs incurred from screening for this anomaly may actually be increased, albeit still cost-effective.[19] Although the largest economic gains in many of the strategies come from not having to treat a chronically physically or mentally challenged person, one study showed that the primary reason for the cost-effectiveness of amniocentesis was the reassurance gained by the patient undergoing the test.[20]

Down Syndrome Screening and Diagnosis

Despite the recent introduction of noninvasive prenatal testing to clinical practice, diagnosis obtained through chorionic villus sampling or amniocentesis is still the gold standard. Although amniocentesis and karyotype for fetal aneuploidy was described almost 50 years ago,[21] it is still not made widely available to all pregnant women.[22] Part of the justification for the National Institute of Child Health and Human Development guidelines limiting routine access to amniocentesis to women aged 35 and older[23] was a CBA of DS screening.[24] Unfortunately, this analysis simply compared costs of a program of receiving amniocentesis to not receiving amniocentesis and determined that beyond age 35, amniocentesis was cost saving. As discussed earlier, this is a much stricter threshold than is commonly used to determine whether an intervention is cost-effective. In fact, a 2004 CUA demonstrated that routinely offering amniocentesis to women of all ages was cost-effective when compared with using an age 35 threshold.[20]

Screening for DS is one of the most common topics for CEAs in prenatal diagnosis. One reason is the development of many different screening strategies beginning with maternal age, followed by maternal serum α-fetoprotein (MSAFP), the "triple screen," which adds estriol and β-human chorionic gonadotropin (β-hCG) to MSAFP, and the "quad screen," which adds inhibin A to the "triple screen." More recently, a battery of first-trimester and either sequential or integrated screening tests has been developed and studied.[25,26] The vast majority of these CEAs demonstrate that screening for DS is cost-effective. In the first CUA of DS screening, first-trimester screening was cost-effective when compared with second-trimester screening.[27] However, it may be that with an increasing number of screens, eventually the marginal gains of an improved screen will be too small to be justified on a cost-effective basis. However, it does not appear that threshold has been reached. Pertinent CEA studies of DS screening that include first-trimester screening are reviewed in later discussion.

ECONOMIC ANALYSES OF FIRST-TRIMESTER SCREENING FOR DOWN SYNDROME

Biggio and coworkers[26] compared the cost-effectiveness of 5 prenatal screening options for DS:

1. Triple screen
2. Quad screen
3. First-trimester only (NT/pregnancy-associated plasma protein-A [PAPP-A]/Free-β-hCG)
4. Integrated (NT/PAPP-A/Free-β-hCG + Quad)
5. Sequential (NT/PAPP-A/Free-β-hCG, then Quad screen)

The analysis was limited to women less than 35 years old and was not from a societal perspective. The denominator or effectiveness was measured in terms of DS cases diagnosed. Importantly, spontaneous losses of DS pregnancies were accounted for in this analysis.

All strategies were less costly and more effective than no screening; thus, screening for DS is economically justified. Sequential was the least costly strategy at 455 million

US dollars (USD) and integrated the most costly at 521 million USD. The most effective strategy, in terms of DS detection, was sequential screening, followed by integrated and first trimester. Sequential screening was associated with the highest number of procedure-related losses, whereas integrated had the lowest number. DS births averted per procedure-related loss is another way to express the tradeoff between efficacy and safety of DS screening.[28] A loss ratio greater than 1 indicated that more DS births will be averted per loss, whereas a loss ratio less than 1.0 suggests that there will be more procedure-related losses than DS cases averted. From the Biggio analysis,[26] the most favorable loss ratio was integrated (loss ratio = 9.3), followed by quad screen (loss ratio = 1.5), and triple screen (loss ratio = 1.3). Sequential screening had the least favorable loss ratio (loss ratio = 0.87).

Another analysis was published in 2005 by Odibo and colleagues.[29] This analysis included the following 9 screening strategies:

1. No screening
2. NT only
3. First-trimester combined screen (NT/PAPP-A/Free-β-hCG)
4. First-trimester serum only (PAPP-A, Free-β-hCG)
5. Quad screen
6. Integrated screening (NT/PAPP-A/Free-β-hCG + quad)
7. Integrated serum screen (PAPP-A/Free-β-hCG + quad)
8. Sequential screening (NT/PAPP-A/Free-β-hCG → quad)
9. Maternal age

This analysis was from a societal perspective. Outcomes analyzed include number of DS cases detected and prevented by each strategy, procedure-related pregnancy losses, and costs. The estimates used were from a systematic review of the literature, and the costs were based on Medicare charges from the United States when available (only direct medical costs are included). These probabilities and costs were similar, although not identical, to those used by Biggio and colleagues.[26] All strategies are less costly than no screening, suggesting that DS screening is justified (**Table 1**). The model results confirmed that sequential screening averts the highest number of DS cases compared with the other strategies, corroborating the report by Biggio and colleagues.[26] The price for this high detection rate is the highest rate of

Table 1
Cost-effectiveness of screening strategies for Down syndrome in Odibo et al

Strategy	Cost (mil)	T21 Live Birth Averted	Euploid Losses	T21 Live Birth/ Euploid Loss
No screen	2382	0	0	—
NT	698	4620	1525	1.4
Quad	1024	3920	2855	3.0
First trimester	968	4920	1082	4.5
First trimester (serum)	739	3600	2088	1.7
Integrated serum	1248	4760	524	9.1
Integrated	1554	5264	579	9.1
Sequential	1715	5320	3767	1.4

Abbreviation: T21, Trisomy 21.
Data from Odibo AO, Stamilio DM, Nelson DB, et al. A cost-effectiveness analysis of prenatal screening strategies for Down syndrome. Obstet Gynecol 2005;106:562–8.

procedure-related losses. Most loss ratios were positive, although the most favorable loss ratios were achieved by integrated and integrated serum testing. The strategies with the most favorable tradeoffs between cost, detection, and safety seem to be first trimester, integrated serum screening, and integrated. Several incremental analyses were also performed.

Interpretation of the analysis of Odibo and coworkers[29] would support the following conclusions. First, screening for DS is economically justified. Second, first trimester, integrated, and integrated serum seem to be the most favorable strategies. There is only small incremental gain when comparing integrated serum to integrated testing.

Cost-Effectiveness of Contingent Screening

Although the studies by Biggio and colleagues[26] and Odibo and colleagues[29] represent an exhaustive exploration of the comparisons, one can make between a wide range of screening regimens, neither considered contingent screening. Contingent screening operates under the assumption that one will use a 3-pronged approach in the first-trimester screening test: (1) positive screen: those women with a high risk (commonly 1 in 50) would proceed to invasive prenatal diagnosis; (2) negative screen: those with a very low risk (perhaps < 1 in 1500 or < 1 in 2000) would not obtain a second-trimester test, thus saving on the additional testing; (3) intermediate screen: those women with a risk between these thresholds would go on to be screened in the second trimester.

In the first cost-effectiveness study to include contingent screening as a strategy, a CUA by Ball and colleagues[30] based on clinical data from the FASTER trial (First and Second Trimester Evaluation of Risk)[31] found that contingent screening was a dominant strategy. This analysis conducted incremental comparisons, conducted the analysis from the societal perspective, and used QALYs as its effectiveness measure.

An important component of the contingent screening protocol is the choice of the risk thresholds of low and high risk. A 2009 analysis by Gekas and colleagues[32] examined just that. Similar to the study by Ball and colleagues, they too found contingent screening to be a dominant strategy.

COST-EFFECTIVENESS OF CHROMOSOMAL MICROARRAY

Amniocentesis with karyotype has been the standard for second-trimester prenatal diagnosis for decades. Recently, CMA (synonymous with comparative genomic hybridization) has been introduced from postnatal diagnosis into the prenatal realm owing to its ability to detect genetic abnormalities with finer precision. One cost-effective analysis investigating the utility of CMA was identified. Performed from a societal perspective, Harper and colleagues[33] compared 4 strategies (**Fig. 1**):

1. Karyotype alone
2. CMA alone
3. Karyotype and CMA
4. Karyotype followed by CMA in the case that karyotype was nondiagnostic or normal

Strategy 2, CMA alone, was the dominant strategy for sonographically detected anomalies, as shown in the Monte Carlo simulation in **Fig. 2**. The incremental cost-effectiveness ratio (ICER) between CMA alone and karyotype alone was $24,712 as CMA alone led to an additional 17 diagnoses per 1000 fetuses. Although this study examined the cost-effectiveness of CMA use for anomalies as a whole, further studies are needed to investigate the cost-effectiveness of CMA use among specific anomalies.

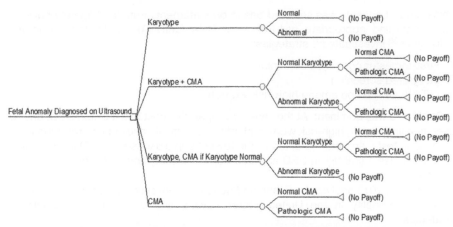

Fig. 1. Decision analytical model incorporating use of CMA. (*From* Harper LM, Sutton AL, Longman RE, et al. An economic analysis of prenatal cytogenetic technologies for sonographically detected fetal anomalies. Am J Med Genet A 2014;164A:1192–7; with permission.)

COST-EFFECTIVENESS OF NONINVASIVE PRENATAL SCREENING

The direct-to-consumer marketing of noninvasive prenatal screening in 2011 led to even more options for patients and providers. Noninvasive prenatal screening is an attractive option, particularly for DS screening, because of high sensitivity, low false positive rates, and the misconception that one can avoid the risks of invasive testing.[34] However, its cost-effectiveness has been questioned by several recent analyses. The cost of noninvasive prenatal screening is more expensive than traditional testing and varies greatly by manufacturer. As of 2014, Harmony was least expensive at $795, whereas MaterniT21 was most expensive at $2762.[35,36]

A 2013 cost-effective analysis by Song and colleagues[36] evaluated noninvasive prenatal screening for the detection of DS in a high-risk cohort defined as women 35 years of age and older, those with a positive screening test, or those with a family history.

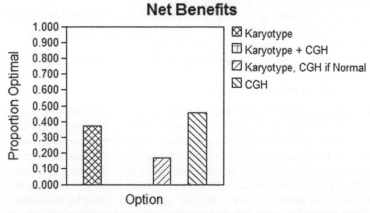

Fig. 2. Monte Carlo simulation CMA. CGH, comparative genomic hybridization. (*From* Harper LM, Sutton AL, Longman RE, et al. An economic analysis of prenatal cytogenetic technologies for sonographically detected fetal anomalies. Am J Med Genet A 2014;164A:1192–7; with permission.)

This group of patients was selected based on statements from leading national societies regarding appropriate cell-free fetal DNA (ccfDNA) candidates. Song and colleagues[36] investigated 3 strategies:

1. First-trimester combined screening
2. Integrated screening
3. cffDNA as first line among high-risk women

Strategy 3 was dominant. At the lowest comparative cost of 3.4 billion USD, cffDNA used first line among high-risk women identified the most cases of DS, required fewer diagnostic tests, and therefore, led to the fewest euploid losses (n = 3) as compared with strategies 1 (3.8 billion USD and 525 euploid losses) and 2 (3.9 billion USD and 525 euploid losses).

Similarly, a 2015 analysis by Evans and colleagues investigated using ccfDNA as a screening modality in the United States. Evans and colleagues[37] evaluated 3 strategies:

1. cffDNA as a screening test for all women
2. Contingent strategy: cffDNA offered if first-trimester screening resulted high risk
3. Hybrid strategy: cffDNA offered to all women 35 years old or older or less than or equal to 35 years old if first-trimester screening resulted in high risk

This analysis drew similar conclusions to that of Song and colleagues.[36] First, primary screening with cffDNA is the most expensive strategy. Second, Evans and colleagues found that cffDNA is cost-effective when used in a contingent strategy with a risk cutoff of 1/1000.

The work by both Song[36] and Evans and their colleagues are methodologically sound. Although ccfDNA does appear to be cost-effective for DS screening, it comes at the expense of lower detection rates for other aneuploidies and structural abnormalities that are detected by traditional measures, factors not accounted for in these analyses.

Kaimal and colleagues[38] addressed this issue in a 2015 decision analytical model that assessed outcomes of prenatal testing strategies across a patient's reproductive lifespan. They explored 6 strategies:

1. Multiple marker screening (NT/PAPP-A/Free-β-hCG + quad) and the option for diagnostic testing after the screening tests resulted
2. Multiple marker screening and the option for diagnostic testing or ccfDNA
3. ccfDNA screening alone followed by the option for diagnostic testing
4. ccfDNA + NT with diagnostic testing if desired
5. Concurrent multiple marker (see strategy 1) and cffDNA with diagnostic testing if desired
6. Diagnostic testing without screening

Kaimal and associates[38] found that multiple marker screening and the option for diagnostic testing (strategy 1) had the highest sensitivity for aneuploidy but also the highest procedure-related losses. As expected, cffDNA detected the most cases of trisomy 21 with the lowest detection rates for other anomalies. Because of the varying baseline incidence of aneuploidy across a women's reproductive life, different strategies were found to be dominant at different maternal ages. At ages 20 and 30, strategy 1 is dominant. This strategy shifted around age 38 as maternal aneuploidy risk increases. This transition yields interesting although not surprising results. At age 40, strategy 2 is least expensive: strategy 1 had an ICER of $1992/QALY, and strategy 3 (ccfDNA as first line) became more cost-effective with an ICER of $73,154/QALY.

It is important to note that ccfDNA becomes cost-effective only in the 40-and-over population.

When studying cost-effective analyses, it is important to determine who the payer is. Walker and colleagues[39] examined the use of first-trimester noninvasive prenatal screening in 4 different strategies and evaluated the cost-effectiveness from 3 perspectives: societal, government, and payer. They found universal cffDNA to be cost-effective from a societal standpoint, but not from a government or payer viewpoint.

Four years into the commercial use of cffDNA, these conclusions can be cautiously drawn: (1) with the current pricing structure, cffDNA is not cost-effective as a primary screening tool; (2) cffDNA appears cost-effective for DS syndrome screening among high-risk women; (3) cffDNA, although sensitive for DS, does not screen for many other chromosomal or structural malformations; these costs are omitted in most cffDNA cost-effective analyses.

LIMITATIONS INHERENT ON ECONOMIC ANALYSES METHODOLOGY

Although CEA is a useful tool in the evaluation of prenatal screening and diagnostic programs, there are several important methodologic issues that need to be emphasized. The first issue seen in some of the analyses discussed earlier is the problem of a useful denominator. From a societal perspective, if one is to compare investment in various programs, a comparable denominator is needed. This comparable denominator is commonly life-years or QALYs. However, this can be challenging in prenatal diagnosis, where the outcomes do not affect maternal life expectancy and the valuation of utilities is limited. Fortunately, there have been several studies that evaluate maternal preferences toward DS by Kuppermann and colleagues,[40,41] so studies of prenatal diagnosis of DS benefit from including these values.

Another methodologic issue that arises is the use of CBA. Although a CBA can demonstrate whether a program will cost more than it will save, it cannot be used to assess whether a program is cost-effective. If the benefits in terms of quality of life are worth the additional expenditures, the program may be cost-effective despite its expense. However, from a cost-effectiveness standpoint, the best way to analyze this question is to determine whether the additional costs are worth the outcomes achieved.[42] Furthermore, even if a program is not cost-effective from a societal perspective, the screening test may be desirable to a subset of individuals based on their particular preferences. In this setting, at the very least, patients should be given information about such screening or diagnostic tests and be allowed to determine for themselves whether they wish to bear the costs and risks of such tests.

The assumption regarding the termination of affected pregnancies is another key methodologic concern in prenatal diagnosis. Although many programs may be cost-effective based on the costs of affected fetuses being averted, if a large proportion of women decide to continue affected pregnancies, these costs may remain. Another important aspect of CEA in prenatal diagnosis is the reassurance gained by women with normal results, which should be accounted for in the outcomes analyzed. How this and other outcomes are valued by other members of the family should be incorporated into future analyses.

Most CEAs in prenatal diagnosis have been modeling studies. Although the insight gained from such analyses is important, before screening programs are made universal, clinical trials or prospective studies to assess the true costs and benefits should be performed. As new programs are analyzed, economies of scale from volume effects and economies of scope from the redundancy of prenatal diagnostic and screening tests should be estimated as an aspect of these studies. With the recent programmatic change in the state of California, as well as the introduction of CMA and noninvasive prenatal screening around the United States and other countries, prospective analysis of these programs is merited.

SUMMARY

It appears in several studies that first-trimester screening for DS is cost-effective. In particular, contingent screening appears to be dominant as compared with other forms of screening. Furthermore, based on one CEA from a societal perspective investigating the use of CMA, CMA is cost-effective in the genetic workup of a sonographically identified anomalous fetus.[33] Last, 4 years into the commercial use of noninvasive prenatal screening, screening for DS among high-risk women appears cost-effective. However, as a population-based screening tool with the current pricing structure, cffDNA is not cost-effective as a primary screening tool in the general population.[43–45]

ACKNOWLEDGMENTS

The authors would like to acknowledge the contributions of Drs Aaron Caughey and Anjali Kaimal to the first edition of this article.

REFERENCES

1. Chernew ME, Hirth RA, Cutler DM. Increased spending on health care: how much can the United States afford? Health Aff (Millwood) 2003;22:15–25.
2. Hartman M, Martin AB, Benson J, et al. National health spending in 2011: overall growth remains low, but some payers and services show signs of acceleration. Health Aff (Millwood) 2013;32:87–99.
3. Weinstein MC, Stason WB. Foundations of cost-effectiveness analysis for health and medical practices. N Engl J Med 1977;296:716–21.
4. Eisenberg JM. Clinical economics. A guide to the economic analysis of clinical practices. JAMA 1989;262:2879–86.
5. Cutler DM, McClellan M. Is technological change in medicine worth it? Health Aff (Millwood) 2001;20:11–29.
6. Shackley P. Economic evaluation of prenatal diagnosis: a methodological review. Prenat Diagn 1996;16:389–95.
7. Caughey AB. Cost-effectiveness analysis of prenatal diagnosis: methodological issues and concerns. Gynecol Obstet Invest 2005;60:11–8.
8. DeShazo J, Cameron TA. The effect of health status on willingness to pay for morbidity and mortality risk reductions. Los Angeles, CA: California Center for Population Research; 2005. Available at: http://escholarship.org/uc/item/9431841p#page-4. Accessed February 25, 2016.
9. Shepard DS. Cost-effectiveness in health and medicine. M.R. Gold, J.E Siegel, L.B. Russell, et al (eds). New York: Oxford University Press, 1996. J Ment Health Policy Econ 1999;2:91–2.
10. Torrance GW. Measurement of health state utilities for economic appraisal. J Health Econ 1986;5:1–30.
11. Torrance GW, Thomas WH, Sackett DL. A utility maximization model for evaluation of health care programs. Health Serv Res 1972;7:118–33.
12. Weinstein MC, Siegel JE, Gold MR, et al. Recommendations of the panel on cost-effectiveness in health and medicine. JAMA 1996;276:1253–8.

13. Detsky AS, Naglie IG. A clinician's guide to cost-effectiveness analysis. Ann Intern Med 1990;113:147–54.

14. Drummond MF, Jefferson TO. Guidelines for authors and peer reviewers of economic submissions to the BMJ. The BMJ Economic Evaluation Working Party. BMJ 1996;313:275–83.

15. Subak LL, Caughey AB, Washington AE. Cost-effectiveness analyses in obstetrics & gynecology. Evaluation of methodologic quality and trends. J Reprod Med 2002;47:631–9.

16. Smith WJ, Blackmore CC. Economic analyses in obstetrics and gynecology: a methodologic evaluation of the literature. Obstet Gynecol 1998;91:472–8.

17. Pinto NM, Nelson R, Puchalski M, et al. Cost-effectiveness of prenatal screening strategies for congenital heart disease. Ultrasound Obstet Gynecol 2014;44:50–7.

18. Layde PM, von Allmen SD, Oakley GP Jr. Maternal serum alpha-fetoprotein screening: a cost-benefit analysis. Am J Public Health 1979;69:566–73.

19. Werner EF, Han CS, Burd I, et al. Evaluating the cost-effectiveness of prenatal surgery for myelomeningocele: a decision analysis. Ultrasound Obstet Gynecol 2012;40:158–64.

20. Harris RA, Washington AE, Nease RF Jr, et al. Cost utility of prenatal diagnosis and the risk-based threshold. Lancet 2004;363:276–82.

21. Steele MW, Breg WR Jr. Chromosome analysis of human amniotic-fluid cells. Lancet 1966;1:383–5.

22. Kuppermann M, Goldberg JD, Nease RF Jr, et al. Who should be offered prenatal diagnosis? The 35-year-old question. Am J Public Health 1999;89:160–3.

23. National Institute of Child Health and Human Development. Antenatal diagnosis: report of a consensus development conference. US Dept of Health, Education and Welfare, Public Health Service, National Institutes of Health; 1979.

24. Hagard S, Carter FA. Preventing the birth of infants with Down's syndrome: a cost-benefit analysis. Br Med J 1976;1:753–6.

25. Wapner R, Thom E, Simpson JL, et al. First-trimester screening for trisomies 21 and 18. N Engl J Med 2003;349:1405–13.

26. Biggio JR Jr, Morris TC, Owen J, et al. An outcomes analysis of five prenatal screening strategies for trisomy 21 in women younger than 35 years. Am J Obstet Gynecol 2004;190:721–9.

27. Caughey AB, Kuppermann M, Norton ME, et al. Nuchal translucency and first trimester biochemical markers for down syndrome screening: a cost-effectiveness analysis. Am J Obstet Gynecol 2002;187:1239–45.

28. Caughey AB, Lyell DJ, Filly RA, et al. The impact of the use of the isolated echogenic intracardiac focus as a screen for Down syndrome in women under the age of 35 years. Am J Obstet Gynecol 2001;185:1021–7.

29. Odibo AO, Stamilio DM, Nelson DB, et al. A cost-effectiveness analysis of prenatal screening strategies for Down syndrome. Obstet Gynecol 2005;106:562–8.

30. Ball RH, Caughey AB, Malone FD, et al. First- and second-trimester evaluation of risk for Down syndrome. Obstet Gynecol 2007;110:10–7.

31. Malone FD, Canick JA, Ball RH, et al. First-trimester or second-trimester screening, or both, for Down's syndrome. N Engl J Med 2005;353:2001–11.

32. Gekas J, Gagne G, Bujold E, et al. Comparison of different strategies in prenatal screening for Down's syndrome: cost effectiveness analysis of computer simulation. BMJ 2009;338:b138.

33. Harper LM, Sutton AL, Longman RE, et al. An economic analysis of prenatal cytogenetic technologies for sonographically detected fetal anomalies. Am J Med Genet A 2014;164A:1192–7.
34. Society for Maternal-Fetal Medicine (SMFM) Publications Committee. #36: prenatal aneuploidy screening using cell-free DNA. Am J Obstet Gynecol 2015;212: 711–6.
35. Lo JO, Cori DF, Norton ME, et al. Noninvasive prenatal testing. Obstet Gynecol Surv 2014;69:89–99.
36. Song K, Musci TJ, Caughey AB. Clinical utility and cost of non-invasive prenatal testing with cfDNA analysis in high-risk women based on a US population. J Matern Fetal Neonatal Med 2013;26:1180–5.
37. Evans MI, Sonek JD, Hallahan TW, et al. Cell-free fetal DNA screening in the USA: a cost analysis of screening strategies. Ultrasound Obstet and Gynecol 2015;45: 74–83.
38. Kaimal AJ, Norton ME, Kuppermann M. Prenatal testing in the genomic age: clinical outcomes, quality of life, and costs. Obstet Gynecol 2015;126:737–46.
39. Walker BS, Nelson RE, Jackson BR, et al. A cost-effectiveness analysis of first trimester non-invasive prenatal screening for fetal trisomies in the United States. PLoS One 2015;10:e0131402.
40. Kuppermann M, Feeny D, Gates E, et al. Preferences of women facing a prenatal diagnostic choice: long-term outcomes matter most. Prenat Diagn 1999;19: 711–6.
41. Kuppermann M, Nease RF, Learman LA, et al. Procedure-related miscarriages and Down syndrome-affected births: implications for prenatal testing based on women's preferences. Obstet Gynecol 2000;96:511–6.
42. Musci TJ, Caughey AB. Cost-effectiveness analysis of prenatal population-based fragile X carrier screening. Am J Obstet Gynecol 2005;192:1905–12 [discussion: 1912–5].
43. Ayres AC, Whitty JA, Ellwood DA. A cost-effectiveness analysis comparing different strategies to implement noninvasive prenatal testing into a Down syndrome screening program. Aust N Z J Obstet Gynaecol 2014;54:412–7.
44. Conner P, Gustafsson S, Kublickas M. First trimester contingent testing with either nuchal translucency or cell-free DNA. Cost efficiency and the role of ultrasound dating. Acta Obstet Gynecol Scand 2015;94:368–75.
45. Fairbrother G, Burigo J, Sharon T, et al. Prenatal screening for fetal aneuploidies with cell-free DNA in the general pregnancy population: a cost-effectiveness analysis. J Matern Fetal Neonatal Med 2016;29(7):1160–4.

Modifying Risk of Aneuploidy with a Positive Cell-Free Fetal DNA Result

A. Ashleigh Long, MD, PhD*, Alfred Z. Abuhamad, MD,
Steven L. Warsof, MD

KEYWORDS

- Prenatal screening • NIPT • Noninvasive • Prenatal diagnosis • Prenatal risk
- Aneuploidy

KEY POINTS

- Despite superior sensitivities and positive predictive values of noninvasive prenatal testing (NIPT) screening beyond traditional screening, a positive cell-free fetal DNA (cfDNA) result should not be considered a diagnostic test and should be verified by karyotyping through an invasive testing method, such as chorionic villous sampling, or amniocentesis.
- NIPT screening should be completed in conjunction with an early ultrasound evaluation, which would incorporate the superior accuracy of cfDNA molecular analyses with the early morphologic evaluation of the fetus.
- The use an early morphology ultrasound examination in conjunction with cfDNA screening in a general obstetrics population has several advantages.
- These advantages include highly accurate dating of gestational age, early detection of multiple gestations, determination of chorionicity and the early detection of twin-twin transfusion syndrome, early detection fetal abnormalities, and early detection of congenital heart disease.

BACKGROUND

Screening and diagnostic testing for chromosomal aneuploidy have been available since the 1970s, when the karyotyping of fetal cells from amniotic fluid obtained through amniocentesis was first performed.[1] Invasive diagnostic procedures and karyotyping could not feasibly be performed on all pregnancies; therefore, screening strategies were developed to determine which pregnancies should be offered diagnostic testing. In general, the most effective screening programs were those with sensitivities

Disclosure Statement: The authors have nothing to disclose.
Department of Obstetrics and Gynecology, Eastern Virginia Medical School, 825 Fairfax Avenue, Suite 500, Hofheimer Hall, Norfolk, VA 23507, USA
* Corresponding author.
E-mail address: longaa@evms.edu

Clin Lab Med 36 (2016) 249–259
http://dx.doi.org/10.1016/j.cll.2016.01.018
0272-2712/16/$ – see front matter
labmed.theclinics.com

as high as possible approaching 100% with false positive or screen positive rates as low as possible.

Initial screening strategies in the 1970s and early 1980s relied on maternal age and family history of aneuploidy. If the patient was aged 35 (Down syndrome [DS] risk of 1:270) or greater at the time of delivery, or had a first-degree family history of aneuploidy, women were offered invasive diagnostic testing either by amniocentesis in the second trimester or with chorionic villous sampling (CVS) using a transcervical or transabdominal approach in the late first trimester. Although this screening was accepted by a large segment of the population, it had poor sensitivity (25%–30%) for aneuploidy detection, and a high selection or false positive rate (15%–20%), resulting in a large number of invasive diagnostic procedures with few aneuploidies detected. This strategy missed 70% to 75% of aneuploidies as most aneuploidies are born to women less than the age of 35. In some countries, maternal age of 38 (1:150 risk of DS) or 40 (1:100 risk of DS) were used as alternate screening criteria based on financial and medical resources to provide genetic screening services in these countries, which led to an even lower sensitivity, but with fewer invasive procedures.

Subsequent development of additional screening methods in the late 1980s focused on the second trimester of gestation with screening strategies that measured serum levels of maternal serum analytes, Maternal Serum Alpha Fetal Protein (MSAFP), Beta Human Chorionic Gonadotrophin (BHCG), serum levels of unconjugated estriol (uE3), and Inhibin. In the late 1990s, additional late first-trimester screening was developed using the combination of ultrasound nuchal translucency measurements and with BHCG and Plasma-Associated Pregnancy Protein A (PAPP-A) serum analytes; this increased the sensitivity of aneuploidy detection to 80% to 85% while decreasing the false positive rate to 5%. Combinations of first- and second-trimester strategies were referred to as integrated, sequential, or contingency screening and increased the sensitivity for aneuploidy to 95% while still maintaining the 5% false positive rate.

Although these developments enhanced sensitivity and detection rates, the 5% false positive rate implied that the positive predictive value (PPV), which varies with the prevalence of the disease in the screened population, remained quite low, especially in the younger pregnant population with low prevalence of aneuploidy. The PPV ranged from 1% in maternal age 15 to 19 with prevalence of aneuploidy of 1:1667 to 20% in the maternal age 40 to 44 when the prevalence of aneuploidy is 1:67 (**Table 1**).

Table 1
Positive predictive value of trisomy 21 screening tests vary by maternal age

Maternal Age	Incidence of DS	No. of Live Births with DS	NIPT	FTS	MSAFP4
—	—	Sensitivity	99	85	75
—	—	False +	0.1%	5%	5%
15–19	1:1667	198	37%	1.0%	0.9%
20–24	1:1448	621	40	1.1	1.0
25–29	1:1118	1008	47	1.5	1.3
30–34	1:742	1328	57	2.2	1.9
35–39	1:239	1937	80.6	6.6	5.9
40–44	1:67	1611	93.7	20	18.4
>45	1:19	366	98.1	48	45

The incidence of trisomy 21 varies dramatically by age, as does the PPV of prenatal screening tests, which include NIPT, first-trimester screening (FTS), and maternal serum markers, such as MSAFP.

CELL-FREE FETAL DNA IN SCREENING FOR ANEUPLOIDY

Noninvasive genomic assessments of the fetus while in utero have been made possible by the analysis of cell-free fetal DNA (cfDNA) fragments from the serum of pregnant woman, as part of a noninvasive prenatal testing (NIPT) screening strategy. Between 7% and 10% of total cell-free DNA in the maternal blood comes from the placental trophoblasts,[2–4] allowing for identification of the DNA associated with the fetal component of the placenta. Using simple venipuncture in the outpatient setting, this cell-free, extracellular fetal DNA can be isolated in the maternal serum from a single blood draw as early as the seventh week of gestation, where it circulates as short fragments of DNA.[3,4] Once collected, both whole genome and targeted chromosomal sequencing approaches can be undertaken using massively parallel sequencing to differentiate fetal from maternal DNA, and to assign a chromosome of origin. Imbalances in the amount of cell free fragments from various chromosomes can be used to screen for chromosomal anomalies such as trisomies and sex chromosome abnormalities. Several clinical trials have validated cfDNA analysis as a screening tool for common aneuploidies, such as trisomy 21, 18, 13, or sex chromosome abnormalities with a high degree of accuracy, making it an ideal screening method for pregnancies at high risk for aneuploidy.[5] Detection and false positive rates have been frequently reported to be at 99% and 0.1%, respectively, for trisomy 21 (DS). Although less data exist for trisomy 18 (Edwards syndrome) and trisomy 13 (Patau syndrome), the detection rates using cfDNA sequencing for these syndromes have been reported greater than 85%.[3,4,6]

Although sensitivities and false positive rates do not vary with disease prevalence, the positive predictive value (PPV) of NIPT, as with all screening strategies, does vary with disease prevalence. Because of its greater precision, however, NIPT has a significantly higher PPV than any other screening strategies, ranging from 37% to 98%, for maternal ages 15 to 45 years (see **Table 1**).

Because of the lower PPV in low-risk populations, present recommendations state that NIPT be used only in pregnancies designated as high risk for aneuploidy, such as maternal age greater than 35, family history of aneuploidy, suspected fetal anomaly by ultrasound, or abnormal traditional first- or second-trimester screening. Recent large studies, including the Non-Invasive Examination of Trisomy (NEXT) clinical trial, have additionally demonstrated the clinical utility of cfDNA use for prenatal screening in the general obstetric population. Recent studies using cfDNA-based prenatal screening in mixed, large populations of both low- and high-risk pregnancies have shown encouraging results. In assessing the possibility of using NIPT as a universal screen for all pregnancies, 2 large population-based studies showed that cfDNA screening revealed higher PPVs and significantly lower false positive rates for detection of trisomies 21 and 18 compared with standard screening approaches involving nuchal translucency and maternal serum analytes.[2,7]

Despite superior sensitivities and PPVs of NIPT screening above traditional screening, a positive cfDNA result should not be considered a diagnostic test and should be verified by karyotyping through an invasive testing method, such as CVS, or amniocentesis, whereby karyotypic analysis of tissue is taken directly from the fetus or placenta. Although these invasive procedures are considered safe, both carry inherent risks, including rupture of membranes, preterm labor, infection, and a small risk of fetal loss following the procedure.[8–10] Recently it was shown that risk of fetal loss from CVS was shown to be 1:455, or 0.22%, and risk of loss from amniocentesis as 1:769, or 0.13%.[11] Given these risks, effectively minimizing false positives in screening tests is considered an important way to limit unnecessary invasive diagnostic procedures and associated fetal loss. In practice, the introduction of cfDNA testing has markedly reduced the number of invasive diagnostic procedures. In our own institution, genetic amniocenteses have decreased 76% and CVS procedures by 83% since the introduction of NIPT in our community between the years of 2004 and 2014 (**Fig. 1**).

DISCORDANT OR FALSE POSITIVE RESULTS WITH CELL-FREE FETAL DNA SCREENING

When an abnormal NIPT result is different from the actual clinical outcome, it is usually classified as a false positive result, but in many instances, there is an underlying biological reason for this result. In these cases, it would be better to be referred to as a discordant result rather than a false positive result. Every attempt should be made to identify the potential for discordant results before any definitive management decisions.

Previously recognized causes of discordant results associated with the use of cfDNA in prenatal screening are listed in **Box 1**. Because NIPT screening is currently recommended only for high-risk pregnancies, patients who are candidates for noninvasive screening should ideally meet with a genetic counselor before the test, and after the cfDNA results have returned. This counseling allows for preliminary assessment of the patient's background risk of chromosomal aneuploidy (eg, that based on maternal age, medical history, family history), and for postscreening readjustment of risk and appropriate counseling. Issues of false positives or discordant results and the need for invasive diagnostic testing can be reviewed before performing the NIPT so that patients will be prepared for the next steps if the need arises.

UNRECOGNIZED MULTIFETAL PREGNANCY

NIPT relies on quantitative analyses of fetal chromosome copy numbers, determined by comparing the absolute number of sequence "reads" or counts derived from the chromosome of interest in the sample, and inferring fetal trisomy when this ratio is greater than a predetermined threshold.[12,13] In their 2015 position statement on noninvasive prenatal screening, the American College of Obstetrics and Gynecology (ACOG) cautioned against the use of cfDNA screening in multifetal gestations, because the presence of additional fetal haplotypes, for example, in unrecognized dizygotic twin pregnancies, would increase the likelihood of a false positive aneuploidy result through the presence of additional fetal haplotypes.[5,12,13] This concern could be easily ruled out in advance of cfDNA testing, with early morphology scan by

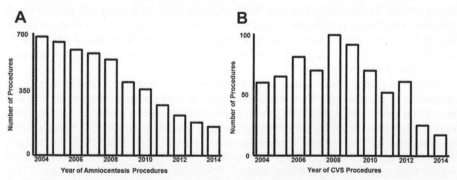

Fig. 1. Effect of first-trimester screening (FTS) and noninvasive prenatal screening (NIPT) on the number of invasive diagnostic prenatal screening procedures between 2004 and 2014. At the authors' institution, the number of amniocentesis procedures dropped by 85% between 2004 and 2014 (*A*), when FTS and NIPT were implemented. The number of CVS decreased by 83% from peak utilization in 2008 (*B*).

Box 1
Etiology of discordant results
Unrecognized multifetal pregnancy
Vanishing twin syndrome
Confined placental mosaicism
Maternal mosaicism
History of maternal organ transplant
Occult maternal malignancy

ultrasound, which would detect the presence of a twin or higher-order gestation and the chorionicity of the gestation.

There are additional ways in which twin gestations may provide false positive aneuploidy results in NIPT. In confirmed multizygous pregnancies, potential problems may arise as one pregnancy may be normal and the other with aneuploidy, with the normal fetus diluting the result from the abnormal pregnancy. In addition, it has been previously shown that in dizygotic twin gestations, the fetal fractions of cfDNA contributed by each twin can be significantly different,[12,13] further complicating the interpretation of the result. In monozygous gestations, whereby each fetus is chromosomally identical, this presents less of a concern; however, only about one-third of twin pregnancies are monozygous in natural conceptions, and 5% or less in patients conceiving with artificial reproductive technology. In addition, several studies have identified other sources of error in the multizygous pregnancy: the first is a "dilutional effect" that maternal obesity may decrease the fetal fraction of DNA, and the second, a smaller overall placental mass associated with IVF conception, especially in twin gestations.[12,13] The rate of aneuploidy is increased in multifetal gestations compared with singleton pregnancies, as is the risk miscarriage from invasive diagnostic testing,[12] further complicating this issue of prenatal screening in multifetal gestation pregnancies.

VANISHING TWIN SYNDROME

Spontaneous loss of an embryo in a twin gestation ("vanishing twin syndrome") occurs in 30% to 40% of all first-trimester twin pregnancies.[13,14] The demise of the embryo has been reported to be frequently associated with chromosomal anomalies.[13,14] Several studies have shown that this phenomenon is a source of false positive cfDNA results,[13–15] whereby the contribution of additional cfDNA from the demised twin can be detected 8 weeks after the demise, creating an additional complement of fetal DNA.[13,14] The recent introduction of single-nucleotide polymorphism–based screening NIPT may provide a solution to this issue.[13] By scanning for the presence of polymorphic loci, this test can detect the presence of different fetal haplotypes, which can help confirm a previously undetected dizygotic vanishing twin when combined with morphology scan.[13] Whenever a confirmed singleton pregnancy with additional haplotypes is noted on single-nucleotide polymorphism NIPT results, the patient should be counseled on proceeding with invasive diagnostic testing before definitive management.[14]

CONFINED PLACENTAL MOSAICISM

Confined placental mosaicism is a well-known biologic phenomenon, affecting 0.8% to 2% of pregnancies, wherein the cytotrophoblastic layer of the placenta contains an aneuploid cell line that has resulted from nondisjunction.[16–18] Because the fetal fraction of cfDNA comes from the trophoblasts of the placenta, this may result in false positive, discordant, NIPT results.[16,18] In this situation, a complete ultrasound study and confirmatory karyotype by amniocentesis would be the most appropriate next step. Direct preparation from chorionic villus sampling would provide the cytotrophoblast karyotype, which would be similar to results from NIPT, but not the fetal karyotype,[16–18] creating an additional source of false positive error. Therefore, if CVS is done, results should be based on cultured cells rather than direct preparations.

MATERNAL MOSAICISM

Alterations in the expected maternal fractions of cfDNA, such as that seen when 2 different maternal genotypes exist at a gene locus or loci, have been shown to skew dependent calculations of the fetal fraction of the cfDNA for a specific chromosome, thereby inaccurately indicating evidence of aneuploidy in the fetus.[19,20] Examples of this include chromosomal translocations and copy number variations, which are not typically noted on NIPT results. Of more concern is maternal mosaicism of the sex chromosomal abnormalities. This phenomenon is increasingly noted in older mothers wherein they seem to develop an increasing number of XO cell lines, which can complicate cfDNA results.

HISTORY OF MATERNAL ORGAN TRANSPLANT

Maternal chimera created from a transplanted organ or bone marrow has previously been documented as a source of additional haplotypes present in the cell-free sample. Interestingly, this has been shown to cause false positives and gender discordance through sex chromosome aneuploidy on NIPT.[21,22] A recent case report reported that transplanted organs from a male donor can lead to the presence of a Y chromosome in the maternal cfDNA pool with a genetically normal female fetus.[21–23] In instances such as these, it is important to counsel the patient with a history of organ transplant on this potential issue during pretest counseling, and to follow-up with a fetal morphology ultrasound scan in the second trimester, or amniocentesis for prenatal karyotype analysis to confirm the gender. Wherein gender discordance occurs with a fetus with XY chromosome and ultrasound shows female genitalia, it is important to reassess the fetus with repeat growth scans and evaluate for other causes of discordant results.

OCCULT MATERNAL MALIGNANCY

Unexplained abnormal cfDNA screening results may also indicate a maternal source of chromosomal anomaly. In a recent study, Bianchi and colleagues[24] examined 125,426 samples from asymptomatic pregnant women who underwent NIPT screening. Of those, 3757 samples (3%) were positive for aneuploidy involving chromosomes 13, 18, 21, X, or Y; from these positively identified samples, 10 cases of undiscovered maternal malignancy were identified. The investigators noted occult maternal cancers were frequently associated with the rare NIPT finding of more than one aneuploidy detected in the cfDNA sample; presumably this discordance in NIPT results is due to the apoptosis of malignant cells into the maternal serum.

From this, it can be seen that there are many potential causes of discordant cfDNA results, in which the NIPT result is discordant to the clinical outcome. In addition, false positive results can be caused by low fetal fraction, maternal obesity, laboratory processing, and human error. Recent studies would indicate that 3% to 8% of specimens may yield false positives, including "no results." This number has fluctuated in different studies dependent on the techniques that laboratories use and their specific algorithms for testing. This issue seems to be decreasing as processing and technology have improved.

SELECTING APPROPRIATE CANDIDATES FOR NONINVASIVE PRENATAL TESTING SCREENING

In a 2015 joint practice bulletin issued by the ACOG and the Society for Maternal Fetal Medicine (SMFM), ideal candidates for NIPT were defined as those women aged 35 years and older, those patients with a history of first-degree relative with chromosomal trisomies or sex chromosome monosomy, a parent carrying a Robertsonian chromosomal translocation with increased risk of trisomy 13 or 21, those with a fetus with ultrasonographic findings that indicate increased risk of aneuploidy, or those with positive first- or second-trimester screening results based on nuchal translucency and analytes in the mother's serum.[5] Restricting cfDNA usage to that of a second line prenatal screening method optimizes the likelihood of identifying the most common aneuploidies in patient populations with the highest incidence of these conditions.[5] Because the PPV of any screening test is directly related to the prevalence of the condition in the population being screened, this approach for selecting patients to receive NIPT increases the PPV of the test results and lowers the chance of false positives. In a patient whose pregnancy is not considered high risk, an abnormal result would have a much lower chance of being a true positive finding when applied incorrectly to a pool of low-risk patients.[5] For example, in a 25-year-old patient, it was reported that the PPV of cfDNA in detecting trisomy 21 was 33% (where 2/3 of patients would have a false positive result), in comparison to that measured in a 40-year-old patient, where the PPV is 87%,[5] leading to significantly fewer false positives. However, the PPV of NIPT is considerably better than that of traditional screening (see **Table 1**).

With improved accuracy of detection compared with traditional screening (ie, screening done by first-trimester ultrasound studies, including nuchal translucency), NIPT screening should be completed in conjunction with an early ultrasound evaluation, which would incorporate the superior accuracy of cfDNA molecular analyses with the early morphologic evaluation of the fetus. In addition, the use of an early morphology ultrasound examination in conjunction with cfDNA screening in a general obstetrics population has several advantages. These advantages include highly accurate determination of gestational age, early detection of multiple gestations, determination of chorionicity, and the early detection of twin-twin transfusion syndrome, early detection fetal abnormalities, and early detection of congenital heart disease. Until more evidence accumulates on the value of the early morphology ultrasound in the low-risk population, current recommendations state that first-trimester ultrasound should be offered based on indications rather than routinely.

USE OF PRENATAL ULTRASOUND SCANS

Sonographic markers may be used for evaluating the fetus for morphologic signs of aneuploidy and may be used to further refine each patient's individual risk of having an affected fetus.[25–28] With a normal ultrasound scan (ie, that which shows no sonographic markers or signs of aneuploidy), the reported associated risk reduction in aneuploidy risk has varied from 60% to 83%.[28–32] In a survey of maternal-fetal medicine (MFM) specialists, 72% of MFM physicians reported using second-trimester ultrasound to decrease aneuploidy risk, where the most frequently cited risk reduction

Table 2
Prediction of aneuploidy risk by the presence of ultrasound markers

Marker	Nyberg et al,[25] 1998	Nyberg et al,[26] 2001	Smith-Bindman et al,[27] 2001	Bromley et al,[28] 2002
Major anomaly	25	—	—	3.3
Nuchal fold	18.6	11	17	—
Short humerus	2.5	5.1	7.5	5.8
Short femur	2.2	1.5	2.7	1.2
Hyperechoic Bowel	5.5	6.7	6.1	—
Pyelectasis	1.6	1.5	1.9	1.5
Echogenic Intercardiac Focus	2	1.8	2.8	1.4

Likelihood ratios of aneuploidy can be adjusted by the presence or absence of structural anomalies and ultrasound "soft markers," as has been shown by the 4 landmark papers noted here.
Data from Refs.[25–28]

in normal ultrasound scans was 50%.[33] Two types of sonographic findings suggestive of fetal aneuploidy can be identified during the second-trimester ultrasound scan; these include structural abnormalities of the fetus (which occur in 3%–5% of all live births), and nonstructural "soft markers," which may be transient, but still have significant utility as a noninvasive screening tool for assessing aneuploidy risk. Soft markers include thickened nuchal fold, echogenic bowel, mild ventriculomegaly, echogenic intracardiac focus, choroid plexus cysts, and renal pyelectasis (**Table 2**).

The presence of soft markers has been shown to increase the risk of fetal aneuploidy at ranges of relative risk (RR) between 1.4 and 12. The presence of a single isolated marker may be of less concern than several markers occurring as aggregates,[28] although as an isolated finding, the presence of a nuchal fold remained a strong predictor of trisomy 21.[26–30] When 2 or more soft markers were seen together, the risk of aneuploidy was increased 12-fold.[28–30] In patients with a positive NIPT, the absence of soft markers or associated structural anomalies on ultrasound can be reassuring, because it lowers the risk of aneuploidy by 50%. Despite this, the risk of aneuploidy after a positive NIPT would remain great enough to offer invasive diagnostic testing.

THE FUTURE

Current advisory recommendations from the American College of Obstetricians and Gynecologists (ACOG) and Society for Maternal Fetal Medicine (SMFM) state that NIPT should only be used in singleton pregnancies predetermined to be at increased risk for aneuploidy.[5] Although NIPT offers increased ability to detect the most common trisomies that affect high-risk pregnancies, concern exists regarding the cost-effectiveness of using this screening in low-risk pregnancies.[5,33–35] The cost of this NIPT technology is predicted to decrease, given increased technologic advances and widespread implementation of NIPT. A decrease in the price of NIPT in the United States from $2500 to $750 has already occurred. Through competitive pricing and contracting, targeted sequencing for trisomy 21, 18, 13 and sex chromosomes may soon drop to $200 per test. At this price, NIPT would be the most cost-effective form of aneuploidy screening with the highest sensitivity, lowest false positive rate, fewest diagnostic procedures, and the lowest rate of fetal loss of normal pregnancies from the invasive procedures (**Table 3**).

Table 3
Cost analysis of prenatal screening per million live births

Test	Screen Cost ($)	Cost ($)	No. Invasive Procedures	Total Costs ($)	Total DS	Detection Rate (%)	Missed Diagnoses	Losses of Normal Fetuses
AMA	0	0	180,000	450M	1428	33	952	900
AFP4	348	348M	50,000	473M	1428	75	350	250
FTS	762	762M	50,000	887M	1428	85	214	250
Seq	1000	1,000M	50,000	1.13B	1428	95	71	250
NIPT-MPSS	1500	1,500M	5000	1.51B	1428	>99	2	25
NIPT-DANSR	200	200M	5000	212.5B	1428	>99	2	25

Abbreviations: AMA, advanced maternal age; AFP4, maternal alpha fetal protein 4; FTS, first trimester screening; Seq, DNA sequencing; NIPT-MPSS, NIPT with massively parallel signature sequencing; NIPT-DANSR, NIPT with digital analysis of selected regions.

SUMMARY

NIPT by cfDNA is a highly specific and sensitive method of screening for common fetal aneuploidies in pregnancies previously designated as high risk for aneuploidies. Several large clinical trials involving the general obstetrics population have additionally proven the superiority of NIPT testing in low-risk pregnancies, with specificities and detection rates greater than the currently used nuchal translucency and biochemical analyte analyses.

The value of cfDNA in noninvasive prenatal screening is considerable in that it decreases unnecessary invasive diagnostic procedures, with a false positive rate of 0.1% and reliable assurance to the patient of chromosomally normal fetus. Recent studies have identified causes of discordant or false positive screening error using this test, which have been summarized. Many times there is a biologic reason for the false positive test, making it more a discordant than false positive result. In the event of a positive cfDNA test, it is important that the patient be referred to a genetic counselor, who can help the patient understand the risk of different aneuploidies and limitations of prenatal testing and to help the patient decide on a complete morphology scan and a confirmatory diagnostic test, such as CVS, or amniocentesis. Thorough ultrasound evaluations can be used to increase or decrease the PPV of the NIPT result. If NIPT is offered to a patient, she should have genetic counseling before and after the test, to ensure complete understanding of the situation and to have options offered before a premature decision for pregnancy termination is considered. An additional advantage of NIPT is that it can be done earlier than other screening techniques, so that in the event of a positive result, further evaluation and diagnostic testing can be completed 2 to 6 weeks earlier than with either first- or second-trimester traditional screening methods, thus making earlier and safer pregnancy terminations available for the patient.

REFERENCES

1. Nadler HL, Gerbie AB. Role of amniocentesis in the intrauterine detection of genetic disorders. N Engl J Med 1970;282(11):596–9.

2. Bianchi DW, Rava RP, Sehnert AJ. DNA sequencing versus standard prenatal aneuploidy screening. N Engl J Med 2014;371(6):578.

3. Gil MM, Quezada MS, Revello R, et al. Analysis of cell-free DNA in maternal blood in screening for fetal aneuploidies: updated meta-analysis. Ultrasound Obstet Gynecol 2015;45:249.

4. Wagner AJ, Mitchell ME, Tomita-Mitchell A. Use of cell-free fetal DNA in maternal plasma for noninvasive prenatal screening. Clin Perinatol 2014;41(4):957–66.

5. Committee Opinion No. 640: cell-free DNA screening for fetal aneuploidy. Obstet Gynecol 2015;126:e31.

6. Evans MI, Sonek JD, Hallahan TW, et al. Cell-free fetal DNA screening in the USA: a cost analysis of screening strategies. Ultrasound Obstet Gynecol 2015;45(1): 74–83.

7. Norton ME, Jacobsson B, Swamy GK, et al. Cell-free DNA analysis for noninvasive examination of trisomy. N Engl J Med 2015;372:1589–97.

8. Hui L, The S, McCarthy EA, et al. Emerging issues in invasive prenatal diagnosis: safety and competency in the post-NIPT era. Aust N Z J Obstet Gynaecol 2015; 55(6):541–6.

9. Warsof SL, Larion S, Abuhamad AZ. Overview of the impact of noninvasive prenatal testing on diagnostic procedures. Prenat Diagn 2015;10:972–9.

10. Wilson RD, Gagnon A, Audibert F, et al. Prenatal diagnosis procedures and techniques to obtain a diagnostic fetal specimen or tissue: maternal and fetal risks and benefits. J Obstet Gynaecol Can 2015;37(7):656–70.

11. American College of Obstetricians and Gynecologists. Prenatal Diagnostic Testing for Genetic Disorders. ACOG Practice Bulletin May 2016.

12. McCullough RM, Almasri EA, Guan X, et al. Non-invasive prenatal chromosomal aneuploidy testing–clinical experience: 100,000 clinical samples. PLoS One 2014;9(10):e109173.

13. Curnow KJ, Wilkins-Haug L, Ryan A, et al. Detection of triploid, molar, and vanishing twin pregnancies by a single-nucleotide polymorphism-based noninvasive prenatal test. Am J Obstet Gynecol 2015;212:79.e1.

14. Grömminger S, Yagmur E, Erkan S, et al. Fetal aneuploidy detection by cell-free DNA sequencing for multiple pregnancies and quality issues with vanishing twins. J Clin Med 2014;3(3):679–92.

15. Thurik FF, Ait Soussan A, Bossers B, et al. Analysis of false-positive results of fetal RHD typing in a national screening program reveals vanishing twins as potential cause for discrepancy. Prenat Diagn 2015;35(8):754–60.

16. Srebniak MI, Diderich KE, Noomen P, et al. Abnormal non-invasive prenatal test results concordant with karyotype of cytotrophoblast but not reflecting abnormal fetal karyotype. Ultrasound Obstet Gynecol 2014;44(1):109–11.

17. Lebo RV, Novak RW, Wolfe K, et al. Discordant circulating fetal DNA and subsequent cytogenetics reveal false negative, placental mosaic, and fetal mosaic cfDNA genotypes. J Transl Med 2015;13:260.

18. Malvestiti F, Agrati C, Grimi B, et al. Interpreting mosaicism in chorionic villi: results of a monocentric series of 1001 mosaics in chorionic villi with follow-up amniocentesis. Prenat Diagn 2015;35(11):1117–27.

19. Wang Y, Chen Y, Tian F, et al. Maternal mosaicism is a significant contributor to discordant sex chromosomal aneuploidies associated with noninvasive prenatal testing. Clin Chem 2014;60:251.

20. Lui YY, Chik KW, Chiu RW, et al. Predominant hematopoietic origin of cell-free DNA in plasma and serum after sex-mismatched bone marrow transplantation. Clin Chem 2002;48:421.

21. Grande M, Jansen FA, Blumenfeld YJ, et al. Genomic microarray in fetuses with increased nuchal translucency and normal karyotype—a systematic review and meta-analysis. Ultrasound Obstet Gynecol 2015;46(6):650–8.

22. Bruno DL, Ganesamoorthy D, Thorne NP, et al. Use of copy number deletion polymorphisms to assess DNA chimerism. Clin Chem 2014;60(8):1105–14.

23. Rupley DM, Janda AM, Kapeles SR, et al. Preconception counseling, fertility, and pregnancy complications after abdominal organ transplantation: a survey and cohort study of 532 recipients. Clin Transplant 2014;28(9):937–45.

24. Bianchi DW, Chudova D, Sehnert AJ, et al. Noninvasive prenatal testing and incidental detection of occult maternal malignancies. JAMA 2015;314:162.

25. Nyberg DA, Luthy DA, Resta RG, et al. Age-adjusted ultrasound risk assessment for fetal Down's syndrome during the second trimester: description of the method and analysis of 142 cases. Ultrasound Obstet Gynecol 1998;2(1):8–14.

26. Nyberg DA, Souter VL, El-Bastawissi A, et al. Isolated sonographic markers for detection of fetal Down syndrome in the second trimester of pregnancy. J Ultrasound Med 2001;20(10):1053–63.

27. Smith-Bindman R, Feldstein VA, Goldberg JD. The genetic sonogram in screening for Down syndrome. J Ultrasound Med 2001;20(11):1153–8.

28. Bromley B, Lieberman E, Shipp TD, et al. The genetic sonogram: a method of risk assessment for Down syndrome in the second trimester. J Ultrasound Med 2002; 21(10):1087–96.

29. Bromley B, Shipp TD, Lyons J, et al. What is the importance of second-trimester "soft markers" for trisomy 21 after an 11- to 14-week aneuploidy screening scan? J Ultrasound Med 2014;33(10):1747–52.

30. Nyberg DA, Luthy DA, Cheng EY, et al. Role of prenatal ultrasonography in women with positive screen for Down syndrome on the basis of maternal serum markers. Am J Obstet Gynecol 1995;173(4):1030–5.

31. Sohl BD, Scioscia AL, Budorick NE, et al. Utility of minor ultrasonographic markers in the prediction of abnormal fetal karyotype at a prenatal diagnostic center. Am J Obstet Gynecol 1999;181(4):898–903.

32. Shipp TD, Benacerraf BR. Second trimester ultrasound screening for chromosomal abnormalities. Prenat Diagn 2002;22(4):296–307.

33. Egan JF, Kaminsky LM, DeRoche ME, et al. Antenatal Down syndrome screening in the United States in 2001: a survey of maternal-fetal medicine specialists. Am J Obstet Gynecol 2002;187(5):1230–4.

34. Walker BS, Nelson RE, Jackson BR, et al. A cost-effectiveness analysis of first trimester non-invasive prenatal screening for fetal trisomies in the United States. PLoS One 2015;10(7):e0131402.

35. Larion S, Warsof SL, Romary L, et al. Uptake of noninvasive prenatal testing at a large academic referral center. Am J Obstet Gynecol 2014;211(6):651.e1–7.

Chromosomal Microarrays for the Prenatal Detection of Microdeletions and Microduplications

Karen Wou, MD[a], Brynn Levy, MSc (Med), PhD[b],
Ronald J. Wapner, MD[c],*

KEYWORDS

- Microarray • Cell-free DNA • Microdeletion • Microduplication
- Copy number variant • Genetic counseling

KEY POINTS

- Compared with karyotype, chromosomal microarray analysis (CMA) allows the detection of submicroscopic deletions and duplications as small as the resolution set by the array design, which is typically in the range of 100 to 300 kb. This range provides an incremental detection rate of potentially significant copy number variants of 3.6%.

- Single nucleotide polymorphism arrays are high-density oligonucleotide-based arrays in which probes are selected with polymorphic alleles (selected DNA segment probes vary by a single base pair).

- CMA is most often criticized for the detection of variants of uncertain significance, estimated around 1%, because it can pose a clinical dilemma and parental anxiety during genetic counseling.

- Genetic counseling should review findings of uncertain significance, predictions of adult-onset disorders, and unanticipated results for comprehensive pretest and posttest counseling.

- Noninvasive prenatal testing–based screening for chromosomal microdeletion syndromes is currently still not recommended by major societies; more scientific evidence is awaited before this can be offered clinically.

Disclosures: None.
[a] Division of Clinical Genetics, Department of Pediatrics, Columbia University Medical Center, 3959 Broadway, CHN 718, New York, NY 10032, USA; [b] Department of Pathology and Cell Biology, Columbia University Medical Center, 3959 Broadway, CHC 406b, New York, NY 10032, USA; [c] Division of Maternal-Fetal Medicine, Department of Obstetrics and Gynecology, Columbia University Medical Center, 622 West 168th Street, PH 16-66, New York, NY 10032, USA
* Corresponding author.
E-mail address: rw2191@cumc.columbia.edu

Clin Lab Med 36 (2016) 261–276
http://dx.doi.org/10.1016/j.cll.2016.01.017
0272-2712/16/$ – see front matter © 2016 Elsevier Inc. All rights reserved.
labmed.theclinics.com

INTRODUCTION

In an era in which advances in molecular cytogenetic techniques have allowed the evaluation of copy number variants (CNV) by chromosomal microarray analysis (CMA), the American Congress of Obstetricians and Gynecologists (ACOG) recommends that all women should be offered invasive testing regardless of risk.[1] Historically, conventional forms of cytogenetic analysis, such as G-banded chromosome analysis and rapid interphase fluorescence in situ hybridization, were the mainstay of diagnosing chromosomal abnormalities.[2–8] For more than 40 years, a G-banded karyotype with a resolution of up to approximately 7 million to 10 million base pairs (bp) has been the standard of care in clinical practice for cytogenetic evaluation. Deletions and duplications that cannot be seen under the microscope because of their small size are referred to as microdeletions and microduplications. These types of imbalances are beyond the diagnostic capacity of conventional karyotype analysis.

Over the last 10 to 15 years, molecular cytogenetic technologies, such as CMA, were developed and introduced into clinical pediatric practice. Compared with metaphase karyotyping, CMA can detect microdeletions and microduplications in the genome that are in the range of hundreds of kilobases.[9–11] In 2010, based on the increased resolution, precision, accuracy, and technical sensitivity of CMA, the American College of Medical Genetics recommended that CMA become the first-line test in the initial postnatal cytogenetic evaluation of children with multiple congenital anomalies, developmental delay, intellectual disability, and autism spectrum disorders.[12] CMA was eventually introduced into prenatal clinical practice allowing the detection of microdeletions and microduplications associated with well-described phenotypes.[13,14] In 2013, ACOG and the Society for Maternal-Fetal Medicine (SMFM) recommended the use of CMA as the first-tier test for the cytogenetic evaluation of fetuses with major structural abnormalities. They also recommended that it be offered to patients with structurally normal fetuses undergoing diagnostic testing for routine reasons, such as positive aneuploidy screening or maternal anxiety. Compared with karyotype, CMA adds additional information in the evaluation of pregnancies with an intrauterine fetal demise or stillbirth.[15] They also emphasized the importance of pretest and posttest genetic counseling, which should comprise the benefits and limitations of the test, including a discussion of the potential to identify variants of uncertain significance (VOUS), nonpaternity, consanguinity, and adult-onset diseases.

This article reviews the basic technology of microarray; the different types of arrays used in clinical practice; the value and clinical significance of the detection of microdeletions, microduplications, and other CNVs; and the importance of pretest and posttest counseling for prenatal diagnosis. It also discusses the current status of noninvasive screening for microdeletion and microduplication syndromes.

BASIC INTRODUCTION TO MICROARRAY

Although karyotyping is an evaluation of the number and structure of the chromosomes under the light microscope, CMA identifies smaller genomic imbalances with the use of molecular technologies.[16] There are 2 approaches to identifying these submicroscopic imbalances: comparative genomic hybridization (CGH) and single nucleotide polymorphisms (SNP).

Comparative Genomic Hybridization–Based Arrays

One approach is based on CGH, in which a patient's DNA is compared with a normal control DNA sample to identify areas that are either under-represented or over-represented in the patient sample.[17] The patient's and control DNA samples are cut into fragments then labeled with different fluorescent colors (usually red and green). Once mixed in equal proportions, they are placed onto a target (glass slide) containing thousands of probes from representative sequences from across the human genome. A CGH array typically contains tens of thousands to a few million probes. The mixture of fragments hybridizes (binds) only to the probes on the array with the exact complimentary sequence. The ratio of fluorescence intensity from the study sample compared with the reference sample is quantified and graphed by digital imaging systems for each of the hybridized regions. This ratio is equal to 1 if contributions from the patient sample and control sample are equal, and this represents the normal copy number at that locus. In the case of excess DNA (a duplication), the ratio of fluorescence intensity is greater than 1, indicating that more of the patient's DNA hybridized compared with the control DNA. In contrast, in a case of loss of genetic

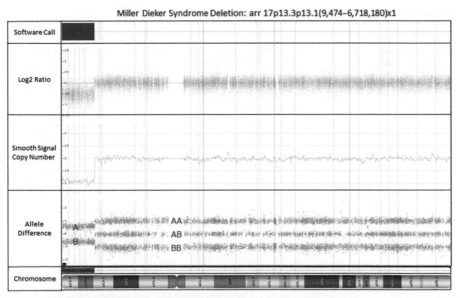

Fig. 1. Screenshot from Affymetrix Chromosome Analysis Suite software (Version 3.1) showing a loss of the terminal region (17p13.3p13.1) of the short arm of chromosome 17, which is associated with a clinical diagnosis of Miller-Dieker syndrome. The precise coordinates of the deletion correspond with chr17: 9,474-6,718,180 using Human Genome Build Hg19. The gene content within the deleted region can be ascertained using the genome coordinates. A deletion is indicated in the Software Call panel by the presence of a red bar. The deletion is identified by a decrease in the log2 ratio from zero as seen in the Log2 Ratio panel. The Smooth Signal Copy Number panel indicates the exact copy number of each probe. This panel is helpful in identifying mosaicism, which is evident when the smooth signal for multiple consecutive probes lies between an integer; for example, between 2 and 3 indicates trisomy mosaicism. The Allele Difference panel indicates the genotype for each SNP probe. For normal copy number of 2, there are only 3 possible SNP combinations, AA, AB, and BB, which are plotted on the Allele Difference graph. When there is a deletion (copy number of 1), the genotype options are either A or B and thus only 2 distinct tracks are visible on the Allele Difference graph. The chromosome ideogram in the Chromosome panel highlights the position (breakpoints) on the chromosome where copy number imbalances are present. The red bar in the Chromosome panel represents a deletion. Gains are typically shown as blue bars. (Affymetrix, Santa Clara, CA.)

material (a deletion), the ratio is significantly less than 1 because there is more hybridization of the control DNA sequences compared with patient's DNA. The location and size of the duplication/deletion can be determined by the number of consecutive probes that show a ratio more than or less than 1.

The resolution and diagnostic capability of the CGH array depends on the number and types of probes used and their distribution across the entire genome.[9] Historically, probes used in array CGH were DNA fragments that were 100 to 200 kb in size. These fragments were representative of specific chromosomal loci across the genome and were cloned as bacterial artificial chromosomes (BACs). BAC probes are rarely used anymore and have been replaced with oligonucleotide probes that are composed of shorter sequences (25–60 bp) of nucleotides that are synthesized directly onto the array surface to match a specific region of DNA. Synthetic oligonucleotide probes offer higher probe density, better reproducibility, and higher accuracy than BAC arrays for the interpretation of CNVs.[9]

Single Nucleotide Polymorphism Arrays

In recent years, a second approach to arrays, based on SNPs, has been used. These arrays are based on high-density oligonucleotides in which target probes are selected having polymorphic alleles, meaning that selected DNA segment probes vary between individuals by a single base pair.[10] SNPs occur naturally in the genome, and currently around 85 million human SNPs have been identified. Arrays of up to ~750,000 SNPs are frequently used in clinical laboratories.

Although the general principle is similar to CGH arrays, only the patient's DNA (fetal) is labeled and hybridized to the SNP array, so copy number changes are determined by measuring the absolute intensity and compared with the intensities of multiple normal controls that were independently hybridized (in silico comparison) (**Fig. 1**). In addition to CNVs, the genotype information in SNP arrays can identify other clinically useful information, such as uniparental disomy (**Fig. 2**), consanguinity, zygosity, parents of origin, and maternal cell contamination. In addition, although triploidy cannot be detected by array CGH, it can easily be identified by assessing the allele patterns on SNP arrays (**Fig. 3**).[11,18]

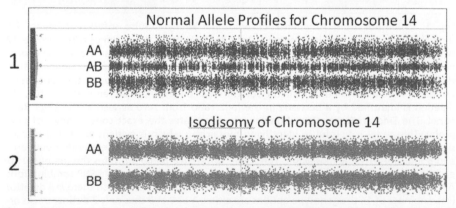

Fig. 2. Screenshot from Affymetrix Chromosome Analysis Suite software (Version 1.1) showing 1 patient with normal SNP patterns across chromosome 14 (*panel 1*) and a second patient with complete absence of all heterozygous (AB) SNPs, indicating isodisomy for chromosome 14 (*panel 2*). (Affymetrix, Santa Clara, CA.)

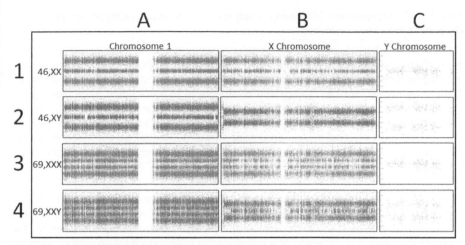

Fig. 3. The allele difference plots show the various SNP genotypes for each SNP locus. In the presence of 2 chromosomes, there are only 3 possible SNP combinations: AA, AB, and BB. The SNP genotype is plotted on the allele difference graph, resulting in 3 distinct tracks (*panels 1A, 2A, 1B, and 4B*). In the presence of 3 chromosomes, there are 4 possible SNP combinations: AAA, AAB, ABB, and BBB, which results in 4 distinct tracks on the allele difference graph (*panels 3A, 4A, and 3B*). In the presence of a single chromosome, the genotype options are either A or B and thus only 2 distinct tracks are visible on the allele difference graph (*panels 2C and 4C*). A normal diploid female patient therefore shows the characteristic 3 tracks for all her chromosomes (*panel 1*), whereas a normal diploid male patient shows the characteristic 3 tracks for all his autosomes and 2 tracks for his X and Y chromosomes (*panel 2*). In a 69,XXX triploid fetus, the 4 characteristic tracks are seen for every autosome as well as the X chromosome (*panel 3*). Triploid fetuses with a 69,XXY constitution show the 4 characteristic tracks for every autosome, 3 tracks representing the 2 X chromosomes, and 2 tracks representing the single Y chromosome (*panel 4*). (Affymetrix, Santa Clara, CA.)

Targeted Versus Whole-Genome Arrays

The number and chromosomal location of the probes determine the diagnostic potential of an array. Targeted arrays can be customized to as many or few microdeletions/duplications syndromes as desired. Specific critical regions associated with disease can be the focus of the array by designing appropriately unique oligonucleotides or SNPs. For example, a targeted array may only include probes that test for copy number imbalances within genes of known pathogenicity. This approach is preferred by some laboratories that wish to minimize the detection of VOUSs or CNVs that may have a variable phenotype or penetrance. However, this approach may miss large and potentially clinically significant CNVs in areas of the genome that lack probe coverage.

Whole-genome arrays include probes spread across the entire genome and provide more complete coverage and thus a higher detection yield. Despite the concerns discussed earlier, Coppinger and colleagues[19] showed that whole-genome arrays provide superior identification of clinically pathogenic syndromes without a higher rate of VOUS. VOUS can be minimized by reporting only large deletions or duplications that are outside the clinically curated targeted regions (often referred to as the backbone regions). At our center, for prenatal samples, we only report CNVs of 1 million base pairs (1 Mb) or larger in the backbone regions.

Benefits of Chromosomal Microarray Analysis Compared with Karyotype for Diagnostic Prenatal Diagnosis

Compared with karyotype, CMA has greater resolution, allowing the detection of submicroscopic deletions and duplications in the kilobase range. In clinical practice, karyotypes routinely identify chromosomal alterations of around 7 to 10 Mb. In addition, CMA does not require cell culture and is amenable to automation, thus resulting in faster turnaround time, reduced failure rate, and a more cost-effective analysis. CMA also allows direct mapping of the alterations to the exact location in the genome sequence to better define marker chromosomes and unbalanced translocations, and to better delineate the start/stop points and gene content of copy number imbalances.

Limitations of Chromosomal Microarray Analysis

Like any other technology, CMA presents some limitations. CMA cannot identify balanced translocations (reciprocal and robertsonian) and inversions, because there is no net loss or gain of genomic material. Although this is only minimally relevant for the current pregnancy, the detection of a translocation is important for counseling with regard to future reproduction. To overcome this, concomitant karyotyping and CMA may be used, although the cost-effectiveness of this approach has not been evaluated.

Triploidies could not be detected by CGH-based arrays in the past but can now be identified by incorporating SNPs into the array. Another limitation of microarray is its inability to detect low-level mosaicism at less than 10% to 20%.[20–24] However, standard karyotyping of 20 cells only detects mosaicism of 14% with 95% confidence.[25] When CMA is performed on DNA extracted directly from uncultured cells, it may reveal mosaicism that may not be apparent in cultured cells because of preferential growth of a normal cell line.[26]

In addition, CMA is most often criticized for the detection of VOUS because it can pose a clinical dilemma and parental anxiety during genetic counseling. A VOUS is described as a genetic aberration for which insufficient or no data exist that link it to a defined clinical phenotype.[27] The occurrence of VOUS must be balanced against the additional information CMA provides. CMA has an incremental detection rate of potentially significant CNVs of 3.6% compared with karyotype.[27] Findings of unknown significance are found in 1.1% of microarray cases and often lead to challenging genetic counseling sessions. However, this rate does not vary from the 1% rate of such findings observed over the past few decades with karyotyping.[28] In the prenatal setting, there is limited clinical and phenotypic information to support any clinical judgment on the possible consequences of some subtle copy number changes, especially when there may be variable expressivity or variable penetrance.[22] However, with increasing experience, the VOUS rate with CMA will continue to decrease, because many previously uncertain findings are reclassified as benign or pathogenic as additional relevant information is gleaned from publically shared clinical databases.[29] It must be noted that some of the available information about CNV-associated phenotypes comes from the postnatal experience of testing affected children, which poses a counseling dilemma for patients and providers in the prenatal setting because postnatal results may be skewed toward the more severe end of the phenotype spectrum.[19]

MICRODELETIONS AND DUPLICATIONS SYNDROMES
Clinical Utility of Chromosomal Microarray Analysis in Prenatal Diagnosis

With the publication of a large prospective, blinded, multicenter, cohort study in the *New England Journal of Medicine* in 2012, it became clear that CMA is superior to karyotyping for prenatal diagnosis, because of its higher resolution and superior yield for genetic abnormalities.[30] Clinically significant CNVs were observed in 6% of patients with a fetus with an ultrasonography abnormality and a normal karyotype result. Clinically relevant CNVs were also shown in 1.7% of fetuses with a normal karyotype and a normal fetal scan in the population of women referred for advanced maternal age, positive biochemical, and nuchal translucency screening, or anxiety. Of the women with a normal scan, 1.5% had VOUS.[30] These data are consistent with the largest published prospective cohort study of the use of CMA in prenatal testing, in which the overall detection rate of clinically relevant significant CNVs was 5.3%.[31] This rate equaled 6.5% when only pregnancies with abnormal ultrasonography findings were considered.[31]

In a meta-analysis including more recent studies, Hillman and colleagues[29] found that CMA for prenatal diagnosis detected an additional 7% of cytogenetic anomalies compared with karyotyping in cases of fetal anomalies. The VOUS rate was higher in this subgroup at 2.1% compared with 1.4% in the general population. Another systematic review of more than 12,000 cases also found similar detection rates of clinically significant copy number changes: 2.4% overall rate, 6.5% in ultrasonography anomalies, and 1% in the general population.[32]

The most common fetal anomalies associated with CNVs occur in the cardiac, skeletal, urogenital, renal, and central nervous systems.[13,14,33,34] In a secondary analysis from the National Institute of Child Health and Human Development microarray trial, it was shown that fetuses with anomalies in multiple systems had a 13% frequency of CNVs compared with 5.1% in fetuses with only a single anomaly.[35] These findings further support the ACOG and SMFM recommendations to offer microarray as the primary diagnostic test in cases with an ultrasonography-detected fetal anomaly.[15] These organizations have also recommended that all women having diagnostic testing for other reasons be offered the opportunity to have microarray analysis of the sample.

CNVs play a major role in human phenotypic variation and disease. In patients of advanced maternal age, positive conventional screening, or diagnostic testing for parental anxiety, approximately 1.0% to 1.7% have a pathogenic CNV; a much higher frequency than the 1:800 population risk of Down syndrome.[29,36] However, CNVs may also be benign familial or population variants that are common in humans throughout the genome.[37,38] Because of this, CNVs are often classified as benign, pathogenic, or (variant) of uncertain significance (VOUS). Although differentiating between these categories can sometimes represent a significant clinical challenge,[39] many CNVs are associated with clearly defined genetic syndromes. Others, not associated with a syndrome, have clear associations with neurocognitive disabilities, including autism and developmental delay. **Tables 1** and **2** list some of the most common and well-described effects of clinically significant CNVs.[40–43]

22q11.2 Deletion syndrome, also known as 22q11 deletion, velocardiofacial syndrome, or DiGeorge syndrome, in which the proximal long arm of chromosome 22 is deleted, seems to be the most common recurrent deletion syndrome. This microdeletion syndrome was found in 1 out of 992 pregnancies from a low-risk population; a higher prevalence than previously estimated.[44] Affected individuals have a wide range of findings, such as congenital heart diseases, particularly conotruncal anomalies; cleft lip and/or palate; specific facial features; renal abnormalities; hearing loss; ophthalmic abnormalities; skeletal problems; immunodeficiency; hypocalcemia; and feeding and swallowing problems. Although many of these findings are detected on prenatal ultrasonography, it is also important to note that children with this microdeletion frequently have autistic spectrum disorder, psychiatric disorders (including

Table 1
Examples of common microdeletion and microduplication syndromes

Microdeletion Syndromes	Incidence	Chromosome Band	Major Phenotypic Features
22q11.2 deletion syndrome	1 in 2000–4000	22q11.2	Cardiac anomalies, cleft palate, distinctive facial features, immunodeficiencies, hypocalcemia, feeding difficulties, developmental delays, mental illnesses, ADHD, autism
DiGeorge syndrome 2 (10p13-p14 deletion)	1 in 200,000	10p13 pter	Genetic heterogeneity of DiGeorge syndrome: cardiac defects, hypoparathyroidism, T-cell immunodeficiency, and facial dysmorphism
Williams syndrome	1 in 7500	7q11.23	Cardiac malformation, psychomotor retardation, a characteristic facial dysmorphism, and a specific cognitive and behavioral profile
Prader-Willi syndrome	1 in 10,000–30,000	15q11.2-q13 (paternal)	Severe neonatal hypotonia, hyperphagia with a risk of morbid obesity, learning difficulties and behavioral problems or severe psychiatric problems, characteristic facial features
Angelman syndrome	1 in 12,000–20,000	15q11.2-q13 (maternal)	Severe intellectual deficit, absent speech, outbursts of laughter with hand flapping, microcephaly, puppetlike gait, ataxia, and epileptic seizures
Smith-Magenis syndrome	1 in 25,000	17p11.2	Variable intellectual deficit, sleep disturbance, craniofacial and skeletal anomalies, psychiatric disorders, and speech and motor delay
Wolf-Hirschhorn syndrome	1 in 50,000	4p16.3	Craniofacial features, growth impairment, intellectual disability, severe delayed psychomotor development, seizures, and hypotonia
Cri du chat syndrome	1 in 20,000–50,000	5p15.2-entire 5p	High-pitched cry, intellectual disability, developmental delay, hypotonia, microcephaly, low birth weight, distinctive facial features, heart defect

(continued on next page)

Table 1
(continued)

Microdeletion Syndromes	Incidence	Chromosome Band	Major Phenotypic Features
Langer-Giedion syndrome	Unknown	8q23.2-8q24.1	Intellectual deficit, redundant skin, multiple cartilaginous exostoses, characteristic facies and cone-shaped phalangeal epiphyses, growth retardation, microcephaly, hypotonia, and hearing problems
Miller-Dieker syndrome	Unknown	17p13.3	Lissencephaly, severe developmental delay, epilepsy, feeding problems, and distinct facial features
1p36 Microdeletion	1 in 5000–10,000	1p36.33/32/31/23	Distinctive facial dysmorphic features, hypotonia, developmental delay, intellectual disability, seizures, heart defects, hearing impairment, and prenatal-onset growth deficiency
3q29 Microdeletion	Unknown	3q29	Mild/moderate intellectual deficit, mild dysmorphic features, autism, gait ataxia; congenital malformations uncommon
Sotos syndrome	1 in 5000–10,000	5q35.3	Overgrowth, macrocephaly, distinctive facial gestalt, feeding issues, hypotonia, developmental delay, learning difficulty, tumor risks
Kleefstra syndrome	<1 in 1 million	9q34.3	Intellectual disability, childhood hypotonia, severe expressive speech delay and a distinctive facial appearance, congenital anomalies
Jacobsen/11q terminal deletion	1 in 100,000	11q24.1/24.3/25	Developmental delay, cognitive impairment, behavioral problems, autism, Paris-Trousseau syndrome, facial features, congenital anomalies
Koolen–de Vries syndrome	1 in 16,000	17q21.31	Developmental delay, childhood hypotonia, facial dysmorphism, and friendly/amiable behavior

Abbreviation: ADHD, attention-deficit/hyperactivity disorder.
Data from Refs.[41–44]

Table 2
Examples of common microduplication syndromes

Microduplication Syndromes	Incidence	Chromosome Band	Major Phenotypic Features
5q35 (NSD1) microduplication	<1 in 1 million	5q35	Microcephaly, short stature, developmental delay, and delayed bone maturation
Williams-Beuren microduplication	Unknown	7q11.23	Cardiac malformations, distinctive facies, connective tissue diseases, mild intellectual disability, a specific cognitive profile, unique personality characteristics, growth abnormalities, and endocrine abnormalities
15q11-q13 Microduplication	<1 in 1 million	15q11-q13	Developmental delay, cognitive impairment, seizures, neurobehavioral disorders of the autistic or psychotic spectrum, subtle dysmorphic features, short stature, macrocephaly, and hypotonia
17p13.3 microduplication	<1 in 1 million	17p13.3	Mild to moderate psychomotor delay, hypotonia, and discrete craniofacial dysmorphic features
Potocki-Lupski syndrome	Unknown	17p11.2	Hypotonia, poor feeding, failure to thrive, mental retardation, developmental delay, pervasive developmental disorders, autism spectrum disorders, and congenital anomalies

Data from Refs.[41–44]

schizophrenia), developmental delay, and learning difficulties, all of which cannot be predicted by ultrasonography alone.

Although most 22q11.2 microdeletions are de novo, 10% to 15% of cases are inherited from one of the parents, although the affected parent may not manifest clinical features. Early prenatal diagnosis enables the expecting parents and involved physicians to prepare for the care of affected children in a multidisciplinary approach. Early treatment of acute problems such as severe hypocalcemia leading to seizures or early intervention for more chronic neurocognitive difficulties can improve long-term prognosis and optimize the health and development of the affected children.[45]

There are other microdeletions with less well-defined phenotypes but with important neurocognitive consequences. For example, the 16p11.2 microdeletion phenotype includes developmental delay, intellectual disability, and autism spectrum disorder. This common microdeletion involves the loss of 1 chromosomal segment harboring 25 annotated genes or transcripts. It is unclear how the deletion of any of these genes causes the clinical findings. Individuals with 16p11.2 microdeletion also seem to be at increased risks for seizures, psychiatric disorders, and obesity. Although these clinical features cannot be identified prenatally by ultrasonography, they can arguably be considered of equal importance to any congenital structural anomaly. Before the advent of prenatal CMA, the 16p11.2 microdeletion syndrome only became evident in the postnatal stage when patients were referred for a work-up because of developmental delay, intellectual disability, or autism. Early detection of this syndrome in the prenatal setting has allowed earlier referral for neurologic and neuropsychological assessment and treatment in early infancy. Provision of therapies like physical, occupational, and speech therapy is likely to facilitate the best outcomes.

PRETEST AND POSTTEST GENETIC COUNSELING

As recommended by ACOG and SMFM, all patients undergoing diagnostic testing by chorionic villus sampling (CVS) or amniocentesis should be informed of the availability and value of microarray analysis of the pregnancy.[15] Genetic counseling should also review findings of uncertain significance, predictions of adult-onset disorders, and unanticipated results. It is important to understand the impact of such findings on both patients and providers and to formulate the appropriate requirements for comprehensive pretest counseling.

Uncertainty and unpredictability are problematic for both the patients and the health care providers.[46,47] Genetic counselors, in particular, experience distress associated with managing informational uncertainty, giving bad news, and interacting with patients who are experiencing intense emotions such as grief.[48] In a survey completed by 193 genetic counselors, only 59% of them felt comfortable counseling patients when VOUS were found on microarray, and only 43% were comfortable helping patients decide about termination of pregnancy.[49] The level of comfort depended on the counselor's experience with prenatal CMA. In contrast, women generally seek prenatal testing for support and reassurance about their pregnancy.[50,51] The time during prenatal testing is often one of distress and anxiety as women wait for test results. These feelings are likely to be exacerbated in cases in which uncertain significance is found on microarray.

NONINVASIVE PRENATAL TESTING

Microdeletions and microduplications can be screened for by noninvasive methods such as cell-free fetal DNA. However, at present this is not recommended by major societies,[15] because present technologies are still limited and have not been appropriately validated for clinical purposes.[52,53] Presently, applicability is restricted to identification of a limited number of specific microdeletions or to microdeletions larger than a certain size.[53–56]

Two approaches have been used to screen for microdeletions. In one, whole-genome sequencing of cell-free fetal DNA in the maternal plasma is performed at the level of 1 billion tags, compared with 10 million to 20 million tags used with current massively parallel sequencing for fetal aneuploidy screening. At this level, DNA copy number imbalances as small as 3 Mb (such as 22q11.2) can be differentiated, but smaller CNVs are missed,[54,57] which overlooks a great proportion of clinically relevant microdeletions. At present, the feasibility of offering routine screening for microdeletions and microduplications by this approach remains a challenge because of the increased costs of sequencing at this level.

In a second method, microdeletions are identified by taking advantage of SNPs. In this approach, the maternal genotype is identified by sequencing cells in the buffy coat of the sample and is then subtracted out to allow detection of smaller fetal genomic abnormalities that are present in the cell-free DNA component of the maternal blood sample. In a recent article, Wapner and colleagues[53] studied 469 samples to estimate the performance of an SNP-based noninvasive prenatal test for 5 microdeletion syndromes. They found detection rates of 97.8% for a 22 q11.2 deletion, and of 100% in the case of Prader-Willi, Angelman, 1p36 deletion, and cri du chat syndromes, with false-positive rates ranging from 0% to 0.76%.[53] Note that most of these samples were not from pregnant woman carrying affected children but from artificial mixtures of maternal DNA spiked with small amounts of cell-free DNA from an affected child. Although this is encouraging, it needs to be prospectively validated in a cohort of pregnant woman. In addition, because clinically relevant microdeletions can occur on any chromosome, SNP probes need to target the entire genome, as opposed to a subset of the genome, before offering comprehensive microdeletion and microduplication screening to the general population.

Some companies have already been offering expanded noninvasive prenatal testing (NIPT) to include a set of 5 to 7 microdeletions: 22q deletion syndrome (DiGeorge), 5p (cri du chat syndrome), 15q (Prader-Willi/Angelman syndromes), 1p36 deletion syndrome, 4p (Wolf- Hirschhorn syndrome), 8q (Langer-Giedion syndrome), and 11q (Jacobsen syndrome). Other companies use higher resolution sequencing to detect microdeletions of 7 Mb or larger. Although no prospective population-based studies have been reported for either approach, detection rates in the range of 60% to 99% are suggested.[53] It is important to reiterate that these microdeletions occur in equal frequencies across all maternal ages and most often without any ultrasonography abnormalities. The rarity of specific microdeletions also needs to be taken into consideration. The population frequency of each microdeletion syndrome ranges from 1 in 4000 (22q11.2) to 1 in 50,000 (cri du chat). Even at the high sensitivities and specificities reported, the positive predictive values are significantly lower than those associated with NIPT for common trisomies.[53] Although detection of whole-genome microdeletions carries a high false-positive rate, which may not be acceptable to some patients, others find the additional information valuable and are willing to accept the need for a diagnostic procedure.

At present, no major national obstetric or genetic organization recommends screening for microdeletions until more robust data are published. The European Society of Human Genetics and the American Society of Human Genetics do not recommend NIPT-based screening for chromosomal microdeletion syndromes in their recent joint statement because "more scientific evidence, such as validation studies as opposed to proof of principle studies, are needed before this can be offered clinically."[58] To date, the ACOG and SMFM do not endorse routine cell-free DNA screening for microdeletion syndromes.[17] Patients who want testing for CNVs should be offered diagnostic testing by CVS or amniocentesis. Recent studies and meta-analysis suggest that the loss rates of these procedures may be as low as 1 in 1000 procedures for amniocentesis and CVS.[59]

REFERENCES

1. American College of Obstetricians and Gynecologists. ACOG practice bulletin no. 88, December 2007. Invasive prenatal testing for aneuploidy. Obstet Gynecol 2007;110(6):1459–67.

2. Tepperberg J, Pettenati MJ, Rao PN, et al. Prenatal diagnosis using interphase fluorescence in situ hybridization (FISH): 2-year multi-center retrospective study and review of the literature. Prenat Diagn 2001;21(4):293–301.

3. Evans MI, Henry GP, Miller WA, et al. International, collaborative assessment of 146,000 prenatal karyotypes: expected limitations if only chromosome-specific probes and fluorescent in-situ hybridization are used. Hum Reprod 1999;14(5):1213–6.

4. Ward BE, Gersen SL, Carelli MP, et al. Rapid prenatal diagnosis of chromosomal aneuploidies by fluorescence in situ hybridization: clinical experience with 4,500 specimens. Am J Hum Genet 1993;52(5):854–65.

5. Hulten MADS, Pertl B. Rapid and simple prenatal diagnosis of common chromosome disorders: advantages and disadvantages of the molecular methods FISH and QF-PCR. Reproduction 2003;126(3):279–97.

6. El Mouatassima S, Becker M, Kuziob S, et al. Prenatal diagnosis of common aneuploidies using multiplex quantitative fluorescent polymerase chain reaction. Fetal Diagn Ther 2004;19:496–503.

7. Mann K, Donaghue C, Fox SP, et al. Strategies for the rapid prenatal diagnosis of chromosome aneuploidy. Eur J Hum Genet 2004;12(11):907–15.

8. Divane A, Carter NP, Spathas DH, et al. Rapid prenatal diagnosis of aneuploidy from uncultured amniotic fluid cells using five-colour fluorescence in situ hybridization. Prenat Diagn 1994;14(11):1061–9.

9. Shearer BM, Thorland EC, Gonzales PR, et al. Evaluation of a commercially available focused aCGH platform for the detection of constitutional chromosome anomalies. Am J Med Genet 2007;143A:2357–70.

10. Beaudet AL, Belmont JW. Array-based DNA diagnostics: let the revolution begin. Annu Rev Med 2008;59:113–29.

11. Bignell GR, Huang J, Greshock J, et al. High-resolution analysis of DNA copy number using oligonucleotide microarrays. Genome Res 2004;14(2):287–95.

12. Manning M, Hudgins L, Professional Practice and Guidelines Committee. Array-based technology and recommendations for utilization in medical genetics practice for detection of chromosomal abnormalities. Genet Med 2010;12(11): 742–5.

13. Shaffer LG, Coppinger J, Alliman S, et al. Comparison of microarray-based detection rates for cytogenetic abnormalities in prenatal and neonatal specimens. Prenat Diagn 2008;28(9):789–95.

14. Kleeman L, Bianchi DW, Shaffer LG, et al. Use of array comparative genomic hybridization for prenatal diagnosis of fetuses with sonographic anomalies and normal metaphase karyotype. Prenat Diagn 2009;29(13):1213–7.

15. American College of Obstetricians and Gynecologists Committee on Genetics. Committee opinion no. 581: the use of chromosomal microarray analysis in prenatal diagnosis. Obstet Gynecol 2013;122(6):1374–7.

16. Aradhya S, Cherry AM. Array-based comparative genomic hybridization: clinical contexts for targeted and whole-genome designs. Genet Med 2007;9(9): 553–9.

17. Snijders AM, Nowak N, Segraves R, et al. Assembly of microarrays for genome-wide measurement of DNA copy number. Nat Genet 2001;29(3):263–4.

18. Zhao X, Li C, Paez JG, et al. An integrated view of copy number and allelic alterations in the cancer genome using single nucleotide polymorphism arrays. Cancer Res 2004;64(9):3060–71.

19. Coppinger J, Alliman S, Lamb AN, et al. Whole-genome microarray analysis in prenatal specimens identifies clinically significant chromosome alterations without increase in results of unclear significance compared to targeted microarray. Prenat Diagn 2009;29:1156–66.

20. Hoang S, Ahn J, Mann K, et al. Detection of mosaicism for genome imbalance in a cohort of 3,042 clinical cases using an oligonucleotide array CGH platform. Eur J Med Genet 2011;54(2):121–9.

21. Ballif BC, Rorem EA, Sundin K, et al. Detection of low-level mosaicism by array CGH in routine diagnostic specimens. Am J Med Genet A 2006; 140(24):2757–67.

22. Cheung SW, Shaw CA, Scott DA, et al. Microarray-based CGH detects chromosomal mosaicism not revealed by conventional cytogenetics. Am J Med Genet A 2007;143A(15):1679–86.

23. Neill NJ, Torchia BS, Bejjani BA, et al. Comparative analysis of copy number detection by whole-genome BAC and oligonucleotide array CGH. Mol Cytogenet 2010;3:11.

24. Scott SA, Cohen N, Brandt T, et al. Detection of low-level mosaicism and placental mosaicism by oligonucleotide array comparative genomic hybridization. Genet Med 2010;12(2):85–92.

25. Hook EB. Exclusion of chromosomal mosaicism: tables of 90%, 95% and 99% confidence limits and comments on use. Am J Hum Genet 1977;29(1): 94–7.

26. Hall GK, Mackie FL, Hamilton S, et al. Chromosomal microarray analysis allows prenatal detection of low level mosaic autosomal aneuploidy. Prenat Diagn 2014;34(5):505–7.

27. Shaffer LG, Dabell MP, Rosenfeld JA, et al. Referral patterns for microarray testing in prenatal diagnosis. Prenat Diagn 2012;32(6):611.

28. Chang YW, Chang CM, Sung PL, et al. An overview of a 30-year experience with amniocentesis in a single tertiary medical center in Taiwan. Taiwan J Obstet Gynecol 2012;51(2):206–11.

29. Hillman SC, McMullan DJ, Hall G, et al. Use of prenatal chromosomal microarray: prospective cohort study and systematic review and meta-analysis. Ultrasound Obstet Gynecol 2013;41(6):610–20.

30. Wapner RJ, Martin CL, Levy B, et al. Chromosomal microarray versus karyotyping for prenatal diagnosis. N Engl J Med 2012;367(23):2175–84.

31. Shaffer LG, Dabell MP, Fisher AJ, et al. Experience with microarray-based comparative genomic hybridization for prenatal diagnosis in over 5000 pregnancies. Prenat Diagn 2012;32(10):976–85.

32. Callaway JL, Shaffer LG, Chitty LS, et al. The clinical utility of microarray technologies applied to prenatal cytogenetics in the presence of a normal conventional karyotype: a review of the literature. Prenat Diagn 2013;33(12):1119–23.

33. Faas BH, van der Burgt I, Kooper AJ, et al. Identification of clinically significant, submicroscopic chromosome alterations and UPD in fetuses with ultrasound anomalies using genome-wide 250k SNP array analysis. J Med Genet 2010;47: 586–94.

34. Shaffer LG, Rosenfeld JA, Dabell MP, et al. Detection rates of clinically significant genomic alterations by microarray analysis for specific anomalies detected by ultrasound. Prenat Diagn 2012;32(10):986–95.

35. Donnelly JC, Platt LD, Rebarber A, et al. Association of copy number variants with specific ultrasonographically detected fetal anomalies. Obstet Gynecol 2014; 124(1):83–90.

36. Van den Veyver IB, Patel A, Shaw CA, et al. Clinical use of array comparative genomic hybridization (aCGH) for prenatal diagnosis in 300 cases. Prenat Diagn 2009;29(1):29–39.

37. Iafrate AJ, Feuk L, Rivera MN, et al. Detection of large-scale variation in the human genome. Nat Genet 2004;36(9):949–51.

38. Sebat J, Lakshmi B, Troge J, et al. Large-scale copy number polymorphism in the human genome. Science 2004;305(5683):525–8.

39. Lee C, Iafrate AJ, Brothman AR. Copy number variations and clinical cytogenetic diagnosis of constitutional disorders. Nat Genet 2007;39(7 Suppl):S48–54.

40. Gross SJ, Bajaj K, Garry D, et al. Rapid and novel prenatal molecular assay for detecting aneuploidies and microdeletion syndromes. Prenat Diagn 2011;31(3): 259–66.

41. Vialard F, Simoni G, Gomes DM, et al. Prenatal BACs-on-Beads™: the prospective experience of five prenatal diagnosis laboratories. Prenat Diagn 2012; 32(4):329–35.

42. Shaffer LG, Coppinger J, Morton SA, et al. The development of a rapid assay for prenatal testing of common aneuploidies and microdeletion syndromes. Prenat Diagn 2011;31(8):778–87.

43. Rosenfeld JA, Morton SA, Hummel C, et al. Experience using a rapid assay for aneuploidy and microdeletion/microduplication detection in over 2,900 prenatal specimens. Fetal Diagn Ther 2014;36(3):231–41.

44. Grati FR, Molina Gomes D, Ferreira JC, et al. Prevalence of recurrent pathogenic microdeletions and microduplications in over 9500 pregnancies. Prenat Diagn 2015;35(8):801–9.

45. Cancrini C, Puliafito P, Digilio MC, et al. Clinical features and follow-up in patients with 22q11.2 deletion syndrome. J Pediatr 2014;164(6):1475–80.e2.

46. Van Zuuren FJ, van Schie EC, van Baaren NK. Uncertainty in the information provided during genetic counseling. Patient Educ Couns 1997;32:129–39.

47. Politi MC, Legare F. Physicians' reactions to uncertainty in the context of shared decision making. Patient Educ Couns 2010;80:155–7.

48. Bernhardt BA, Rushton CH, Carrese J, et al. Distress and burnout among genetic service providers. Genet Med 2009;11:527–35.

49. Bernhardt BA, Kellom K, Barbarese A, et al. An exploration of genetic counselors' needs and experiences with prenatal chromosomal microarray testing. J Genet Couns 2014;23(6):938–47.

50. Bernhardt BA, Soucier D, Hanson K, et al. Women's experiences receiving abnormal prenatal chromosomal microarray testing results. Genet Med 2013; 15(2):139–45.

51. Hunt LM, de Voogd KB, Castaneda H. The routine and the traumatic in prenatal genetic diagnosis: does clinical information inform patient decision-making? Patient Educ Couns 2005;56:302–12.

52. Benn P, Cuckle H. Theoretical performance of non-invasive prenatal testing for chromosome imbalances using counting of cell-free DNA fragments in maternal plasma. Prenat Diagn 2014;34(8):778–83.

53. Wapner RJ, Babiarz JE, Levy B, et al. Expanding the scope of noninvasive prenatal testing: detection of fetal micro deletion syndromes. Am J Obstet Gynecol 2015;212(3):332.e1–9.

54. Jensen TJ, Dzakula Z, Deciu C, et al. Detection of micro deletion 22 q11.2 in a fetus by next-generation sequencing of maternal plasma. Clin Chem 2012; 58(7):1148–51.

55. Yatsenko SA, Peters DG, Saller DN, et al. Maternal cell-free DNA-based screening for fetal micro deletion and the importance of careful diagnostic follow-up. Genet Med 2015;17(10):836–8.

56. Rabinowitz M, Savage M, Pettersen B, et al. Noninvasive cell-free DNA-based prenatal detection of micro deletions sing single nucleotide polymorphism-targeted sequencing. Obstet Gynecol 2014;123(Suppl 1):167S.

57. Peters D, Chu T, Yatsenko SA, et al. Noninvasive prenatal diagnosis of a fetal microdeletion syndrome. N Engl J Med 2011;365(19):1847–8.

58. Dondorp W, de Wert G, Bombard Y, et al. Non-invasive prenatal testing for aneuploidy and beyond: challenges of responsible innovation in prenatal

screening. Summary and recommendations. Eur J Hum Genet 2015. [Epub ahead of print].

59. Akolekar R, Beta J, Picciarelli G, et al. Procedure-related risk of miscarriage following amniocentesis and chorionic villus sampling: a systematic review and meta-analysis. Ultrasound Obstet Gynecol 2015;45(1):16–26.

Genetic Carrier Screening in the Twenty-first Century

Ruofan Yao, MD, MPH, Katherine R. Goetzinger, MD, MSCI*

KEYWORDS

- Ashkenazi Jewish • Carrier screening • Cystic fibrosis • Spinal muscular atrophy
- Tay-Sachs disease

KEY POINTS

- Carrier screening for cystic fibrosis should be offered to all patients in the preconception or prenatal period regardless of ethnicity.
- Population-based carrier screening for Tay-Sachs disease should be performed using enzymatic assay, with molecular methods reserved for those patients with abnormal or inconclusive enzymatic results.
- The American College of Medical Genetics currently supports a carrier screening panel for 9 disorders for persons of Ashkenazi Jewish descent; however, expanded panels are available.
- Although the carrier detection rate for spinal muscular atrophy is greater than 90%, there is currently no test available to predict the severity of the disorder once a mutation is identified.
- Pretest and posttest genetic counseling, including residual risk estimation, should be made available to all couples undergoing carrier screening.

INTRODUCTION

The purpose of carrier screening is to identify individuals who carry a disease-causing genetic mutation that places them at risk for having a child with a serious disorder. Typically, these individuals are asymptomatic and have a negative family history for the disorder. Most conditions included in carrier screening panels are single-gene disorders that are inherited in an autosomal recessive pattern; therefore, both parents must be carriers in order to produce an affected offspring. The ultimate goal of this screening process is to provide reproductive counseling and family planning options to at-risk couples, ideally in the preconception period.

The authors have no conflicts of interest to disclose.
Department of Obstetrics, Gynecology and Reproductive Medicine, University of Maryland School of Medicine, 22 S Greene Street, Baltimore, MD 21201, USA
* Corresponding author. Division of Maternal Fetal Medicine, Department of Obstetrics, Gynecology and Reproductive Medicine, University of Maryland School of Medicine, 22 South Greene Street, Room N6W104F, Baltimore, MD 21201.
E-mail address: kgoetzinger@fpi.umaryland.edu

Clin Lab Med 36 (2016) 277–288
http://dx.doi.org/10.1016/j.cll.2016.01.003
0272-2712/16/$ – see front matter © 2016 Elsevier Inc. All rights reserved.

labmed.theclinics.com

A paradigm of carrier screening is provided by the near eradication of Tay-Sachs disease since the introduction of carrier screening for this disorder in the Ashkenazi Jewish population in the 1970s.[1] Since that time, carrier screening for other single-gene disorders, such as cystic fibrosis (CF) and hemoglobinopathies, has been integrated into preconception and prenatal care. Historically, carrier screening has been focused on specific disorders that cluster in particular racial/ethnic communities; however, with advancing genetic technology, population-based expanded carrier screening panels are gaining more widespread use in reproductive medicine. This article reviews recommendations for ethnicity-based carrier screening for common disorders as well as considerations for expanded carrier screening.

CYSTIC FIBROSIS

CF is a multisystem disease that is characterized by chronic airway infection, pancreatic insufficiency, gastrointestinal dysfunction, and male infertility. It is one of the most common single-gene disorders in the white population, with an incidence ranging between 1 in 3000 and 1 in 3300 individuals.[2,3] Symptoms typically present in early childhood, but, in a minority of cases, the diagnosis is not evident until adulthood. CF is inherited in an autosomal recessive pattern with the responsible gene located on chromosome 7. This gene encodes the protein known as CF transmembrane conductance regulator (CFTR), a 170-kD cyclic AMP–regulated chloride channel located on the apical membrane of epithelial cells. Absence of, or mutation in, CFTR leads to abnormal fluid and electrolyte membrane transport, resulting in dehydrated secretions, decreased mucus clearance in the lung, deficient secretion of pancreatic enzymes, gut dysmotility, and increased sodium chloride levels in sweat.[2,4] More than 1000 different CFTR mutations have been identified with an expansive racial and ethnic distribution. This sizable number of mutations coupled with extreme phenotypic variation has presented a challenge in carrier screening and prenatal diagnosis.

The most common mutation is ΔF508, which is a frameshift mutation caused by a 3-base-pair deletion at codon 508 in exon 10 of CFTR, resulting in the absence of a phenylalanine residue. Other common mutations include G542X, R553X, W1282X, N1303K, 621+1G-to-T, 1717-1G-to-A, and R117H.[2,5] The ΔF508 mutation accounts for 70% of CF mutations in the white population, whereas W1282X is the most common mutation in the Ashkenazi Jewish population, followed by ΔF508.[6] Both the white and Ashkenazi Jewish populations have the highest incidence of disease and also the highest carrier detection rate. Although Hispanic people have a high incidence of disease, the sensitivity of carrier testing remains only 57% to 72%, because detectable alleles account for only slightly more than half of the CF mutations observed in this population. In contrast, African Americans have a lower incidence of disease, and current screening only detects approximately 65% to 69% of carriers[3] (Table 1).

In 1997, the National Institutes of Health (NIH) held a consensus conference to address the complex issues associated with CF carrier screening in a panethnic population. This conference was followed, in 1998, by an additional NIH conference directed at the implementation of this committee's recommendations. Based on these recommendations, CF carrier screening was to be offered to (1) adults with a positive family history of CF, (2) partners of known CF carriers, (3) couples currently planning a pregnancy, and (4) couples seeking prenatal care.[7] In 2001, recommendations were issued from another steering committee composed of representatives from the American College of Medical Genetics (ACMG), the American College of Obstetricians and Gynecologists (ACOG), and the National Human Genome Research Institute. This

Table 1
Sensitivity of carrier screening for CF by ethnicity

Ethnic Group	Incidence of CF	Carrier Frequency	Detection Rate (%)	[a]Estimated Carrier Risk After Negative Screen
White	1 in 3300	1 in 25	80–88	1 in 166 (1 in 125–1 in 208)
African American	1 in 15,300	1 in 65	65–69	1 in 198 (1 in 186–1 in 210)
Ashkenazi Jewish	1 in 3970	1 in 24	94–97	1 in 600 (1 in 400–1 in 800)
Hispanic	1 in 8900	1 in 46	57–72	1 in 135 (1 in 107–1 in 164)
Asian	1 in 35,000	1 in 94	30–49	1 in 159 (1 in 134–1 in 184)

[a] Approximate numbers based on ranges in detection rate.
Data from Refs. [7,9]

group recommended narrowing the screening population to non-Jewish white people and Ashkenazi Jews, although testing was still made available to other ethnic groups with informed consent and recognition of limitations of screening.[8] In addition, in 2005, ACOG revised its recommendations to state that it is reasonable to offer CF carrier screening to all patients, with the caveat that screening is most efficacious in the non-Hispanic white and Ashkenazi Jewish populations. This recommendation is based on the fact that it is becoming increasingly difficult to assign an individual to any particular ethnic group. Patients electing carrier screening for CF should undergo both pretest and posttest counseling, with particular attention paid to ethnic background, detection rate, and residual risk estimate.[9]

The current CF carrier screening panel was introduced by the ACMG/ACOG steering committee in 2001, and was initially composed of 25 mutations. These mutations were chosen based on an allele frequency of greater than or equal to 0.1% in the general US population, regardless of their phenotypic expression of mild versus severe disease.[8] In 2004, the ACMG conducted a second review of the standard mutation panel, which specifically evaluated mutation distribution among various ethnic groups. Based on this review, 2 mutations (1078delT and I148T) were removed from the standard screening panel, narrowing it to include only 23 mutations. These 2 mutations were selected for removal based on observed frequencies of less than 0.1%. Although this review also identified other mutations that were observed at a frequency of greater than 0.1%, no additions were made to the panel because the investigators did not think that these would substantially increase the sensitivity of the screening test.[10]

At present, there are 4 reflex mutations included as part of the standard screening panel as well. When a patient is positive for R117H, a reflex test for the 5T/7T/9T variant is sent. If positive for 5T, determination as to whether the polymorphism is in cis or in trans with the R117H allele is undertaken.[8] R117H in combination with the 5T variant in trans manifests as congenital bilateral absence of the vas deferens (CBAVD), but if in cis with the 5T variant, classic CF is expressed. Given that 5% of the general population tests positive for the 5T polymorphism alone, this test is recommended only as a reflex to a positive R117H result.[8,10] Non-CF-causing variants, including I506V, I507V, and F508C, can mistakenly cause false-positives results based on laboratory and testing methodologies. For example, in patients who screen positive for ΔF508 carrier status and also screen positive for one of the mutations mentioned earlier, a false-positive test for ΔF508 homozygosity may be obtained, although the patient is an otherwise healthy individual.[8] Although F508C has been associated with CBAVD, neither I506V nor I507V have been associated with any phenotypic manifestations of classic CF or CBAVD.[11] Therefore, reflex testing for I506V, I507V, and F508C should be performed in any healthy individual who tests positive for ΔF508 or ΔI507 homozygosity. Otherwise, these mutations should not be used for a priori testing.

In patients with a personal or family history of CF or in male patients with CBAVD, identification of the disease-causing mutation should be pursued by reviewing medical records and, if unattainable, proceeding with DNA sequencing of the CFTR gene in the proband. If the proband is unavailable, DNA sequencing of the CFTR gene in the fetus can be performed, although time constraints in the setting of prenatal diagnosis must be considered. Extended CF mutation panels may also be available at select laboratories, but their use should be reserved for particular clinical circumstances, including patients with reproductive partners with CF or CBAVD and no identified mutation, family history of CF with no identified mutation, or a positive newborn screening test with none or only 1 identified CF mutation.[3] There has been considerable debate over whether to routinely offer extended panel screening to couples who test positive/negative for CF carrier status using the standard 23-mutation panel. The ACMG consensus is that this should not be offered as a standard of care, because it is likely to yield little additional information. For couples who request supplementary material, the existence of extended panels should be made known.[8,10]

CARRIER SCREENING FOR JEWISH GENETIC DISORDERS

There are several autosomal recessive disorders that occur at a higher frequency in individuals of eastern European Jewish descent, specifically in the Ashkenazi Jewish community. Individually, these disorders are rare, with incidences ranging from 1 in 900 to 1 in 40,000; however, approximately 1 out of every 4 Ashkenazi Jews is a carrier for at least 1 of these disorders, making screening efficient in this population.[12] This high carrier frequency can be attributed to genetic drift, resulting from (1) a bottleneck effect in which a small number of genetic variants were transmitted within the population, and (2) a founder effect in which a few rare alleles present in an individual in the original population were passed on to a homogenous population of descendants. Together, these effects have resulted in a genetically homogenous population with a high frequency of recessive alleles compared with the general population.[13]

Tay-Sachs disease was one of the first diseases for which carrier screening was available. This autosomal recessive lysosomal storage disorder is caused by a mutation in the alpha subunit of the HEXA gene on chromosome 15. This mutation causes a deficiency of the hexosaminidase A enzyme, which results in intralysosomal accumulation of ganglioside GM2 and subsequent neuronal death. The classic phenotype of Tay-Sachs disease is one of progressive neurodegenerative change beginning at 3 to 6 months of life, leading to death by 2 to 4 years of life. Juvenile-onset and adult-onset forms have also been described and are associated with more variable deficiencies in hexosaminidase A production. At present, there is no effective treatment available.[14,15] Through the International Tay-Sachs Disease Data Collection Network, a rigorous program of education, voluntary carrier screening, and genetic counseling was instituted for prospective control of this lethal disease. Since the program institution in 1970, more than 1 million young adults have been screened, and the incidence of Tay-Sachs disease has decreased by greater than 90% in the Ashkenazi Jewish population.[1]

The carrier frequency for Tay-Sachs disease is 1 in 30 in the Ashkenazi Jewish population.[15] Carrier frequencies are also disproportionately higher in individuals of Cajun and French-Canadian descent, and screening is recommended in these populations as well.[16] The current paradigm for carrier screening is serum or leukocyte determination of hexosaminidase A activity, given that heterozygotes have decreased levels of enzymatic activity compared with noncarriers. Pregnancy, use of oral conceptive pills, and chronic disease falsely decrease serum levels of hexosaminidase; therefore, leukocyte testing must be performed in these populations.[17] DNA-based molecular analysis should be used when enzymatic analysis is abnormal or inconclusive to confirm the diagnosis. More than 100 disease-causing mutations have been identified; however, 3 mutations account for 93% of carriers in the Ashkenazi Jewish population (+TAC1278 and +1 IVS 12 associated with classic phenotype and G269S associated with adult onset).[17] Other mutations included in the standard 6-mutation molecular panel include +1 IVS 9, which is associated with classic Tay-Sachs in non-Jewish populations, as well as 2 pseudodeficiency alleles (R247W and R249W). Individuals who are heterozygotes for these pseudodeficiency alleles show an apparent deficiency in hexosaminidase A activity when tested against the synthetic substrate but not against the natural substrate; therefore, these mutations are of no biological consequence. These pseudodeficiency alleles are present in 2% to 3% of the Ashkenazi Jewish population and 35% to 45% of the non-Jewish population.[18-20]

The sequential approach of enzymatic testing followed by molecular testing detects 98% of all carriers, whereas DNA-based mutation analysis only identifies 92% to 94% of carriers in the Ashkenazi Jewish population and 23% to 46% of non-Jewish carriers. In contrast, approximately 35% of non-Jewish and 4% of Jewish enzymatically identified carriers reveal no identifiable mutation by molecular analysis.[15,18] In 2009, Schneider and colleagues[21] compared the test performance characteristics of enzymatic versus molecular screening in more than 1000 individuals who self-identified as Ashkenazi Jewish. Of the 35 carriers identified by enzymatic screening, 4 would have been missed using molecular analysis alone, yielding a false-negative rate of 11.4%. Given the demographic changes in the Ashkenazi Jewish population with increasing rates of intermarriage and mixed ancestry, enzymatic testing remains superior as first-line carrier screening for Tay-Sachs disease.

In addition to CF and Tay-Sachs disease, ACOG also recommends carrier screening for Canavan disease and familial dysautonomia for individuals of Ashkenazi Jewish descent.[15] These disorders were selected based on their severity, high carrier frequency, and high sensitivity to detect most carriers with available screening modalities. The carrier frequency is as high as 1 in 40 for Canavan disease and 1 in 32 for familial dysautonomia in the Ashkenazi Jewish population. Both disorders cause profound neurologic deficits and shortened life span.[13] Greater than 99% of carriers can be detected with molecular testing, using a standard 3-mutation panel for Canavan disease and 2-mutation panel for familial dysautonomia.[22,23] Despite available carrier testing, ACOG does not support routine screening for the following 5 disorders: Gaucher disease type 1, Fanconi anemia, Niemann-Pick disease, Bloom syndrome, and mucolipidosis type IV. Instead, ACOG suggests that patient education material should be given to those who inquire about additional carrier screening to allow informed decision making. This decision is based on the lower carrier frequencies and/or lower severity of these disorders. For example, the carrier frequency is 1 in 107 for Bloom syndrome and 1 in 127 for mucolipidosis type IV. These disorders do not meet the greater than or equal to 1% allele frequency considered as a prerequisite for inclusion in carrier screening panels. In contrast, Gaucher disease is the most common autosomal recessive disorder in the Ashkenazi Jewish population with a carrier frequency of 1 in 18. However, clinical manifestations of this disorder are heterogeneous, the primary disease type affecting the Ashkenazi Jewish population is not lethal and has non-neuronal sequelae, and effective treatment with enzyme replacement therapy is available.[13] Despite these shortcomings, there are few mutations that account for these disorders in the Ashkenazi Jewish population; therefore, carrier detection rates exceed 95% using DNA mutation analysis. Based on this high degree of screening efficiency coupled with community preference, the ACMG issued guidelines in 2008 that recommend inclusion of these additional 5 disorders in the carrier screening panel for the Ashkenazi Jewish population (**Table 2**).[12]

Both ACOG and ACMG endorse the following general recommendations for the execution of carrier screening in the Ashkenazi Jewish population. Family history should be obtained for any individual contemplating pregnancy to determine whether either partner is of Ashkenazi Jewish descent, defined as having at least 1 grandparent of this ancestry. Ideally, testing should be performed before conception so that appropriate reproductive decisions can be made based on results. Genetic counseling should be made available to all carrier couples. If only 1 member of a couple is of Ashkenazi Jewish descent, that person should be screened first. If positive for any of the recessive alleles, partner screening should be pursued with the caveat that carrier frequency and detection rate in the non–Ashkenazi Jewish population is largely unknown for most disorders included in the panel; therefore, residual risk may be inaccurate. In addition, carrier screening should always be voluntary and requires informed consent for all conditions included in the panel.[12,15]

SPINAL MUSCULAR ATROPHY

Spinal muscular atrophy (SMA) is characterized by progressive motor neuron degeneration in the spinal cord leading to proximal muscle weakness and, ultimately, respiratory depression. SMA has an autosomal recessive inherence pattern. It affects 1 in 10,000 births, with a carrier frequency of 1 in 35 to 1 in 117 in the general population.[24–27]

There are 4 clinically recognized phenotypes of SMA. SMA type I (Werdnig-Hoffmann) presents before 6 months of age with severe hypotonia, with no ability to

Table 2
Ashkenazi Jewish screening panel recommendations

Disorder	Carrier Frequency	Detection Rate (%)	Screening Recommendations
CF	1 in 29	97	ACOG, ACMG
Tay-Sachs disease	1 in 30	98 by enzymatic assay 94 by molecular assay	ACOG, ACMG
Canavan disease	1 in 40	98	ACOG, ACMG
Familial dysautonomia	1 in 32	99	ACOG, ACMG
Gaucher disease	1 in 15	95	ACMG
Niemann-Pick disease	1 in 90	95	ACMG
Bloom Syndrome	1 in 100	95–97	ACMG
Mucolipidosis IV	1 in 127	95	ACMG
Fanconi anemia	1 in 89	99	ACMG

Data from Gross SJ, Pletcher BA, Monaghan KG. Carrier screening in individuals of Ashkenazi Jewish descent. Genet Med 2008;10(1):54–6; and American College of Obstetricians and Gynecologists. Preconception and prenatal carrier screening for genetic diseases in individuals of eastern European Jewish descent. ACOG Committee Opinion #442. Washington, DC: American College of Obstetricians and Gynecologists; 2009.

sit or gain head control. It is the most severe form of SMA, with life expectancy of less than 2 years. SMA type II presents before 18 months of age. Patients are able to sit but cannot walk without assistance. SMA type III presents after 18 months of age with variable severity. Affected individuals with SMA type III are generally expected to reach adulthood with minor muscle weakness. SMA type IV presents in adulthood with minor muscle weakness and is the mildest form of the disease. Types I and II account for nearly 90% of all cases of SMA.[28]

SMA is caused by mutations in the survival motor neuron (SMN) locus located on chromosome 5. There are 2 nearly identical SMN genes at this locus, denoted as SMN1 and SMN2. The 2 genes are very similar and encode for the same gene product, with the main difference being that SMN2 has a single base change on exon 8. This change results in 50% to 90% exon skipping at this location and leads to reduced gene function.[29]

Recombination occurs at the SMN locus at a rate of 1 in 10,000. The result of genetic recombination leads to gene conversion or copy number variation in either SMN gene.[30] Ninety-five percent of SMA cases are caused by loss-of-function mutations in SMN1 as a result of exon 7 deletion or missing SMN1 gene entirely. Most remaining cases are compound heterozygotes with an intragenic mutation in the remaining SMN1 gene.[24–27,30] The variable severity in SMA is modulated by the copy number of SMN2 genes inherited by the patient, with an inverse relationship observed between disease severity and SMN2 copy number.[30–32]

Because 95% of cases of SMA are caused by SMN1 deletion mutations, DNA analysis is highly sensitive in the diagnosis of SMA in affected individuals (95% sensitivity, 100% specificity).[27] However, this technique is inadequate as a carrier screening test because it cannot distinguish heterozygotes with at least 1 copy of normal SMN1.

Quantitative polymerase chain reaction (PCR) assay is currently the best available method for screening SMA carriers. This method uses exon-specific DNA probes that target regions of the SMN1 and SMN2 exons. The result can then be compared with reference genes to determine the copy numbers of both SMN1 and SMN2 genes in a patient. This method can provide a carrier detection rate of greater than 90% to 95%; however, this method also has limitations.[23,31] Because of crossing-over mutation events, 3% to 4% of SMA carriers carry 2 copies of the SMN1 gene (2 + 0) on one chromosome and none on the other. In addition, another 2% of carriers have a SMN1 gene with an intragenic mutation, which is not detected by quantitative PCR. Carriers with these type of configurations would be falsely screened as negative.[26,27]

The frequency of SMA carriers with a 2 + 0 configuration is race dependent. According to a nationwide study of more than 72,000 subjects, 27% of African Americans carry a 2 + 0 configuration SMN1 allele compared with 3.6% for white people and 7.8% for Hispanic people. As a result, the carrier detection rate using current screening methods is significantly reduced, estimated at 70% among African Americans compared with more than 91% for all other races studied.[25]

Because of the wide variation in SMA phenotype and the limitations of screening technology, various professional governing bodies have differing opinions regarding carrier screening. Although no clear clinical or health policy standards exist in defining high carrier frequency in the general population, the ACMG noted that the carrier frequency of SMA in the general population is comparable with that of Tay-Sachs disease, which has a carrier frequency of 1 in 30 among Ashkenazi Jews and 1 in 73 among French Canadians. In addition, the 90% to 95% carrier detection rate using quantitative PCR test meets ACMG standards for inclusion of a disorder in a carrier screening panel. Based on these considerations, the ACMG supports population-based screening for SMA using current testing methods.[27]

In contrast, ACOG currently does not recommend population-wide screening, citing the lack of pilot programs, cost-effectiveness analysis, population awareness, and laboratory assay standards as some of the key limitations preventing implementation of a successful screening program.[26] In addition, although SMA is most commonly a clinically severe disease, more than 10% of patients with SMA have milder phenotypes. At this time, there is no available test to predict SMA phenotype.[33,34] ACOG currently recommends that SMA carrier screening be offered only to patients with a family history of SMA or SMA-like disease. Couples who request SMA carrier screening should undergo genetic counseling regarding the sensitivity, specificity, and limitations of the test before undergoing screening.[26]

EXPANDED CARRIER SCREENING PANELS

With advancing technology and the development of multiplex platforms, the ease and speed at which mutation analysis can be performed have been optimized, leading to the creation of expanded carrier screening panels. These expanded panels have been introduced not only into Ashkenazi Jewish communities but also into the general population. In 2008, the ACMG published criteria for the consideration of inclusion of additional disorders into the Ashkenazi screening panel. These criteria include (1) the natural history of the disease should be well understood, (2) the disorder should carry the potential for significant morbidity and/or mortality in the homozygous or compound heterozygous state, and (3) there should be either a greater than 90% detection rate or greater than or equal to 1% allele frequency in the Ashkenazi Jewish population.[12]

In 2010, Scott and colleagues[35] published their experience with an expanded 16-disorder Ashkenazi Jewish carrier screening panel, including 118 mutations and variants. All mutations in the panel had a greater than 90% detection rate except for Usher syndrome type 1, which had only a 75% detection rate. The highest residual risk (1 in 281) was for Gaucher disease, whereas the lowest residual risk (1 in 13,301) was for Bloom syndrome. Among a random subset of 466 Ashkenazi Jewish patients who underwent pretest genetic counseling, 82% elected to have the expanded panel performed. Excluding CF, greater than 95% of these patients chose to include screening for all available disorders. These results show acceptance and desire for expanded carrier screening panels in the Ashkenazi Jewish population.[35]

With advancing technology, many laboratories now include more than 25 disorders in their Ashkenazi Jewish carrier screening panels. Proponents of expanded carrier screening panels argue that inclusion of a broader range of disorders, especially those with milder phenotypes, could provide more opportunity for early diagnosis and intervention. After sequencing 128 Ashkenazi Jewish genomes, Baskovich and colleagues[36] identified a panel of 163 mutations for 76 autosomal recessive, 24 autosomal dominant, and 3 X-linked disorders that could serve as genotyping targets in expanded Ashkenazi Jewish carrier screening panels. Of note, these disorders include those with variable expressivity, incomplete penetrance, and presymptomatic diagnosis. However, there remain significant concerns regarding the incorporation of this advancing genetic technology into clinical practice. Not only will the complexity of pretesting and posttesting counseling increase but also the sheer volume of patients requiring genetic counseling. Scott and colleagues[35] showed that, by moving from a 9-disorder to a 16-disorder panel, the number of identified carriers increased from 1 in 5 to 1 in 3. This finding presents significant economic and liability ramifications. It is also important to note that calculated carrier frequencies are often derived from small studies. In a recent study comparing reported carrier rates in the literature with screening data from 6 laboratories, the laboratory carrier frequency of Walker-Warburg syndrome was nearly double that reported in the literature.[37] The accuracy of the carrier frequency and detection rate is paramount in accurate residual risk calculation and appropriate posttest counseling. Furthermore, this study also showed the disparity in Ashkenazi Jewish panel composition among laboratories, highlighting the need for updated professional standards for screening.

With regard to panethnic screening panels, these are being justified by the increasing amount of mixed ancestry in North America and the growing inability for individuals to identify themselves as members of a single ethnicity. Critics of ethnicity-specific screening also argue that this method requires health care providers to be proficient in screening by family history and understanding which diseases should be targeted in specific ethnic populations. Furthermore, it must be recognized that genetic conditions do not occur solely in specific ethnic groups; therefore, limiting screening to these groups may put other at-risk individuals at a disadvantage.[38] Using a multiplex platform to screen for more than 100 Mendelian disorders, Srinivasan and colleagues[39] identified 35% of subjects as carriers for at least 1 deleterious mutation and 0.6% to 0.8% of couples as carrier couples, which is a high yield for a carrier screening panel. **Table 3** summarizes the potential advantages and limitations of introducing expanded carrier screening panels on a population-wide level.

In 2013, the ACMG published a position statement outlining the following 5 criteria that are essential for a disorder to be included on a carrier screening panel: (1) disorders should be severe enough for carrier couples to consider prenatal diagnosis to make reproductive decisions; (2) patients must provide consent for any adult-onset disorders included on a screening panel; (3) the causative genes, mutations, and mutation frequencies should be known in the population being tested in order to calculate a meaningful residual risk; (4) there must be a validated clinical association between the mutations and the severity of the disorder; and (5) there must be compliance with the ACMG *Standards and Guidelines for Clinical Genetics Laboratories*, including quality control and proficiency testing.[40] These criteria were affirmed in a joint consensus statement issued by ACOG, ACMG, the National Society of Genetic Counselors, the Perinatal Quality Foundation, and the Society for Maternal Fetal Medicine in 2015.[41] Despite these recommendations, many laboratories continue to operate independently from these guidelines, thereby creating additional layers of

Table 3
Advantages and limitations of expanded carrier screening panels

Advantages	Limitations
Community preference	Need for pretest and posttest genetic counseling; volume and financial implications
Technologic ease in screening for multiple disorders using multiplex platforms	
Recognizes mixed ancestry in North America	Panels include disorders with incomplete penetrance, variable expressivity, and adult-onset
Does not require provider proficiency in taking a genetic history and in targeted ethnicity-based screening	
	Rarity of some included disorders makes residual risk estimation inaccurate
	Disparity in composition of expanded panels by laboratory
	Downstream effects of cost savings and improved medical outcomes remain unknown

complexity for patient counseling. In addition, the downstream effects of cost savings and, more importantly, improved medical outcomes remain unknown.

REFERENCES

1. Kaback M, Lim-Steele J, Dabholkar D, et al. Tay-Sachs disease-carrier screening, prenatal diagnosis and the molecular era. An international perspective, 1970-1993. The International TSD Data Collection Network. JAMA 1993; 270(19):2307–15.

2. Boucher RC. Cystic fibrosis. In: Harrison TR, Kasper DL, editors. Harrison's principles of internal medicine. 16th edition. New York: McGraw-Hill; 2005. p. 1543–6.

3. Wapner RJ, Jenkins TM, Khalek M. Prenatal diagnosis of congenital disorders. In: Creasy RK, Resnik R, Iams JD, editors. Maternal-fetal medicine. principles and practice. 6th edition. Philadelphia: Saunders Elsevier; 2009. p. 221–74.

4. Nussbaum RL, McInnes RR, Willard HL. The molecular, biochemical, and cellular basis of genetic disease. In: Thompson & Thompson genetics in medicine. 7th edition. Philadelphia: Saunders Elsevier; 2007. p. 364–7.

5. Tsui L-C. Mutations and sequence variations detected in the cystic fibrosis transmembrane conductance regulator (CFTR) gene: a report from the Cystic Fibrosis Genetic Analysis Consortium. Hum Mutat 1992;1(3):197–203.

6. Shoshani T, Augarten A, Gazit E, et al. Association of a nonsense mutation (W1282X), the most common mutation in the Ashkenazi Jewish cystic fibrosis patients in Israel, with presentation of severe disease. Am J Hum Genet 1992;50(1): 222–8.

7. Genetic testing for cystic fibrosis. National Institutes of Health Consensus Development Conference Statement on genetic testing for cystic fibrosis. Arch Intern Med 1999;159(14):1529–39.

8. Grody WW, Cutting GR, Klinger KW, et al. Laboratory standards and guidelines for population-based cystic fibrosis carrier screening. Genet Med 2001;3(2): 149–54.

9. American College of Obstetricians and Gynecologists. Update on carrier screening for cystic fibrosis. ACOG Committee Opinion #486. Washington, DC: American College of Obstetricians and Gynecologists; 2011.

10. Watson MS, Cutting GR, Desnick RJ, et al. Cystic fibrosis population carrier screening: 2004 revision of American College of Medical Genetics mutation panel. Genet Med 2004;6(5):387–91.

11. Dork T, Dworniczak B, Aulehis-Schotz C, et al. Distinct spectrum of CFTR gene mutations in congenital absence of vas deferens. Hum Genet 1997;100(3–4): 365–77.

12. Gross SJ, Pletcher BA, Monaghan KG. Carrier screening in individuals of Ashkenazi Jewish descent. Genet Med 2008;10(1):54–6.

13. Ferreira JC, Schreiber-Agus N, Carter SM, et al. Carrier testing for Ashkenazi Jewish disorders in the prenatal setting: navigating the genetic maze. Am J Obstet Gynecol 2014;211(3):197–204.

14. Nussbaum RL, McInnes RR, Willard HL. Tay-Sachs disease. In: Thompson & Thompson genetics in medicine. 7th edition. Philadelphia: Saunders Elsevier; 2007. p. 310–1.

15. American College of Obstetricians and Gynecologists. Preconception and prenatal carrier screening for genetic diseases in individuals of eastern European Jewish descent. ACOG Committee Opinion #442. Washington, DC: American College of Obstetricians and Gynecologists; 2009.

16. American College of Obstetricians and Gynecologists. Screening for Tay-Sachs disease. ACOG Committee Opinion #318. Washington, DC: American College of Obstetricians and Gynecologists; 2005.

17. O'Brien JS, Okada S, Chen A, et al. Tay-Sachs disease: detection of heterozygotes and homozygotes by serum hexosaminidase assay. N Engl J Med 1970; 283:15–20.

18. Kaback MM. Population-based genetic screening for reproductive counseling: the Tay-Sachs model. Eur J Pediatr 2000;159:S192–5.

19. Cao Z, Natowicz MR, Kaback MM, et al. A second mutation associated with apparent beta-hexosaminidase A pseudo frequency estimation. Am J Hum Genet 1993;53:1198–205.

20. Triggs-Raine BL, Mules EH, Kaback MM, et al. A pseudodeficiency allele common in non-Jewish Tay-Sachs carriers: implications for carrier screening. Am J Hum Genet 1992;51:793–801.

21. Schneider A, Nakagawa S, Keep R, et al. Population-based Tay-Sachs screening among Ashkenazi Jewish young adults in the 21st century: hexosaminidase A enzyme assay is essential for accurate testing. Am J Med Genet A 2009; 149A:2444–7.

22. Kaul R, Gao GP, Aloya M, et al. Canavan disease: mutations among Jewish and non-Jewish patients. Am J Hum Genet 1994;55:34–41.

23. Dong J, Edelmann L, Bajwa AM, et al. Familial dysautonomia: detection of the IKBKAP IVS20 (+6T to C) and R696P mutations and frequencies among Ashkenazi Jews. Am J Med Genet 2002;110:253–7.

24. MacDonald WK, Hamilton D, Kuhle S. SMA carrier testing: a meta-analysis of differences in test performance by ethnic group. Prenat Diagn 2014;34(12): 1219–26.

25. Sugarman Ea, Nagan N, Zhu H, et al. Pan-ethnic carrier screening and prenatal diagnosis for spinal muscular atrophy: clinical laboratory analysis of >72,400 specimens. Eur J Hum Genet 2012;20(1):27–32.

26. American College of Obstetricians and Gynecologists. ACOG Committee Opinion #432. Washington, DC: American College of Obstetricians and Gynecologists; 2009.

27. Prior TW. Carrier screening for spinal muscular atrophy. Genet Med 2008;10(11): 840–2.

28. Lunn MR, Wang CH. Spinal muscular atrophy. Lancet 2008;371(9630):2120–33.

29. Lefebvre S, Bürglen L, Reboullet S, et al. Identification and characterization of a spinal muscular atrophy-determining gene. Cell 1995;80(1):155–65.

30. Larson JL, Silver AJ, Chan D, et al. Validation of a high resolution NGS method for detecting spinal muscular atrophy carriers among phase 3 participants in the 1000 genomes project. BMC Med Genet 2015;16(1):100.

31. Prior TW, Snyder PJ, Rink BD, et al. Newborn and carrier screening for spinal muscular atrophy. Am J Med Genet A 2010;152A(7):1608–16.

32. Su YN, Hung CC, Lin SY, et al. Carrier screening for spinal muscular atrophy (SMA) in 107,611 pregnant women during the period 2005-2009: a prospective population-based cohort study. PLoS One 2011;6(2):e17067.

33. Chen WJ, He J, Zhang Q, et al. Modification of phenotype by SMN2 copy numbers in two Chinese families with SMN1 deletion in two continuous generations. Clin Chim Acta 2012;413(23–24):1855–60.

34. Feldkötter M, Schwarzer V, Wirth R, et al. Quantitative analyses of SMN1 and SMN2 based on real-time LightCycler PCR: fast and highly reliable carrier testing

and prediction of severity of spinal muscular atrophy. Am J Hum Genet 2002; 70(2):358–68.

35. Scott SA, Edelmann L, Liu L, et al. Experience with carrier screening and prenatal diagnosis for 16 Ashkenazi Jewish genetic diseases. Hum Mutat 2010;31(11): 1240–50.

36. Baskovich B, Hiraki S, Upadhyay K, et al. Expanded genetic screening panel for the Ashkenazi Jewish population. Genet Med 2015. [Epub ahead of print]. http:// dx.doi.org/10.1038/gim.2015.123.

37. Hoffman JD, Park JJ, Schreiber-Agus N, et al. The Ashkenazi Jewish carrier screening panel: evolution, status quo and disparities. Prenat Diagn 2014;34: 1161–7.

38. Rose NC. Expanded carrier screening: too much of a good thing? Prenat Diagn 2015;35:936–7.

39. Srinivasan BS, Evans EA, Flannick J, et al. A universal carrier test for the long tail of Mendelian disease. Reprod Biomed Online 2010;21:537–51.

40. Grody WW, Thompson BH, Gregg AR, et al. ACMG position statement on prenatal/preconception expanded carrier screening. Genet Med 2013;15(6):482–3.

41. Edwards JG, Feldman G, Goldberg J, et al. Expanded carrier screening in reproductive medicine – points to consider. Obstet Gynecol 2015;125(3):653–62.

Screening and Testing in Multiples

Mark I. Evans, MD[a,b,c],*, Stephanie Andriole, MS, CGC[a],
Shara M. Evans, MSc, MPH[b,d]

KEYWORDS

- Prenatal screening • Cell-free fetal DNA • Free β- hCG • Amniocentesis • CVS
- Fetal reduction • Multiple pregnancy risks

KEY POINTS

- Both prenatal screening and testing are more complicated in multiples than in singletons.
- The risks of reproduction are directly related to chorionicity and for monochorionic twins (identical twins), the chromosomes and mendelian status of both twins are the same and the risk equals that of a singleton; for structural abnormalities the risks are considerably more than twice those for singletons.
- For dichorionic twins (fraternal) the risks of all are approximately additive.
- Screening is less effective in multiples than in singletons and it is difficult to distinguish which is which; diagnostic tests require more skill to determine which fetus is which.
- Fetal reduction, in experienced hands, has been shown to improve pregnancy outcomes in dichorionic twins but has high complication rates for monochorionic twins.

MULTIPLE PREGNANCIES

Over the past 35 years, infertility treatment has gone from fundamentally little more than providing encouragement to highly sophisticated pharmacologic and surgical interventions allowing millions of couples to have their own children.[1] However, of all babies born following in vitro fertilization (IVF), more than half are part of multiple pregnancies. In the United States the twin pregnancy rate, commonly quoted for decades to be 1 in 90, has more than doubled to nearly 1 in 30.[2] About 67% of all twins in the United States emanate from infertility treatments. Furthermore, the rate of monozygotic (MZ) twinning, per se, and as part of higher order multiples has continued

This article is an update of an article previously published in Clinics in Laboratory Medicine, Volume 30, Issue 3, September 2010.

[a] Fetal Medicine Foundation of America, USA; [b] Comprehensive Genetics, 131 East 65th Street, New York, NY 10065, USA; [c] Mt. Sinai School of Medicine, New York, NY, USA; [d] University of Colorado, Aurora, CO, USA
* Corresponding author. Comprehensive Genetics, 131 East 65th Street, New York, NY 10065.
E-mail address: evans@compregen.com

to increase, with its associated dramatically increased risks of anomalies, loss, and prematurity.[1]

The increasing rate of multiple pregnancies that is associated with advanced maternal age has expanded the need for prenatal diagnosis in twins and higher order gestations.[2] The same principles for diagnosis and screening in singleton pregnancies apply to multiples. However, there can be significant differences in the safety and efficacy of all approaches.[3] Furthermore, screening for aneuploidy in multiple gestations with the possibility of discordant karyotypes bears significant clinical, technical, and ethical issues, such as:

1. Lower performance of serum screening protocols compared with singleton pregnancies[4]
2. Inability of cell-free DNA screening to distinguish which fetus is which
3. The complexity of invasive diagnostic procedures
4. The risk of loss of an unaffected twin caused by the sequelae of the invasive procedures

Risks of Anomalies

Certain structural abnormalities, such as neural tube defects and cardiac defects, are more commonly seen in twin gestations than in singletons.[5] Chromosomal risks are the same per fetus, but given that there are 2 chances per dizygotic (DZ) pregnancy, the effective rate seems double (**Table 1**). MZ twins are especially prone to defects of laterality, such as situs inversus, but they are identical for chromosomal or mendelian disorders.

For DZ twins the risk of either twin being aneuploid is an independent probability. For example, the risk of having a baby with a traditional chromosome abnormality at maternal age 35 years is approximately 1 in 190. If there are 2 fetuses, the risk is essentially doubled (ie, 2 in 190 or 1 in 95). A 1 in 95 risk corresponds with the risk of a singleton for a 38-year-old woman. Similarly, the risk for a 30-year-old woman with a singleton is 1 in 380. With twins the risk is approximately 2 in 380 (ie, 1 in 190), which is the risk for a 35-year-old woman. Overall, the risk of at least 1 DZ twin having a serious problem is about 7%, but for an MZ twin the number is about 10%. Monoamniotic twins have an even higher incidence of structural abnormalities than do monochorionic (MC)/diamniotic (DA) fetuses.

Counseling

Counseling for prenatal diagnosis should include appreciation of the differences between screening and diagnosis, including the risks and benefits of each. For multiple pregnancies, most of which are conceived after long-standing infertility and treatment, patients' attitudes and choices regarding invasive prenatal diagnosis might differ from

Table 1			
Incidence of chromosomal abnormalities in at least 1 fetus in a multifetal gestation			
Maternal Age (y)	Singleton	Twin	Triplet
20	1 in 526	1 in 263 ≈ age 34 y	1 in 175 ≈ age 36 y
25	1 in 476	1 in 238 ≈ age 34 y	1 in 150 ≈ age 36 y
30	1 in 385	1 in 192 ≈ age 35 y	1 in 128 ≈ age 37 y
35	1 in 192	1 in 96 ≈ age 38 y	1 in 64 ≈ age 40 y
40	1 in 66	1 in 33 ≈ age 43 y	1 in 22 ≈ age 45 y

those of patients conceiving naturally.[6,7] Likewise, because of the high percentage of patients using eggs from donors much younger than themselves, the numerically greater risk based on egg age and the patient's tolerance of risk are often at odds. The authors have found that, for patients in their 40s and 50s, although the traditional chromosomal risks are often the age of an egg donor, the tolerance of risk is based on their own age.[8,9] Specifically, patients state that they would rather take the risk of diagnostic procedures even with a low abnormality incidence to avoid the chance of being in their 60s and having a special-needs child. This finding emphasizes the special issues in counseling such a selected population.

Historically, evaluations of the risks of definitive diagnosis (eg, chorionic villus sampling [CVS] and amniocentesis) in twins have varied widely but were usually quoted as a risk of procedure-associated fetal loss of 0.5% to 2% for CVS and 0.5% to 1% for amniocentesis.[10–12] With improvements in ultrasonography and a cadre of physicians highly experienced in such procedures, risks have significantly diminished. Several recent studies have shown that, in experienced hands, CVS is just as safe as amniocentesis.[11–13] Procedure versus natural history data in multiples have been limited, but generally have shown low risks with experienced operators. Most of the studies conclude that the spontaneous total pregnancy loss rate is about 6% to 7%.[14] Patients considering which diagnostic test to have should be counseled regarding the specific risks (and benefits) of such procedures in twins; for example, the risk of fetal loss after having either procedure, specifically in twin pregnancies. Issues such as sampling errors and the certainty of concordant or discordant results, in each test, should be addressed during counseling. The need for a second procedure, because of placental mosaicism, inappropriate sampling, and laboratory failures, or for selective feticide, should also be discussed. In our experience, in the most experienced of hands, the procedure risks are equal and therefore strongly favor CVS both for the privacy available and the lower risk of fetal reduction when chosen.[3]

Documentation and identification
The initial step before any diagnostic procedure in multifetal pregnancies is evaluation and documentation of the chorionicity, ideally at 8 to 12 weeks, followed by identification of each fetus and placenta (**Fig. 1**). Although chorionicity is best evaluated during the first trimester,[15] second-trimester scanning can detect chorionicity with an accuracy of 94% to 100%.[16] The location of both (or more) sacs, fetuses, placentas, cord

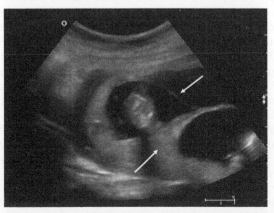

Fig. 1. Chorionicity determination in triplet pregnancy. Top arrow indicates the thin monochorionic membrane. Bottom arrow indicates the thick lambda sign of dichorionic twins.

insertions, and fetal genders at sufficient gestational age should be evaluated and clearly documented using text and diagram. Because any women undergoing genetic amniocentesis or CVS are also potential candidates for selective termination, incorrect documentation, sampling, or labeling might bring about a termination of the wrong fetus.[3] In general, the authors think that multiple pregnancy diagnosis is best done by operators who are also skilled in reduction, because too many mistakes can happen when 1 person does the diagnosis and then relies on a second physician doing the reduction to make sure which is which.

Aneuploidy Screening

Screening for genetic disorders in pregnancies has evolved over multiple decades. Space does not permit a comprehensive approach here, or even the citing of an appropriate number of references, but many aspects are covered in other articles here and in other publications.[17] Furthermore, this article only focuses on those issues specifically related to multiple pregnancies. Maternal carrier detection of mendelian disorders is generally unaffected by multiple gestation, but those conditions (eg, aneuploidy) in which fetal status is key are subject to the uncertainty of determination of which fetus contributed what component to the observed value in the mother. Those assessments, such as nuchal translucency (NT), which are fetal specific are less likely to be influenced than those that involve maternal serum blending of multiple fetal contributions.

Over the past 2 decades, several investigators used the term pseudorisks for Down syndrome from second-trimester screening recognizing that differentiation between one normal and one abnormal twin was problematic.[18] It was thought that maternal serum levels should be approximately double those of singleton pregnancies. However, it was appreciated even in the 1980s and 1990s that, for second-trimester biochemical screening, such was not the case. O'Brien and colleagues[19] showed in more than 4000 twins that alpha fetoprotein levels were more than doubled, human chorionic gonadotropin (hCG) was slightly less than doubled, and estriol considerably less than doubled. Thus, using a mere doubling as expected would bias the data and be suboptimal. Furthermore, the well-appreciated ethnic and racial differences known for second-trimester screening still needed to be evaluated by ethnic group in multiples. The same questions still remain in the first trimester.

NT measurements have also been used extensively in multiple pregnancies. The general conclusion is that, in DZ twins and higher, there is effectively no influence of one fetus on the other. In MZ twins, in which, by definition they are both the same, how to interpret differences in NT is problematic at the least. The general consensus has been to use the largest value for communication to the patient.[20]

The interpretation of biochemistry in multiples is even more problematic for reasons exactly paralleling that in the second trimester: what is the contribution of each fetus to the overall value?[17] There is no clear answer to that question. Overall data suggest that screening efficiency is decreased at least 10% in twins and that biochemistry is not effective in triplets or higher.[21] Furthermore, several studies suggest that the patterns of biochemistry in natural versus IVF pregnancies are different, with assisted cases having higher free β-hCG and lower Pregnancy Associated Plasma Protein - A (PAPP-A) levels, building in an increased risk for Down syndrome when actuarial data do not show an increase.[20]

In the past few years, there has been dramatic shift in the manner of prenatal chromosome screening as cell-free fetal DNA, otherwise called noninvasive prenatal testing or more appropriately NIP screening (NIPS), has greatly increased in use in the United States and elsewhere. NIPS has gone through several phases of development. First, complex counting techniques such as digital polymerase chain reaction were used to quantify the amount of chromosome 21–specific DNA compared with other chromosomes. These lacked the statistical power needed to discriminate between abnormal and normal cases.[22,23] The focus then turned to analysis of placental-specific RNAs so that there would be no background maternal DNA to confuse the diagnosis.[22] Investigators also attempted to use epigenetic and size differences between placental and maternal DNA fragments to enrich the fetal proportion.[24] There was then a rush toward commercialization despite limited population-based evaluation and peer-reviewed literature. In 2009 a data fraud was discovered that severely impugned the field.[24]

In 2011, a new approach using massive parallel shotgun sequencing showed that identification and counting of a large number of DNA fragments was both feasible and practical. Algorithms were developed that were capable of quantifying the contribution of DNA from specific chromosomes, making possible the identification of cases at high risk for trisomy 21 and 18.[25–29] Alternative methods such as the use of single nucleotide polymorphism probes to differentiate the maternal and fetal contributions, and the specific use of preselected fragments of interest before sequencing to reduce cost, have also been introduced.[26,30] After initial publications of the experience in populations of woman at high risk for aneuploidy, the test was brought to the market by multiple companies.

Most of the initial publications focused on screening high-risk patients or used populations enriched with excess Down syndrome cases.[26] There has been confusion among patients, and some providers, who do not realize that, although the sensitivity and specificity of the test do not depend on prevalence, the positive and negative predictive values do. Patients have difficulty understanding the difference, and many assume that a positive NIPS result is a diagnosis of aneuploidy. Even in high-risk cases, the risk (ie, positive predictive value [PPV]) is often no more than 75%, and in low-risk cases can be as low as 15%.[27] The extension of NIPS to selected rare microdeletions has further decreased the overall statistical performance, with considerably increased false-positive cases. For some microdeletion/duplication syndromes, the PPV can be as low as 5%.[27] Failure to understand these statistical realities has led to a general misconception among the public that NIPS effectively replaces amniocentesis and CVS, resulting in as much as a 50% decrease in the use of those diagnostic tests in favor of NIPS.[28]

Many clinicians using NIPS as their primary screening tool are also often eschewing NT and combined serum screening. For many patients, their first ultrasonography scan is at 18 to 20 weeks. Therefore, in addition to losing the advantage of establishing accurate dates and diagnosing multiple gestations in the first trimester, many major structural anomalies easily detected at 12 to 13 weeks are not being discovered until 2 months later.

The application of NIPS to multiples has been problematic; in the absence of ultrasonography findings (more likely if the NT examination is discontinued) it is impossible to determine which twin is at risk. Furthermore, the performance characteristics for conditions other than Down syndrome could be poor. For examples, the PPV for DiGeorge syndrome has been found to be less than 5%. Thus, for twins, the expected yield could be 2.5% or less. For both singletons and multiples, a common response to abnormal combined screening (free β-hCG, PAPP-A, and NT) has been to run NIPS. However, if the results are abnormal, they have to be confirmed by a diagnostic procedure. If they are normal, the same diagnostic procedure is needed to determine the abnormality. Thus, NIPS adds delay with no benefit in these situations.

The growth of first-trimester NIPS has had 2 competing effects on the preference for early prenatal diagnosis and its use. Many cytogenetic laboratories have noticed a

30% to 50% decrease in karyotypes requested for prenatal diagnosis because more and more patients are relying on these screening methods.[29] Some centers have reported high detection rates for diminished use of invasive procedures, but other reports have suggested that the net effect has not improved, and in some cases has even worsened.[28,29]

There is a large literature on the competing methods for determining genetic risks on which patients make decisions about whether to have definitive results by diagnostic tests or to rely on screening methods that provide odds adjustments only.[30] The literature has delved into both issues concerning the measurements, quality control, and statistical manipulation of NT measurements and the interpretation of the various laboratory results.[31] These matters are beyond the scope of this article but form an important aspect of the overall picture of risks and benefits of diagnostic procedures that cannot be completely separated from the procedure-specific results.

Diagnostic Procedures

Amniocentesis

Overall, amniocentesis has been the mainstay of diagnostic procedures since the late 1960s. Its use in twin pregnancies has been established for about 30 years,[32] but the exact methodology varies between centers. Furthermore, different views are held on specific issues, such as using dye to mark the sampled sac and the need for 2 punctures in MC pregnancies.

Three techniques have been described for amniocentesis in twins. The most common technique is the use of 2 different needles (usually 20-gauge or 22-gauge spinal needles) inserted separately and sequentially into each amniotic cavity under ultrasonography guidance. After the insertion of the first needle, about 2 mL are drawn into a small syringe to clear out any maternal cell contamination. Then 20 mL of fluid are aspirated for cytogenetic evaluation. The authors then reattach the discard syringe, draw back to fill about 5 mL, and then plunge back the contents into the uterine cavity. This technique produces a snowstorm of the debris lying in the cavity (**Fig. 2**). It

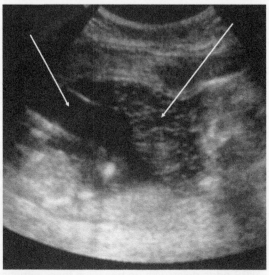

Fig. 2. Twin amniocentesis snowstorm. Right arrow shows reinjection of amniotic fluid creating bubbles of debris. Left arrow indicates the clear side.

outlines the cavity nicely. The other sac is clear. A second needle is then inserted into one of the clear areas. In earlier years, some investigators advocated the use of methylene blue, but this is now considered contraindicated because of associated risks of small bowel atresia, hemolytic anemia, and fetal death.[33] Indigo carmine has been widely used and has not been related to any adverse effects.[34] Using the plunge technique, the authors believe that dye is almost never needed in twins. In triplets or more, there are not enough data to be certain. It could be reserved for cases in which it is difficult to clearly show the septum (eg, in amniotic fluid volume discordance).

Two other approaches have occasionally been used: using the same needle and going directly from one sac to the other, and using 2 needles simultaneously into both sacs. The authors have discussed these topics elsewhere, and these are rarely used.[35]

Amniocentesis in monochorionic twins MC pregnancies can be diagnosed with high specificity and sensitivity even in later stages of pregnancy. Such pregnancies are by definition monozygotic, and carry identical sets of chromosomes (and are referred to as identical twins). Therefore, to karyotype MC/DA pregnancies, only 1 sac should generally be tapped. However, many case reports have described identical twins with discordant phenotype and karyotype. The causes of the phenotypic discordance are varied and include rare karyotypic differences, mosaicism, skewed X-inactivation, differential gene imprinting, and small-scale mutations.[36] Cases of MC twins with discordant phenotype include mosaicism for Turner syndrome, Down syndrome, Patau syndrome, trisomy 1, and 22q11 deletion syndrome.[9] The exact prevalence of heterokaryotypic MZ pregnancies is unknown, but it is a rare phenomenon. The authors' opinion, as well as others',[9,37] is that, if 1 or both of the fetuses has an ultrasonography abnormality (or marker of aneuploidy), both sacs should be sampled, even if the twins are apparently MC. When chorionicity is certain, both fetuses do not have any anatomic abnormality, and fetal growth is not severely discordant, sampling a single amniotic sac is sufficient. Although the risk of a single puncture in twins should theoretically be lower than tapping both amniotic cavities, data regarding such a comparison in MC twins are limited.

Fetal loss rate The postprocedural loss rate should be evaluated compared with a natural history cohort of such pregnancies or, ideally, compared with a control group. In singleton pregnancies, Evans and Wapner[38] analyzed the literature and found a general consensus of amniocenteses risks of about 1 in 300 to 1 in 350 when done by experienced operators, and rates much higher with occasional operators. Eddleman and colleagues[39] from the FASTER (First And Second Trimester Evaluation of Risk) consortium suggested a 1 in 1600 procedure risk, but there were multiple methodologic problems with their conclusions. Wapner and colleagues[40] showed that, with proper design, loss rates were close to the 1 in 300 figure quoted earlier. For example, the loss rate in Eddleman and colleagues'[39] high-risk unsampled group was 3.76%, whereas in the high-risk sampled group it was only 1.06%. No one believes that performing amniocentesis is protective. The same inverse ratio is seen with advanced maternal age, in which the amniocentesis group had a lower loss rate than the control group. Alfirevic and Tabor[12] showed that, had the original Tabor and colleagues[41] study used the same loss classifications (only counting losses and deaths before 24 weeks) as the Eddleman and colleagues[39] study, then Tabor and colleagues[41] would have found a loss rate difference of 0.21%, which would have been statistically nonsignificant.

The natural history of twin pregnancies carries a pregnancy loss rate up to 24 weeks of about 6.3% and severe prematurity (24–28 weeks) rate of about 8%.[14] The data regarding the pregnancy loss rate after amniocentesis are comparable with these background loss rates.

Chorionic villus sampling

Multiple studies over 25 years, including national and collaborative trials, have shown that CVS in singleton pregnancies is safe, with an acceptable rate of fetal loss of about 0.5% to 3%.[10] The advantages of early prenatal diagnosis by CVS, providing rapid karyotyping, enzyme analysis, and DNA analysis, in twin pregnancies are similar to those related to singleton pregnancies; for example, early diagnosis allowing earlier termination of pregnancy, if indicated. However, in multifetal pregnancies, early diagnosis by CVS also facilitates early selective reduction of the affected fetus with fewer psychological and medical complications.[42–44]

Specific issues concerning CVS in multifetal pregnancies include (1) the methodology and safety of CVS in these pregnancies; (2) the sampling error rates for twins; and (3) issues concerning the impact of CVS on subsequent procedures, such as selective termination.

The technique of CVS in multiple pregnancies is considerably more complicated than in singletons and it should be done by experienced operators to ensure accurate mapping of the fetuses and placentas and correct ultrasonography-guided placement of the instruments into each placenta (**Fig. 3**). It is crucial to evaluate and document the chorionicity (based on first-trimester ultrasonography using the lambda sign), location of the fetuses, their related placentas, and the location of the cord insertions (specifically important for CVS). The description of the fetal and placental locations should be detailed in such a manner that it allows proper identification of the affected fetus; especially when feticide might be considered.

The contamination rate (of one sample with villi from the other fetus) reported in the literature is usually based on cases with incorrect gender determination or XX/XY mosaicism (which is ruled out). With experience and careful methodology, the sampling error rates reported earlier[36] of about 4% to 5% have decreased to almost

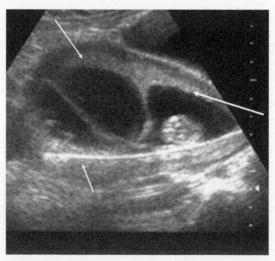

Fig. 3. Triplet CVS approach. Arrow at bottom shows catheter in posterior fundal placenta. Arrow at right shows path for catheter in low anterior placenta. Arrow at left shows path for needle to anterior fundal placenta.

none.[45] DNA fingerprinting can be used to determine zygocity when required in same-sex twins with placental findings that are not conclusive.

CVS in multifetal pregnancies can be achieved by either a transabdominal or trans-cervical approach.[3] Operators must be familiar with both approaches. Technique is even more critical in multiples, because operators must make sure that a needle or catheter does not go through one placenta to reach another.

Fetal loss rate The estimated risk of spontaneous abortion and fetal loss after CVS in singletons has varied widely over the years (0.5%–4.3%). Early studies suggested that 2 or more samplings during 1 procedure might be associated with an increased risk of fetal loss.[46] The mean number of samplings per twin pregnancy reported in the literature ranges between 2.02 and 2.2 but some cases underwent up to 5 needle insertions.[44] However, those studies that have compared fetal loss rates in singletons and twins within the same institution found that CVS was not associated with an increased risk of either total pregnancy losses or single fetal losses.[47] Several articles have addressed the questions of procedure risks and reached different conclusions. Caughey and colleagues[48] from the University of California, San Francisco, performed a retrospective cohort study of nearly 10,000 CVS and 30,000 amniocenteses with normal cytogenetic results over a 30-year period and documented reduced complication rates in both groups over time but a greater decrease in CVS losses. When the data were adjusted for maternal age, indication for procedure, provider, year of procedure, gestational age at procedure, race, ethnicity, and parity, the ratio of losses for CVS to losses for amniocentesis decreased from a 1983 to 1987 cohort at 4.23 to 1.03 from 1998 to 2003. The differences were nonsignificant in the years since 1993.

Overall, in the most experienced of hands, CVS on multiples is no different than in singletons and no different than amniocentesis. Furthermore, because of the clear advantage of doing fetal reductions in the first trimester compared with the second, for patients who desire definitive answers, the authors think that CVS has clear advantages.

In an attempt to coordinate the published data, Mujezinovic and Alfirevic[13] performed a meta-analysis of CVS and amniocentesis complications. They found 29 studies since 1995 that met their criteria for amniocenteses performed after 14 weeks and 16 studies for CVS. Pooled, total pregnancy losses were classified as being (1) within 14 days of procedure, (2) before 24 weeks of gestation, or (3) total. For amniocenteses the results were 0.6%, 0.9%, and 1.9%. For CVS, the corresponding rates were virtually identical at 0.7%, 1.3%, and 2.0% (**Table 2**). More recent studies have replicated these conclusions.[49,50] It is important to remember that an earlier gestational age at which CVS is performed translates into higher likely rates at all data points, because more cases that are destined to die will still be in the viable pool at the time of CVS that would be gone before amniocentesis.

Table 2 Loss rates after procedures		
	Meta-analysis	
	Amniocentesis (%)	**CVS (%)**
14 d	0.6	0.7
24 wk	0.9	1.0
Total	1.9	2.0

Data from Mujezinovic F, Alfirevic Z. Procedure related complications of amniocentesis and chorionic villus sampling. Obstet Gynecol 2007;110:687–94.

However, in our experience, the transcervical procedure requires considerably more skill and experience for the operator to become competent, but, for optimal outcomes, both procedures need to be in the armamentarium of prenatal diagnostic centers.

Microarrays Standard cytogenetic resolution is limited by light microscopy such that the minimum discrimination ability for classic cytogenetics is about 7 Mb. There are numerous serious microdeletion and microduplication disorders, such as Williams syndrome, Angelman, Prader-Willi, and cri du chat, that have copy number variants (CNVs) too small to see by these methods.[9] Array comparative genomic hybridization (aCGH) has the ability to identify microdeletions or duplications (CNVs) less than 200,000 base pairs (200 Kb), but in clinical prenatal practice findings of 500 kb to 1 Mb are routinely reported. Over the past decade, aCGH has virtually replaced the karyotype in the evaluation of dysmorphic neonates because the yield of finding a cause for the clinical findings is essentially double that of the karyotype.[12,14]

Prenatally, aCGH was initially used when structurally abnormal fetuses were seen on ultrasonography, finding a clinically relevant CNV, not seen on karyotype, in 6% to 8% of patients.[15,51] In patients who have no ultrasonography findings, collaborative data suggest that at least 1% of all patients have a significant CNV not determinable by any other method.[51] Given that 1% of all children develop neurodevelopmental delays and about 1% have autism, the authors now offer CVS and aCGH to all patients regardless of age.[3] Although specific microdeletions or duplications are individually rare, collectively they are more common than the classic trisomies and can have equally concerning phenotypes. Given that the standard for offering diagnostic procedures has been considered the 1 in 190 risk of standard aneuploidy in 35-year-olds, the 1 in 100 risk of an abnormal CNV in everybody now means that, to us, everyone is a candidate for diagnostic procedures and aCGH.[52–56] In twins, the minimal risk of a significant problem is now 1 in 50. These concepts have revolutionized the field.[3,9]

FETAL REDUCTION

FR has been used for more than 2 decades to improve the clinical outcome of high-order multiple pregnancies.[57,58] In multiple, collaborative publications from around the world, the world's most experienced centers have shown that, with multiples, if success is defined as a healthy mother and health family, fewer is always better. The specifics depend on starting and finishing numbers (**Fig. 4**). Furthermore, recent data suggest that, for women who start with twins, using the same definition of success, it is safer to reduce to a singleton than keep the twins. The improvement is not as great as going down from quintuplets, but the improvement is real.

The selection process in experienced hands is hierarchical. In inexperienced hands, the criteria are essentially empirical/technical (such as fetal location). Some operators use sonographic screening by NT measurement, presence of nasal bone, or complete anatomic survey (by transvaginal or transabdominal scanning).[1,42]

CHORIONIC VILLUS SAMPLING AND FETAL REDUCTION

Our approach in most cases is to offer CVS before reduction. Typically, we sample 1 more fetus than we are planning to keep; that is, if we are keeping 2, we sample all 3 triplets or 3 of 4 quadruplets. We then run a fluorescence in situ hybridization analysis

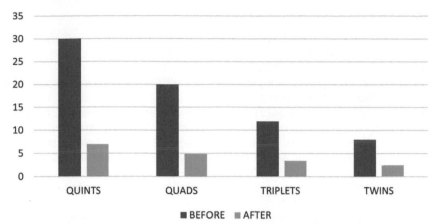

Fig. 4. Fetal Reduction risk reduction. QUADS, quadruplets; QUINTS, quintuplets.

overnight and use those data in the overall evaluation of which fetuses to preserve. We use the following hierarchy[59,60]:

1. A documented abnormality
2. Suspicion and concern such as smaller crown rump length (CRL) or larger NT
3. Other technical factors of serious concern
4. If nothing else matters, then we consider gender differences

The last criterion was only added in the past several years when it became apparent that patients' wishes for gender information now no longer include the significant male preference seen in earlier decades. For couples reducing to twins, the most common preference is for 1 of each.[1,43,60]

Several reports have shown that genetic analysis by CVS before selective early fetal reduction does not increase the risk of miscarriage or early delivery (compared with reduction without CVS). As expected, Brambati and colleagues[61] showed that the pre-term delivery rate was associated with the eventual number of fetuses; having CVS did not increase the risk of fetal losses (including perinatal losses) or early deliveries. Furthermore, in a review by Jenkins and Wapner,[62] the rate of miscarriage in a group that had CVS and fetal reduction (5.5% total pregnancy loss) was similar to the rate in a group that did not have CVS (5.6%).

SUMMARY

The choice of screening or invasive procedure in twin pregnancies depends on several factors, but ultimately is a personal choice of where the patient wishes to put her risk; that is, a small risk of having a baby with a serious disorder versus a small risk of having a complication because she wishes to avoid that. In our experience, these are personality issues and there is no clear answer that applies to every patient. The advantages in early diagnosis are clear.[9,11,63]

Given that the past 20 years have not settled the question of true risks of amniocentesis and CVS or the differences between them, how to interpret such risks has profound effects on the perceived value of techniques, either leading to a decision to screening or going directly to CVS. There are profound practice, economic, and patent issues surrounding the data and the implications of the interpretation of the data. No single short review can exhaustively examine all of the issues.

REFERENCES

1. Evans MI, Britt DW. Selective reduction in multifetal pregnancies. In: Paul M, Grimes D, Stubblefield P, et al, editors. Management of unintended and abnormal pregnancy. London: Wiley-Blackwell; 2009. p. 312–8.
2. Available at: https://www.sartcorsonline.com/rptCSR_PublicMultYear.aspx?Clinic PKID=0. Accessed February 2, 2016.
3. Evans MI, Wapner RJ, Berkowitz RL. Non invasive prenatal screening vs. advanced diagnostic testing: caveat emptor. Am J Obstet Gynecol 2016, in press.
4. Spencer K, Nicolaides KH. Screening for trisomy 21 in twins using first trimester ultrasound and maternal serum biochemistry in a one-stop clinic: a review of three years' experience. BJOG 2003;110:276–80.
5. Luke B. Monozygotic twinning as a congenital defect and congenital defects in monozygotic twins. Fetal Diagn Ther 1990;5(2):61–9.
6. Holmes A, Jauniaux E. Prospective study of parental choice for aneuploidy screening in assisted conception versus spontaneously. Reprod Biomed Online 2004;8(2):243–5.
7. Geipel A, Berg C, Katalinic A, et al. Different preferences for prenatal diagnosis in pregnancies following assisted reproduction versus spontaneous conception. Reprod Biomed Online 2004;8:119–24.
8. Evans MI, Curtis J, Andriole SA, et al. Invasive procedures in the first trimester. In: Abramowicz J, editor. First trimester ultrasound – a comprehensive guide. Berlin (Germany): Springer; 2016. p. 367–82.
9. Evans MI, Andriole S, Birenbaum R, et al. Prenatal diagnosis in the molecular age – indications, procedures, and laboratory techniques. In: MacDonald MG, Seshis MMK, editors. Avery's neonatology: pathophysiology and management of the newborn. 7th edition. Philadelphia: Wolters Kluwer/Lippincott Williams & Wilkins; 2016. p. 113–33.
10. Brambati B, Tului L, Alberti E. Prenatal diagnosis by chorionic villus sampling. Eur J Obstet Gynecol Reprod Biol 1996;65:11–6.
11. Alfirevic Z, Sundberg K, Brigham S. Amniocentesis and chorionic villus sampling for prenatal diagnosis. Cochrane Database Syst Rev 2003;(3):CD003252.
12. Alfirevic Z, Tabor A. Pregnancy loss rates after midtrimester amniocentesis. Obstet Gynecol 2007;109:1203–4.
13. Mujezinovic F, Alfirevic Z. Procedure related complications of amniocentesis and chorionic villus sampling. Obstet Gynecol 2007;110:687–94.
14. Yaron Y, Bryant-Greenwood PK, Dave N, et al. Multifetal pregnancy reductions of triplets to twins: comparison with nonreduced triplets and twins. Am J Obstet Gynecol 1999;180:1268–71.
15. Sepulveda W, Sebire NJ, Hughes K, et al. The lambda sign at 10-14 weeks of gestation as a predictor of chorionicity in twin pregnancies. Ultrasound Obstet Gynecol 1996;7:421–3.
16. Vayssiere CF, Heim N, Camus EP, et al. Determination of chorionicity in twin gestations by high-frequency abdominal ultrasonography: counting the layers of the dividing membrane. Am J Obstet Gynecol 1996;175:1529–33.
17. Evans MI, Galen RS, Drugan A. Biochemical screening. In: Evans MI, Johnson MP, Yaron Y, et al, editors. Prenatal diagnosis: genetics, reproductive risks, testing, and management. New York: McGraw-Hill; 2006. p. 277–88.
18. Sebire NJ, Snijders RJM, Hughes K, et al. Screening for trisomy 21 in twin pregnancies by maternal age and fetal nuchal translucency thickness at 10-14 weeks of gestation. Br J Obstet Gynaecol 1996;103:999–1003.

19. O'Brien JE, Dvorin E, Yaron Y, et al. Differential increases in AFP, hCG, and uE3 in twin pregnancies: impact on attempts to quantify Down syndrome screening calculations. Am J Med Genet 1997;73:109–12.

20. Cleary-Goldman J, Berkowitz RL. First trimester screening for Down syndrome in multiple pregnancy. Semin Perinatol 2005;29:395–400.

21. Krantz D, Hallahan T, He K, et al. First trimester screening in triplets. Am J Obstet Gynecol 2011;205:364.e1–5.

22. Lo YM. Noninvasive prenatal detection of fetal chromosomal aneuploidies by maternal plasma nucleic acid analysis: a review of the current state of the art. BJOG 2009;116:152–7.

23. Evans MI, Wright DA, Pergament E, et al. Digital PCR for noninvasive detection of aneuploidy: power analysis equations for feasibility. Fetal Diagn Ther 2012;31:244–7.

24. Pollack A. Biotech company fires chief and others over handling of data. NY Times 2009. Available at: http://www.nytimes.com/2009/09/29/business/29drug.html?_r=0.

25. Ehrich M, Deciu C, Zwiefehofer T, et al. Noninvasive detection of trisomy 21 by sequencing of DNA in maternal blood: a study in a clinical setting. Am J Obstet Gynecol 2011;204:205.e1–11.

26. Sparks AB, Struble CA, Wang ET, et al. Noninvasive prenatal detection and selective analysis of cell-free DNA obtained from maternal blood: evaluation for trisomy 21 and trisomy 18. Am J Obstet Gynecol 2012;206:319.e1–9.

27. Bianchi DW, Platt LD, Goldberg JD, et al. Genomewide fetal aneuploidy detection by maternal plasma DNA sequencing. Obstet Gynecol 2012;119:890–901.

28. Benn P, Cuckle H. Theoretical performance of non-invasive prenatal testing for chromosome imbalances using counting of cell-free DNA fragments in maternal plasma. Prenat Diagn 2014;34:778–83.

29. Henry GP, Britt DW, Evans MI. Screening advances and diagnostic choice: the problem of residual risk. Fetal Diagn Ther 2008;23:308–15.

30. Gonce A, Borrell A, Fortuny A, et al. First trimester screening for trisomy 21 in twin pregnancy: does the addition of biochemistry make an improvement? Prenat Diagn 2005;25:1156–61.

31. Evans MI, van Decruyes H, Nicolaides KH. Nuchal translucency (NT) measurements for 1st trimester screening: the "price" of inaccuracy. Fetal Diagn Ther 2007;22:401–4.

32. Bang J, Nielsen H, Philip J. Prenatal karyotyping of twins by ultrasonically guided amniocentesis. Am J Obstet Gynecol 1975;123:695–6.

33. Nicolini U, Monni G. Intestinal obstruction in babies exposed in utero to methylene blue. Lancet 1990;336:1258–9.

34. Cragan JD, Martin ML, Khoury MJ, et al. Dye use during amniocentesis and birth defects. Lancet 1993;341:1352.

35. Jeanty P, Shah D, Roussis P. Single-needle insertion in twin amniocentesis. J Ultrasound Med 1990;9:511–7.

36. Machin GA. Some causes of genotypic and phenotypic discordance in monozygotic twin pairs. Am J Med Genet 1996;61:216–28.

37. Nieuwint A, Zalen-Sprock R, Hummel P, et al. 'Identical' twins with discordant karyotypes. Prenat Diagn 1999;19:72–6.

38. Evans MI, Wapner RJ. Invasive prenatal diagnostic procedures 2005. In: Reddy U, Mennuti MT, editors. Seminars in perinatology, vol. 29. Philadelphia: Elsevier Publishing Company; 2005. p. 215–8.

39. Eddleman KA, Malone FD, Sullivan L, et al. Pregnancy loss rates after mid-trimester amniocentesis. Obstet Gynecol 2006;108:1067–72.

40. Wapner RJ, Evans MI, Platt LD. Pregnancy loss rates after midtrimester amniocentesis. Obstet Gynecol 2007;109:780.

41. Tabor A, Philip J, Madsen M, et al. Randomised controlled trial of genetic amniocentesis in 4606 low-risk women. Lancet 1986;1:1287–93.

42. De Catte L, Foulon W. Obstetric outcome after fetal reduction to singleton pregnancies. Prenat Diagn 2002;22:206–10.

43. Evans MI, Kaufman M, Urban AJ, et al. Fetal reduction from twins to a singleton: a reasonable consideration. Obstet Gynecol 2004;104:102–9.

44. Wapner RJ, Johnson A, Davis G, et al. Prenatal diagnosis in twin gestations: a comparison between second-trimester amniocentesis and first-trimester chorionic villus sampling. Obstet Gynecol 1993;82:49–56.

45. Antsaklis A, Souka AP, Daskalakis G, et al. Second-trimester amniocentesis vs. chorionic villus sampling for prenatal diagnosis in multiple gestations. Ultrasound Obstet Gynecol 2002;20:476–81.

46. Rhoads GG, Jackson LG, Schlesselman SE, et al. The safety and efficacy of chorionic villus sampling for early prenatal diagnosis of cytogenetic abnormalities. N Engl J Med 1989;320:609–17.

47. Brambati B, Tului L, Guercilena S, et al. Outcome of first-trimester chorionic villus sampling for genetic investigation in multiple pregnancy. Ultrasound Obstet Gynecol 2001;17:209–16.

48. Caughey AB, Hopkins LM, Norton ME. Chorionic villus sampling compared with amniocentesis and the difference in the rate of pregnancy loss. Obstet Gynecol 2006;108:612–6.

49. Akolekar R, Beta J, Picciarelli G, et al. Procedure related risk of miscarriage following amniocentesis and chorionic villus sampling: a systematic review and meta-analysis. Ultrasound Obstet Gynecol 2015;45:16–26.

50. Wulff CB, Gerds TA, Rode L, et al. Risk of fetal loss associated with invasive testing following combined firsts trimester screening for Down syndrome: a national cohort study of 147 987 singleton pregnancies. Ultrasound Obstet Gynecol 2016;47:38–44.

51. Wapner RJ, Martin CL, Levy B, et al. Chromosomal microarray versus karyotyping for prenatal diagnosis. N Engl J Med 2012;367:2175–84.

52. Wilson RD, Ledbetter DH, Pergament E. Current controversies in prenatal diagnosis 3: the ethical and counseling implications of new genomic technologies: all pregnant women should be offered prenatal diagnostic genome-wide testing for prenatally identified fetal congenital anomalies. Prenat Diagn 2015;35:19–22.

53. American College of Obstetricians and Gynecologists Committee on Genetics. Committee opinion No. 581: the use of chromosomal microarray analysis in prenatal diagnosis. Obstet Gynecol 2013;122:1374–7.

54. Saldarriaga W, Garcia-Perdoma HA, Arango-Pineda J, et al. Karyotype versus genomic hybridization for the prenatal diagnosis of chromosomal abnormalities: a metaanalysis. Am J Obstet Gynecol 2015;212:330.e1–10.

55. Dale RC, Grattan-Smith P, Nicholson M, et al. Microdeletions detected using chromosome microarray in children with suspected genetic movement disorders: a single-centre study. Dev Med Child Neurol 2012;54:618–23.

56. Vallespin E, Palomares Bralo M, Mori MA, et al. Customized high resolution CGH-array for clinical diagnosis reveals additional genomic imbalances in previous well-defined pathological samples. Am J Med Genet A 2013;161A:1950–60.

57. Shaffer LM, Dabell MP, Fisher AJ, et al. Experience with microarray-based comparative genomic hybridization for prenatal diagnosis in over 5000 pregnancies. Prenat Diagn 2012;32:976–85.
58. Gebb J, Dar P, Rosner M, et al. Long term neurologic outcomes after common fetal interventions. Am J Obstet Gynecol 2015;212:527.e1–9.
59. Rosner M, Pergament E, Andriole S, et al. Detection of genetic abnormalities using CVS and FISH prior to fetal reduction in sonographically normal appearing fetuses. Prenat Diagn 2013;33:940–4.
60. Evans MI, Rosner M, Andriole S, et al. Evolution of gender preferences in multiple pregnancies. Prenat Diagn 2013;33:935–9.
61. Brambati B, Tului L, Baldi M, et al. Genetic analysis prior to selective fetal reduction in multiple pregnancy: technical aspects and clinical outcome. Hum Reprod 1995;10:818–25.
62. Jenkins TM, Wapner RJ. The challenge of prenatal diagnosis in twin pregnancies. Curr Opin Obstet Gynecol 2000;12:87–92.
63. Evans MI, Andriole SA, Evans SM. Genetics: update on prenatal screening and diagnosis. Obstet Gynecol Clin North Am 2015;42:193–208.

Inverted Pyramid of Care

Jiri D. Sonek, MD, RDMS[a],*, Karl Oliver Kagan, MD, PhD[b],
Kypros H. Nicolaides, MD[c]

KEYWORDS

- First trimester • Screening • Diagnosis • Anomalies • Maternal complications
- Preeclampsia

KEY POINTS

- Most fetal chromosomal and structural anomalies can be diagnosed by the end of the first trimester of pregnancy.
- Cell free fetal DNA is a significant advance in screening for fetal aneuploidy; however, its use is limited and is best used in combination with first-trimester ultrasound and maternal serum screening.
- The risk of some pregnancy complications that become clinically evident only later in pregnancy can be established in the first trimester; the incidence of some of these disorders, such as preeclampsia, can be reduced if treatment is instituted early in pregnancy.
- First-trimester screening also shows some promise in other pregnancy-related problems (eg, spontaneous preterm birth, small for gestational age without preeclampsia, macrosomia, gestational diabetes) and represents a fertile field for future research.

INTRODUCTION

Pregnancy management typically involves reacting to maternal and fetal problems only after they develop. Because most fetal and maternal complications become apparent late in pregnancy, it has been traditionally thought that is when the most intensive surveillance should be implemented. Indeed, the initial prenatal care guidelines as put forth by the Ministry of Health in the United Kingdom in the early twentieth century reflects this fact.[1] In this schema, which has been accepted throughout the world, the frequency of antenatal visits progressively increases with advancing gestation and is recommended to be on a weekly basis from 36 weeks' gestation onwards.

Recent decades have seen a movement of fetal and maternal investigations to the first trimester of pregnancy.[2] The impetus for this phenomenon can be traced to the

No disclosures.
[a] Center for Maternal-Fetal Medicine, Ultrasound, and Genetics, Fetal Medicine Foundation of USA, Wright State University, Berry Pavilion, 1 Wyoming Street, Dayton, OH 45409, USA; [b] Department of Gynecology and Obstetrics, Universitäts-Frauenklinik, Calwerstrasse, Tübingen 772076, Germany; [c] Harris Birthright Research Centre for Fetal Medicine, King's College Hospital, 16-20 Windsor Walk, London SE5 8BB, UK
* Corresponding author.
E-mail address: jdsonek@premierhealth.com

development of first-trimester ultrasound screening for fetal aneuploidy using nuchal translucency (NT) measurement.[3,4] This screening was quickly followed by the realization that NT thickening can be associated with a whole host of other fetal abnormalities.[5,6] Furthermore, the increased use of ultrasound in the first trimester revealed that many fetal structural problems can already be accurately diagnosed at this point.[7]

The use of maternal serum biochemical screening followed a similar pattern. Free beta–human chorionic gonadotropin (hCG) and pregnancy-associated plasma protein A (PAPP-A) were first used to screen for trisomy 21, but subsequently they were also found to be useful in screening for trisomies 18 and 13 and for triploidy.[8,9] The use of first-trimester biochemistries was then further expanded to predict pregnancy complications that become apparent only later on in pregnancy, such as preeclampsia (PE) and severe intrauterine growth restriction.[10]

The recent introduction of screening using maternal plasma cell-free (cf) DNA represents a significant advance in antenatal detection of aneuploidy.[11] Even though this test analyzes fetal DNA, it still is a screening test, not a diagnostic one. Furthermore, its limited scope and high cost makes it impractical as a primary screening test.[12]

In this article, the authors aim to review the benefits of early pregnancy evaluation and how to best use the tests currently available. The authors also aim to show that some very important complications that occur later in pregnancy can be predicted in the first trimester; therefore, it is worthwhile to increase the focus of clinical evaluations in early pregnancy, thus, inverting the pyramid of prenatal care (**Fig. 1**). By selecting pregnancies that are at the highest risk for complications that become apparent only later in gestation and by identifying those that are at very low risk, a prenatal care plan can be developed that is tailored to individual patients.[13]

FIRST-TRIMESTER SCREENING FOR FETAL ANEUPLOIDY

Fetal aneuploidy is a major cause of perinatal morbidity and mortality as well as long-term disabilities. All diagnostic prenatal tests used to diagnose fetal aneuploidy carry a risk of miscarriage and are expensive.[14] Therefore, starting with a screening test that has the highest possible detection rate and lowest false-positive rate is of critical importance. However, because funds for health care are limited, from the standpoint of public health policy, a screening test that is deemed to be too expensive (ie, is not cost-effective) cannot be universally implemented.

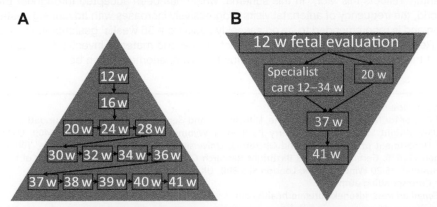

Fig. 1. Traditional pyramid of prenatal care (*A*) and a possible new pyramid (*B*). w, weeks. (*Adapted from* Nicolaides KH. Turning the pyramid of prenatal care. Fetal Diagn Ther 2011;29:184; with permission.)

Until the advent of cfDNA technology, first-trimester combined screening (maternal age and history, gestational age, NT measurement, PAPP-A, and free beta-hCG) performed at 11^{+0} to 13^{+6} weeks' gestation was arguably the most robust screening test for fetal aneuploidy available. For a positive rate of 3% to 5%, screening the combined test can identify more than 90% of fetuses with trisomy 21. The detection rate of trisomies 18 and 13 is about 95% for the same false-positive rate.[15]

The effectiveness of the first-trimester combined screen can be further augmented by the addition of other fetal markers, such as nasal bone evaluation and Doppler evaluations of the ductus venosus and blood flow across the tricuspid valve.[16–18] The additional ultrasound markers can be either obtained at the time of the combined screen or on a contingent basis.[19,20] The contingent protocol calls for patients to be initially divided into 3 categories based on the traditional combined screen: high risk ($\geq$1:50), intermediate risk (1:51–1:1000), and low risk ($\leq$1:1000). Patients in the high-risk category are offered an invasive procedure, and those in the low-risk category are reassured. Patients in the intermediate category then undergo stage-2 screening using the additional ultrasound markers. If the final risk assessment in this group is 1:100 or greater, an invasive test is offered. Those whose risk is less than 1:100 are reassured. The screening performance of both approaches is similar: the detection rate is approximately 93% to 96% for a 2.5% false-positive rate.

There is evidence that the effectiveness of first-trimester screening could also be further enhanced by including additional maternal serum markers, such as placental growth factor (PIGF) and maternal serum alpha-fetoprotein (AFP).[15,21]

First-Trimester Screening for Down Syndrome: Performance and Cost-Benefit

All of the currently available cfDNA tests have a higher detection rate (>99%) for trisomy 21 for a much lower false-positive rate (about 0.1%) than the first-trimester combined test. The performance of cfDNA in screening for trisomy 18 (detection: 96.4%–99.9%), trisomy 13 (detection: 91.7%–99.0%), and monosomy X (detection: 92.9%–96.6%) is lower but is still very good.[11] Despite the good test results, the positive predictive values are such (50%–90%) that it is imperative to confirm each positive result with a diagnostic test.[22]

Many laboratories have expanded the testing panel to include trisomy 9, trisomy 16, trisomy 22, 22q11 deletion (DiGeorge/velocardiofacial syndrome), 1p36 del, 4p- (Wolf-Hirschhorn syndrome), 5p- (Cri-du-chat syndrome), 8qdel (Langer-Giedion syndrome), 11qdel (Jacobsen syndrome), and 15qdel (Angelman/Prader-Willi syndrome).[23] It must be stressed that the true detection and false-positive rates of these diseases remains to be established. Additionally, it is questionable whether the low prevalence of these uncommon conditions justifies screening in the general population. The manner in which cfDNA is to be used in population screening continues to be a subject of debate. However, the most significant impediment to universal implementation is its current cost.

Ultimately, the discussion regarding screening for aneuploidy centers on trisomy 21 because it is the most common type of aneuploidy and, compared with trisomies 18 and 13, it is more difficult to differentiate from euploid fetuses using ultrasound markers. Additionally, survival of fetuses with the other 2 types of aneuploidy is greatly diminished both during fetal life and after delivery, making the timing of the delivery slightly less critical.

Currently, the evaluation of cost-effectiveness of various prenatal screening protocols for trisomy 21 can be derived only from statistical modeling.[24] One such analysis was published recently, and the results are listed in **Table 1**.[25] It contains both the predicted screening performance and costs of screening protocols, 3 of which are

Table 1

Example comparing 3 existing and 4 cell-free DNA testing protocols: model-predicted screening performance and cost per Down-syndrome birth avoided under a set of particular conditions, unit costs and uptake

Protocol	Model-Predicted Screening Performance			Cost per Down Syndrome Birth Prevented ($)	
	DR (%)	FPR (%)	PPV (%)	Average	Marginal[a]
Existing					
Combined test	81.7	2.4	4.3	220,000	—
Contingent test	89.2	1.6	6.7	199,000	—
Combined test & NB	90.2	1.3	8.2	190,000	—
cfDNA					
Routine test	99.3	0.11	54	770,000	3,300,000
Contingent test	94.5	0.09	58	300,000	770,000
Contingent test, PlGF & AFP	96.6	0.09	59	290,000	690,000
AMA & contingent test	94.8	0.06	68	320,000	960,000

Maternal age distribution was standardized. Test conditions: Term (midtrimester) risk cutoff for combined test with or without nasal bone, 1 in 250 (1 in 190), for contingent test, 1 in 50 per 2500 (1 in 38 per 1900), and for contingent cfDNA test with or without PlGF and AFP, 1 in 10 per 2500 (1 in 8 per 1900); advanced maternal age cutoff, 35 years; hCG isoform, free beta; gestational age determined by serum markers at 10 weeks' gestation and NT at 11 weeks. Unit cost: combined test with or without nasal bone, $200; Quad markers, $50; cfDNA test, $1000; PlGF and AFP levels, $50; invasive prenatal diagnosis, $1500; uptake of screening, invasive prenatal diagnosis, and termination of Down syndrome pregnancies, 100%.

Abbreviations: AMA, advanced maternal age; DR, detection rate; FPR, false-positive rate; NB, nasal bone; PPV, positive predictive value.

[a] Cost of each additional birth prevented compared with combined test.

Adapted from Sonek JD, Cuckle HS. What will be the role of first-trimester ultrasound if cell-free DNA screening for aneuploidy becomes routine? Ultrasound Obstet Gynecol 2014;44:622; with permission.

existing traditional protocols and 4 include the addition of cfDNA. The conditions, unit costs, and uptake that were used for these calculations are specified in the footnote. The average cost applies to the cost of screening per case of Down syndrome detected. The marginal cost specifically refers to the cost of detection of each case of Down syndrome through the use of cfDNA that would not have been detected by traditional screening. When cfDNA is used as a primary screen, the average cost of preventing a Down syndrome birth is increased between 3- and 4-fold and the marginal cost is increased 15-fold (approximately $3,300,000). Using any of the approaches whereby cfDNA testing is done on a contingent basis, that is, using cfDNA only in those patients who are determined to be at an increased risk based on traditional screening, the average cost is less than doubled and the marginal cost is less than 4-fold. This approach retains much of the improved performance of routine cfDNA: The false-positive rate remains essentially the same with only a slightly diminished detection rate. This finding seems to be especially true if additional serum markers, PlGF and AFP, are included. Of note is that the approach of selecting older women (≥35 years of age) to undergo primary screening with cfDNA increases the cost without any apparent improvement in the overall screening performance (see **Table 1**).[25]

Another published cost-effectiveness assessment arrived to a similar conclusion. In this study, the most cost-effective approach was to use a contingent strategy whereby the initial risk assessment was based on maternal age, NT measurement, PAPP-A, free beta-hCG, and nasal bone with a 1 per 1000 risk cutoff.[26]

FIRST-TRIMESTER DETECTION OF FETAL STRUCTURAL ABNORMALITIES

About half of the congenital structural defects can now be diagnosed in the first trimester[27,28] because of improvements in ultrasound technology, NT thickening and the presence of other ultrasound markers can herald the presence of structural defects, and detailed evaluation of fetal anatomy is becoming widely recognized as an integral part of the first-trimester ultrasound.

Screening and Diagnosis of Structural Congenital Defects

It has been recognized now for more than 15 years that a thickened NT increases the risk of congenital fetal defects even in the absence of aneuploidy.[5] An evaluation of 4697 euploid fetuses that had an NT measurement greater than the 95th percentile revealed that 7% of them had a major abnormality. This risk increases significantly for an NT greater than 3.5 mm. In fetuses with an NT of 6.5 mm or greater, this risk is almost 50%. Since that time, case reports and case-control studies have confirmed that an increased NT can be associated with a large variety of genetic syndromes and structural defects, such as diaphragmatic hernia, omphalocele, facial clefts, body-stalk anomaly, skeletal defects, congenital adrenal hyperplasia, fetal akinesia deformation sequence, Noonan syndrome, Smith-Lemli–Opitz syndrome, and spinal muscular atrophy.[29]

A recent population-based study of 75,899 pregnancies also demonstrated a correlation between the prevalence of fetal structural defects and NT measurement.[30] After excluding fetuses with aneuploidy and critical cardiac defects, the analysis showed that an NT *greater than* the 95th percentile increased the risk of central nervous system, pulmonary, gastrointestinal, genitourinary, and musculoskeletal defects 1.6 to 2.7-fold. Certain anomalies had an increased risk that was 3-fold or greater: congenital hydrocephalus; agenesis, hypoplasia and dysplasia of the lung; atresia and stenosis of the small intestine; osteodystrophies; and diaphragmatic anomalies.

A recently published meta-analysis by Rossi and Prefumo[27] looked at the detection rates of fetal anomalies in the first trimester. The meta-analysis included 19 studies and a total of 78,002 fetuses, of which 996 has a structural anomaly. The overall detection rate was 51%. Detection rates were higher (62%–65%) in cases whereby both transabdominal and transvaginal ultrasound were used and in cases with a thickened NT.

A prospective analysis of 3094 fetuses confirmed that major fetal abnormalities can be diagnosed with a great reliability in the late first trimester even in a low-risk population (prevalence of major fetal anomalies was 2.8%). The overall detection rate of major anomalies, including congenital heart defects (CHDs), was 84%. In those cases whereby the NT measurement was 2.5 mm or greater, the detection rate was 98%.[31]

First-Trimester Detection of Congenital Cardiac Defects

The association between CHDs and NT measurement is well documented. In a meta-analysis that included 20 studies, the detection rate for major CHDs based on NT measurement alone was estimated at 44% for a 5.5% false-positive rate.[32] The risk of CHDs increases progressively with increasing NT measurement. Analysis that included combined data from 5 studies showed a risk of 3% for NTs 3.5 to 4.4 mm, 7% for NTs 4.5 to 5.4 mm, 20% for NTs 5.5 to 6.4 mm, and 30% for NTs 6.5 mm or greater.[5] Doppler evaluation of blood flow across the tricuspid valve and ductus venosus further improves screening for CHDs.[32–34]

In a first-trimester screening study involving almost 41,000 normal fetuses and 85 with major cardiac defects, Pereira and colleagues[34] found tricuspid regurgitation (TR) and a reversed flow in the ductus venosus each in about 30% of the affected cases. They showed that the combination of 3 markers (NT >99th percentile, TR, and abnormal a-wave) resulted in a detection rate of 52% for a false-positive rate of 4.1%.

First-Trimester Detection of Open Neural Tube Defects

Once it was recognized that the appearance of anencephaly is different in the first trimester from that in the second trimester, early diagnosis of this defect has become routine. However, the diagnosis of open spina bifida has remained a challenge. This situation changed when it was recognized that examination and measurements of structures located in the posterior fossa can provide clues to the presence of open neural tube defects (ONTDs) even in the first trimester. This relies mainly on changes in the appearance of the fourth ventricle (in this context, termed *intracranial translucency* [IT]) and the size of the brainstem (BS) in the sagittal section.[35] It was noted that in fetuses with an ONTD the IT is often obliterated. This is accompanied by other posterior fossa anomalies, such as an increase in the anteroposterior diameter of the BS. In order to assess changes in the posterior fossa objectively, a ratio of the thickness of the BS estimated by a measurement from the sphenoid bone to the floor of the fourth ventricle to a measurement from the floor of the fourth ventricle to the inner edge of the occipital bone (BSOB) was developed. A ratio that is greater than the 95th percentile of a gestational age–adjusted normal range was associated with the presence of ONTDs in 97% of the cases. In a prospective, multicenter first-trimester screening study including about 15,500 normal fetuses and 11 fetuses with open spina bifida, all affected cases were identified or at least suspected by a detailed assessment of the posterior fossa at 11 to 13 weeks' gestation.[36]

Other markers that may be helpful are narrowing of the frontomaxillary angle (detection rate of approximately 90%), biparietal diameter (BPD) measurement less than the fifth percentile (detection rate of approximately 50%), or a small BPD to transabdominal diameter ratio (detection rate of approximately 75%).[37–39]

The use of the BS/BSOB ratio has now expanded beyond simply screening of ONTDs. It has been suggested that if the ratio is less than the fifth percentile (ie, the opposite of what occurs with ONTDs), the risk of abnormalities that originate in the posterior fossa (Dandy-Walker malformation, partial vermian dysgenesis, and Blake cyst) is increased; but further research is necessary in this field.[40]

FIRST-TRIMESTER ASSESSMENT OF MULTIPLE GESTATIONS

Perinatal risk of morbidity and mortality is always increased in multiple gestations. However, the level of risk depends greatly on chorionicity.[41] This assessment is best accomplished in the first trimester, as at this time the ultrasound appearance of a dichorionic/diamniotic dividing membrane is vastly different from that of a monochorionic/diamniotic membrane. This difference becomes more blurred as the pregnancy progresses. Estimation of chorionicity in the first trimester allows accurate counseling regarding the risk of the pregnancy. In monochorionic-diamniotic twin pregnancies, a large difference between the NT measurements of the 2 fetuses or the presence of ductus venosus blood flow abnormalities may be helpful in identifying pregnancies with an increased risk for twin-twin transfusion syndrome.[42,43] All these evaluations allow the most appropriate plan of prenatal care to be outlined and implemented.[44] This aspect for first-trimester ultrasound evaluation has especially gained in importance recently as the incidence of twins has increased significantly in the past few decades.[45]

FIRST-TRIMESTER PREDICTION OF MATERNAL-FETAL COMPLICATIONS

Discussion regarding first-trimester screening often focuses on fetal aneuploidy and structural anomalies. However, maternal and fetal complications that are related to abnormal placentation are much more common than both of these problems combined.

Most placental architecture, including placental maternal blood circulation, is established by the end of the first trimester; no further anatomic modifications are evident after the fourth month of pregnancy. These 2 facts serve to support the 2 following assertions. First, the validity of methods used at the end of the first trimester in screening for placental dysfunction has a sound physiologic basis. Second, in order for any treatment to be successful in reducing the risk of complications related to placental dysfunction, it must be instituted early in pregnancy.

The 2 often-interrelated complications of pregnancy that are major causes of maternal-fetal morbidity and mortality are PE and small-for-gestational-age (SGA) fetuses. A meta-analysis of 9 published studies has shown that the use of low-dose aspirin (75 mg/d) reduces the risk of PE but only if treatment is initiated before 16 weeks' gestation.[46] This finding was confirmed in a more recent meta-analysis.[47]

As a result of these studies, it is now recommended that prophylactic low-dose aspirin treatment should be initiated before 12 weeks' gestation in women who are found to be at an increased risk of PE based on a combination of factors, such as body mass index, parity, and personal as well as family history.[48] However, these factors alone are not adequate to achieve a high enough detection rate and they are nonspecific.

First-trimester screening for these complications can be improved by using additional markers.[49] One is the estimation of downstream resistance by measuring the pulsatility index (PI) in the uterine arteries.[50] Second is maternal blood pressure measurement in the late first trimester. Third is evaluation of certain placental product levels in maternal serum, such as PAPP-A and PIGF. Modeling using the Fetal Medicine Foundation (FMF) algorithm suggests that, for a false-positive rate of 10%, detection of early PE (requiring delivery before 34 weeks' gestation) would be approximately 90% based only on historical factors, maternal blood pressure measurement, and uterine artery PI. The addition of PAPP-A and PIGF levels increases the detection rates to 96%.[51]

The performance of the FMF PE algorithm was validated in a recent Australian study.[52] The algorithm was subsequently used by the same group to evaluate the effectiveness of aspirin treatment (150 mg at night) in those women who were screen positive. There were 12 women (incidence 0.4%) who developed PE in the observation cohort. Of those, 11 (92%) were screen positive. In the intervention group, only one (0.04%) developed PE. Based on the prevalence in the observational group, it was estimated that 10 women in the intervention group should have developed PE. There were 264 (9.9%) women in the intervention cohort who screened positive for PE. Therefore, for every 29 women advised to take aspirin, one case of PE was prevented. There were no apparent adverse effects of this therapy identified. Of note is that the screening algorithm included measurement of PAPP-A but not PIGF, which was not available for their use at that time.[53]

It has also been shown that early administration of low-dose aspirin reduces the incidence of intrauterine growth restriction as well as its related pregnancy and neonatal complications.[54] Using the same FMF screening algorithm mentioned earlier, the estimated detection rates for early onset PE, late-onset PE, preterm SGA, and term SGA were 95%, 46%, 56%, and 44%, respectively, with an overall false-positive rate of 11%.[47,54]

Gestational hypertensive disorders are not only a major cause of perinatal morbidity and mortality but they are also responsible for a large proportion of expenditure for pregnancy and neonatal care. In 2011, the state of California looked at the cost of treating women and their neonates who are affected by hypertensive complications. Using the Medi-Cal fee-for-service fee schedule and reimbursement to private hospitals, they found that the annual incremental cost for gestational hypertensive disorders over that of unaffected pregnancies was $226 million. This number does not even include the lifetime medical costs of treating complications due to prematurity, such as neurologic and developmental disabilities.[55] It is clear that a robust screening program and prophylaxis with low-dose aspirin instituted early in pregnancy has the potential to result in a significant cost saving.

FUTURE APPLICATIONS OF FIRST-TRIMESTER SCREENING PROTOCOLS

Screening for SGA without PE has shown some promise. The risk is increased with an increase in the uterine PI and maternal mean arterial pressure. Decreased maternal serum PAPP-A, free beta-hCG, PIGF, placental protein 13 (PP13), and A disintegrin and metalloproteinase 12 (ADAM12) also increase the risk of SGA.[56,57] For a false-positive rate of 10%, the combination of these markers along with maternal characteristics could identify approximately 75% of SGA fetuses delivering before 37 weeks' gestation and 45% that deliver at term.[58]

The fact that risk of *spontaneous preterm delivery* is associated with cervical shortening is well established in the second trimester, and the same seems to hold in the first trimester.[59,60] Cervical length measurement obtained transvaginally and adhering to strict guidelines in combination with maternal characteristics is likely to be used in the future to select a high-risk group that may benefit from close follow-up and possible treatment. Preterm delivery prediction does not seem to be improved by the use of either maternal serum biochemistries or uterine artery PI.[56]

First-trimester screening for *gestational diabetes mellitus* (GDM) is possible using maternal serum biochemistries. Adiponectin and sex hormone–binding globulin are reduced and visfatin is increased in association with increased risk for GDM. Combination of maternal characteristics and biochemical markers can identify about 75% of pregnancies that will develop GDM for a 20% false-positive rate.[57,61,62]

Screening fetal *macrosomia/large for gestational age (LGA)* using first-trimester parameters has shown some promise. The risk of LGA increases with increased NT measurement, increased levels of maternal serum free beta-hCG and PAPP-A, and a decreased level of adiponectin.[63] For a 10% false-positive rate, the combination of these factors and maternal characteristics can detect approximately 40% of LGA fetuses.[57]

FIRST-TRIMESTER ESTIMATION OF GESTATIONAL AGE

Finally, first-trimester crown-rump length measurement represents the most accurate method for establishing the gestational age in the general population.[64] Accurate gestational age is a critical piece of information that influences essentially all decisions throughout the pregnancy, including such basic aspects of prenatal care as evaluating fetal growth and timing of delivery.

SUMMARY

There are several arguments that can be made to encourage pregnancy evaluation in the late first trimester. This evaluation is not only to benefit patients but also in order to implement a responsible public health policy.

The benefit of first-trimester screening and diagnosis of fetal anomalies is clear. Patients become aware of these conditions early in pregnancy when they can make their decisions in the greatest degree of privacy. In those cases whereby termination is elected, it can be done at a point where it is safest for patients and the least expensive.[65] Furthermore, in many countries, including the United States, attempts are being made by the state legislatures to limit access to termination, especially those done beyond midgestation, making an early diagnosis of fetal problems that much more important.

A responsible public health approach must take into account not only the benefits of any new technology but also the potential disruptive effect that a new technology may have on those that are currently in use. It also needs to take into account all of the benefits of each technology rather than comparing a single aspect of their performance in isolation. Even though both combined screening and cfDNA technology provide an efficient screen for aneuploidy early in pregnancy, cfDNA is more accurate. However, combined first-trimester screening casts a much wider net in terms of the variety of fetal defects it can detect. Therefore, it does not make sense to think of cfDNA technology as a replacement for traditional first-trimester screening. Rather, it should be implemented in a logical and cost-effective manner that complements existing technologies.

Screening for gestational hypertensive disorders and SGA in the first trimester has 2 significant advantages. One is that those patients who are at an increased risk can be monitored more closely later in pregnancy. Second is the fact that treatment with a fairly benign medication (low-dose aspirin), if instituted early in pregnancy, can lead to a significant reduction in the incidence of these conditions. This treatment, in turn, cannot only result in a reduction of perinatal morbidity and mortality but also in a significant cost saving.

First-trimester ultrasound evaluation provides a very accurate estimation of gestational age. In those pregnancies whereby multiple fetuses are identified, the first trimester represents an ideal time to determine the chorionicity. Both of these bits of information are invaluable in designing a plan of management for the rest of the pregnancy.

Aside from all of these applications of first-trimester pregnancy evaluations that have a proven benefit in management for the rest of the pregnancy, there are others, such as screening for SGA without PE, spontaneous preterm delivery, GDM, and fetal macrosomia, that show some promise. It is likely that with time these will also be perfected to make them more clinically pertinent.

REFERENCES

1. Ministry of Health Report. 1929 Memorandum on antenatal clinics: their conduct and scope. London: His Majesty's Stationery Office; 1930.

2. Nicolaides KH. A model for a new pyramid of prenatal care based on the 11 to 13 weeks' assessment. Prenat Diagn 2011;31:3–6.

3. Snijders R, Noble P, Sebire N, et al. UK multicentre project on assessment of risk of trisomy 21 by maternal age and fetal nuchal-translucency thickness at 10–14 weeks of gestation. Lancet 1998;352:343–6.

4. Kagan KO, Wright D, Baker A, et al. Screening for trisomy 21 by maternal age, fetal nuchal translucency thickness, free beta-human chorionic gonadotropin and pregnancy-associated plasma protein-A. Ultrasound Obstet Gynecol 2008; 31:618–24.

5. Souka AP, Kaisenberg Von CS, Hyett JA, et al. Increased nuchal translucency with normal karyotype. Am J Obstet Gynecol 2005;192:1005–21.

6. Hyett J, Perdu M, Sharland G, et al. Using fetal nuchal translucency to screen for major congenital cardiac defects at 10-14 weeks of gestation: population based cohort study. BMJ 1999;318:81–5.

7. Syngelaki A, Chelemen T, Dagklis T, et al. Challenges in the diagnosis of fetal non-chromosomal abnormalities at 11-13 weeks. Prenat Diagn 2011;31:90–102.

8. Kagan KO, Wright D, Valencia C, et al. Screening for trisomies 21, 18 and 13 by maternal age, fetal nuchal translucency, fetal heart rate, free -hCG and pregnancy-associated plasma protein-A. Hum Reprod 2008;23:1968–75.

9. Kagan KO, Anderson JM, Anwandter G, et al. Screening for triploidy by the risk algorithms for trisomies 21, 18 and 13 at 11 weeks to 13 weeks and 6 days of gestation. Prenat Diagn 2008;28:1209–13.

10. Sharp AN, Alfirevic Z. First trimester screening can predict adverse pregnancy outcomes. Prenat Diagn 2014;34:660–7.

11. Gil MM, Quezada MS, Revello R, et al. Analysis of cell-free DNA in maternal blood in screening for fetal aneuploidies: updated meta-analysis. Ultrasound Obstet Gynecol 2015;45:249–66.

12. Benn P, Cuckle H, Pergament E. Non-invasive prenatal diagnosis for Down syndrome: the paradigm will shift, but slowly. Ultrasound Obstetrics Gynecol 2012; 39:127–30.

13. Nicolaides KH. Turning the pyramid of prenatal care. Fetal Diagn Ther 2011;29: 183–96.

14. Akolekar R, Beta J, Picciarelli G, et al. Procedure-related risk of miscarriage following amniocentesis and chorionic villus sampling: a systematic review and meta-analysis. Ultrasound Obstetrics Gynecol 2015;45:16–26.

15. Wright D, Syngelaki A, Bradbury I, et al. First-trimester screening for trisomies 21, 18 and 13 by ultrasound and biochemical testing. Fetal Diagn Ther 2014;35: 118–26.

16. Maiz N, Wright D, Ferreira AFA, et al. A mixture model of ductus venosus pulsatility index in screening for aneuploidies at 11–13 weeks' gestation. Fetal Diagn Ther 2012;31:221–9.

17. Kagan KO, Staboulidou I, Cruz J, et al. Two-stage first-trimester screening for trisomy 21 by ultrasound assessment and biochemical testing. Ultrasound Obstetrics Gynecol 2010;36:542–7.

18. Kagan KO, Cicero S, Staboulidou I, et al. Fetal nasal bone in screening for trisomies 21, 18 and 13 and Turner syndrome at 11-13 weeks of gestation. Ultrasound Obstet Gynecol 2009;33:259–64.

19. Abele H, Wagner P, Sonek J, et al. First trimester ultrasound screening for Down syndrome based on maternal age, fetal nuchal translucency and different combinations of the additional markers nasal bone, tricuspid and ductus venosus flow. Prenat Diagn 2015;35(12):1182–6.

20. Wright D, Bradbury I, Benn P, et al. Contingent screening for Down syndrome is an efficient alternative to non-disclosure sequential screening. Prenat Diagn 2004;24:762–6.

21. Kagan KO, Hoopmann M, Abele H, et al. First-trimester combined screening for trisomy 21 with different combinations of placental growth factor, free β-human chorionic gonadotropin and pregnancy-associated plasma protein-A. Ultrasound Obstet Gynecol 2012;40:530–5.

22. Norton ME, Jacobsson B, Swamy GK, et al. Cell-free DNA analysis for noninvasive examination of trisomy. N Engl J Med 2015;372:1589–97.

23. Wapner RJ, Babiarz JE, Levy B, et al. Expanding the scope of noninvasive prenatal testing: detection of fetal microdeletion syndromes. Am J Obstet Gynecol 2015;212:332.e1–9.

24. Cuckle H, Cuckle H, Benn P, et al. Multianalyte maternal serum screening for chromosomal defects. In: Milunsky A, Milunsky JM, editors. Genetic disorders and the fetus: diagnosis, prevention and treatment. 6th edition. Chichester (United Kingdom): Wiley-Blackwell; 2010. p. 771–818, 1998.

25. Sonek JD, Cuckle HS. What will be the role of first-trimester ultrasound if cell-free DNA screening for aneuploidy becomes routine? Ultrasound Obstetrics Gynecol 2014;44:621–30.

26. Evans MI, Sonek JD, Hallahan TW, et al. Cell-free fetal DNA screening in the USA: a cost analysis of screening strategies. Ultrasound Obstetrics Gynecol 2015;45: 74–83.

27. Rossi AC, Prefumo F. Accuracy of ultrasonography at 11-14 weeks of gestation for detection of fetal structural anomalies: a systematic review. Obstet Gynecol 2013;122:1160–7.

28. Van Mieghem T, Hindryckx A, Van Calsteren K. Early fetal anatomy screening: who, what, when and why? Curr Opin Obstet Gynecol 2015;27:143–50.

29. Timmerman E, Pajkrt E, Maas SM, et al. Enlarged nuchal translucency in chromosomally normal fetuses: strong association with orofacial clefts. Ultrasound Obstetrics Gynecol 2010;36:427–32.

30. Baer RJ, Norton ME, Shaw GM, et al. Risk of selected structural abnormalities in infants after increased nuchal translucency measurement. Am J Obstet Gynecol 2014;211:675.e1–19.

31. Becker R, Wegner RD. Detailed screening for fetal anomalies and cardiac defects at the 11–13-week scan. Ultrasound Obstet Gynecol 2006;27:613–8.

32. Chelemen T, Syngelaki A, Maiz N, et al. Contribution of ductus venosus Doppler in first-trimester screening for major cardiac defects. Fetal Diagn Ther 2011;29: 127–34.

33. Papatheodorou SI, Evangelou E, Makrydimas G, et al. First-trimester ductus venosus screening for cardiac defects: a meta-analysis. BJOG 2011;118:1438–45.

34. Pereira S, Ganapathy R, Syngelaki A, et al. Contribution of fetal tricuspid regurgitation in first-trimester screening for major cardiac defects. Obstet Gynecol 2011; 117:1384–91.

35. Chaoui R, Nicolaides KH. Detecting open spina bifida at the 11-13-week scan by assessing intracranial translucency and the posterior brain region: mid-sagittal or axial plane? Ultrasound Obstet Gynecol 2011;38:609–12.

36. Chen FCK, Gerhardt J, Entezami M, et al. Detection of spina bifida by first trimester screening - results of the prospective multicenter Berlin it-study. Ultraschall Med 2015. http://dx.doi.org/10.1055/s-0034-1399483.

37. Lachmann R, Picciarelli G, Moratalla J, et al. Frontomaxillary facial angle in fetuses with spina bifida at 11-13 weeks' gestation. Ultrasound Obstet Gynecol 2010;36:268–71.
38. Khalil A, Coates A, Papageorghiou A, et al. Biparietal diameter at 11-13 weeks' gestation in fetuses with open spina bifida. Ultrasound Obstet Gynecol 2013; 42:409–15.
39. Simon EG, Arthuis CJ, Haddad G, et al. Biparietal/transverse abdominal diameter ratio ≤1: potential marker for open spina bifida at 11-13-week scan. Ultrasound Obstetrics Gynecol 2015;45:267–72.
40. Volpe P, Contro E, Fanelli T, et al. Appearance of the fetal posterior fossa at 11-14 weeks in foetuses with Dandy-Walker complex or chromosomal anomalies. Ultrasound Obstet Gynecol 2015. [Epub ahead of print].
41. Sebire NJ, Snijders RJ, Hughes K, et al. The hidden mortality of monochorionic twin pregnancies. Br J Obstet Gynaecol 1997;104:1203–7.
42. Kagan KO, Gazzoni A, Sepulveda-Gonzalez G, et al. Discordance in nuchal translucency thickness in the prediction of severe twin-to-twin transfusion syndrome. Ultrasound Obstet Gynecol 2007;29:527–32.
43. Maiz N, Staboulidou I, Leal AM, et al. Ductus venosus Doppler at 11 to 13 weeks of gestation in the prediction of outcome in twin pregnancies. Obstet Gynecol 2009;113:860–5.
44. Khalil A, Rodgers M, Baschat A, et al. ISUOG practice guidelines: the role of ultrasound in twin pregnancy. Ultrasound Obstetrics Gynecol 2016;47(2):247–63.
45. Martin JA, Hamilton BE, Osterman MJK. Three decades of twin births in the United States, 1980–2009. NCHS Data Brief 2012;(80):1–8.
46. Bujold E, Roberge S, Lacasse Y, et al. Prevention of preeclampsia and intrauterine growth restriction with aspirin started in early pregnancy: a meta-analysis. Obstet Gynecol 2010;116:402–14.
47. Roberge S, Nicolaides KH, Demers S, et al. Prevention of perinatal death and adverse perinatal outcome using low-dose aspirin: a meta-analysis. Ultrasound Obstet Gynecol 2013;41:491–9.
48. World Health Organization. WHO recommendations for: prevention and treatment of pre-eclampsia and eclampsia. 2011. Available at: http://www.who.int/reproductivehealth/publications/maternal_perinatal_health/9789241548335/en/. Accessed January 19, 2016.
49. Poon LC, Nicolaides KH. First-trimester maternal factors and biomarker screening for preeclampsia. Prenat Diagn 2014;34:618–27.
50. Velauthar L, Plana MN, Kalidindi M, et al. First-trimester uterine artery Doppler and adverse pregnancy outcome: a meta-analysis involving 55,974 women. Ultrasound Obstet Gynecol 2014;43:500–7.
51. Wright D, Akolekar R, Syngelaki A, et al. A competing risks model in early screening for preeclampsia. Fetal Diagn Ther 2012;32:171–8.
52. Park FJ, Leung CHY, Poon LCY, et al. Clinical evaluation of a first trimester algorithm predicting the risk of hypertensive disease of pregnancy. Aust N Z J Obstet Gynaecol 2013;53:532–9.
53. Park F, Russo K, Williams P, et al. Prediction and prevention of early-onset preeclampsia: impact of aspirin after first-trimester screening. Ultrasound Obstetrics Gynecol 2015;46:419–23.
54. Roberge S, Villa P, Nicolaides K, et al. Early administration of low-dose aspirin for the prevention of preterm and term preeclampsia: a systematic review and meta-analysis. Fetal Diagn Ther 2012;31:141–6.

55. Shmueli A, Meiri H, Gonen R. Economic assessment of screening for pre-eclampsia. Prenat Diagn 2012;32:29–38.

56. Beta J, Akolekar R, Ventura W, et al. Prediction of spontaneous preterm delivery from maternal factors, obstetric history and placental perfusion and function at 11-13 weeks. Prenat Diagn 2011;31:75–83.

57. Nanda S, Akolekar R, Sarquis R, et al. Maternal serum adiponectin at 11 to 13 weeks of gestation in the prediction of macrosomia. Prenat Diagn 2011;31: 479–83.

58. Poon LCY, Karagiannis G, Staboulidou I, et al. Reference range of birth weight with gestation and first-trimester prediction of small-for-gestation neonates. Prenat Diagn 2011;31:58–65.

59. Greco E, Gupta R, Syngelaki A, et al. First-trimester screening for spontaneous preterm delivery with maternal characteristics and cervical length. Fetal Diagn Ther 2012;31:154–61.

60. Retzke JD, Sonek JD, Lehmann J, et al. Comparison of three methods of cervical measurement in the first trimester: single-line, two-line, and tracing. Prenat Diagn 2013;33:262–8.

61. Ferreira AFA, Rezende JC, Vaikousi E, et al. Maternal serum visfatin at 11-13 weeks of gestation in gestational diabetes mellitus. Clin Chem 2011;57:609–13.

62. Thadhani R, Powe CE, Tjoa ML, et al. First-trimester follistatin-like-3 levels in pregnancies complicated by subsequent gestational diabetes mellitus. Diabetes Care 2010;33:664–9.

63. Poon LCY, Karagiannis G, Stratieva V, et al. First-trimester prediction of macrosomia. Fetal Diagn Ther 2011;29:139–47.

64. Committee opinion no 611: method for estimating due date. Obstet Gynecol 2014;124:863–6.

65. Bartlett LA, Berg CJ, Shulman HB, et al. Risk factors for legal induced abortion-related mortality in the United States. Obstet Gynecol 2004;103:729–37.

Aspirin for the Prevention of Preeclampsia and Intrauterine Growth Restriction

Stephanie Roberge, MSc[a], Anthony O. Odibo, MD, MSCE[b],
Emmanuel Bujold, MD, MSc[a,c],*

KEYWORDS

- Pregnancy • Preeclampsia • Intrauterine growth restriction • Aspirin • Placenta

KEY POINTS

- Low-dose aspirin (LDA) (80–160 mg) reduces the risk of preeclampsia (PE) and intrauterine growth restriction by approximately half when started in early pregnancy.
- LDA reduces mainly the preterm and severe forms of PE when started in early pregnancy.
- Women with chronic hypertension and those with prior PE should begin taking LDA in early pregnancy.
- First-trimester screening programs should be implemented to identify women at high-risk for preterm or severe PE.
- Further studies should evaluate the optimal dosage of aspirin and the benefit of adding low molecular weight heparin in women at very-high risk, such as those with prior early onset PE.

INTRODUCTION

Preeclampsia (PE) is a hypertensive disorder of pregnancy characterized by high blood pressure and proteinuria that affects 2% to 5% of pregnant women in developed countries and up to 8% of pregnant women in developing countries.[1,2] It is a major contributor to maternal and fetal morbidity and mortality worldwide, with more than 100,000 maternal deaths every year.[3]

Disclosure: None of the authors have a conflict of interest.
[a] Department of Social and Preventive Medicine, Faculty of Medicine, Université Laval, 2705 Boulevard Laurier, Quebec G1V 4G2, Canada; [b] Division of Maternal Fetal Medicine, Department of Obstetrics & Gynecology, University of South Florida Morsani College of Medicine, 2 Tampa General Circle, 6th Floor, Tampa, FL 33606, USA; [c] Department of Obstetrics and Gynecology, Faculty of Medicine, Université Laval, 2705 Boulevard Laurier, Québec City, Quebec G1V 4G2, Canada
* Corresponding author. Department of Obstetrics and Gynecology, Faculty of Medicine, Université Laval, 2705 Boulevard Laurier, Québec City, Quebec G1V 4G2, Canada.
E-mail address: emmanuel.bujold@crchudequebec.ulaval.ca

Clin Lab Med 36 (2016) 319–329
http://dx.doi.org/10.1016/j.cll.2016.01.013
0272-2712/16/$ – see front matter © 2016 Elsevier Inc. All rights reserved.

The origins of PE are multifactorial, but it is well accepted that abnormal invasion of the placenta and systemic endothelial dysfunction play key roles in the development of the disease. Transformation of uterine spiral arteries by the cytotrophoblasts, which occur mainly in the first-trimester of pregnancy, is typically missing in PE, particularly in preterm PE.[4–8] Such a deep placentation disorder leads to the production of angiogenic factors by the placenta, systemic endothelial cell dysfunction, maternal underperfusion, and ultimately the signs and symptoms of PE.[5,9] Endothelial dysfunction is worsened by other factors such as advanced maternal age, high blood pressure, and obesity. In severe PE, placental disorders are also associated with intrauterine growth restriction (IUGR), preterm birth, and in the worst cases, fetal death, and/or eclampsia.

Numerous therapies have been used to prevent PE, including low-dose aspirin (LDA), calcium, unfractionated heparin, low molecular weight heparin (LMWH), progesterone, antioxidants, and physical activity with inconsistent results.[10–19] Recently, there has been a renewed interest in LDA when meta-analyses showed that PE and other adverse placenta-mediated outcomes of pregnancy could be significantly reduced with LDA started before 16 weeks' gestation.[13,20] The authors reviewed the literature regarding prevention of hypertensive disorders and related perinatal outcomes with LDA started in early pregnancy.

Preeclampsia

According to the American College of Obstetricians and Gynecologists (ACOG), PE is defined by the combination of a high blood pressure (140 mm Hg systolic or higher or 90 mm Hg diastolic or higher that occurs after 20 weeks of gestation in a woman with previously normal blood pressure) and proteinuria (urinary excretion of 0.3 g protein or higher in a 24 hour urine specimen or 2 + protein on dipstick) but the definition can vary between countries.[10,21] PE is associated with placental disease in most cases, with the severity of the disease being more important with early gestational age at delivery.[22] Data from placental bed biopsies showed that most cases of PE are associated with incomplete transformation of uterine spiral arteries.[4] However, deep placentation disorders are also observed mainly in the preterm and severe forms of the disease and are not necessarily specific to the disease.[6,23,24]

Low-Dose Aspirin for the Prevention of Preeclampsia

In 1978, Goodlin and colleagues[25] suggested that recurrent PE can be prevented using LDA and unfractionated heparin. A year later, Crandon and Isherwood reported that primigravidae who were taking LDA during pregnancy were less likely to develop PE than those who did not.[26] The same year, Masotti and colleagues[27] reported that 2 to 5 mg of aspirin per kilogram were associated with a differential inhibition of platelets and vessel-wall cyclooxygenase that could potentially explain the impact of LDA on placentation and PE. Following those studies, Beaufils and colleagues[28] evaluated the benefits of 150 mg of aspirin combined with 300 mg of dipyridamole from 12 weeks of gestation in women at high risk for PE or intrauterine growth restriction (IUGR) on the basis of the obstetric history. In this randomized trial, PE (12%) and major complications (18%, including severe IUGR and fetal death) occurred more frequently in the control group than in the LDA + dipyridamole group, in which no case of PE or major complications was observed. Following that publication, more than 60 randomized trials were published with controversial results.

In 2007, Askie and colleagues[29] reported that LDA could prevent 10% of PE cases. However, they showed high heterogeneity between the studies. In 2010, another meta-analysis from Bujold and colleagues,[13] looking specifically at the time of initiation of LDA, demonstrated that randomized trials that initiated LDA before 16 weeks' gestation showed a high homogeneity and demonstrated that, when started in early pregnancy, LDA was associated with a 53% reduction of PE. Subsequently, subgroup analyses performed by Roberge and colleagues[15,16] revealed that LDA started before 16 weeks was especially efficient for the prevention of the preterm and severe forms of the disease. These observations are in agreement with the hypothesis that the severe and preterm forms of the disease are those related to deep placentation disorders that occur mainly at or before 16 weeks gestation and that LDA improved deep placentation. **Table 1** reports the characteristics of the randomized trials that evaluated the impact of LDA before 16 weeks' gestation for the prevention of PE including the most recent published trials, and **Fig. 1** reports the forest plot of all of them. Overall, when started before 16 weeks, LDA reduces the risk of PE by approximately half (relative risk [RR]: 0.49; 95% confidence intervals [CI]: 0.38–0.64), $P<.01$. Few randomized trials have evaluated the impact of LDA started before 16 weeks on the risk of preterm or severe PE, but the most recent meta-analyses by Roberge and colleagues[15,16] suggest that they could be reduced by 90% (RR: 0.11; 95% CI: 0.04–0.33) and 80% (RR: 0.18; 95% CI: 0.08–0.41), respectively. However, some questions remain unanswered, including the population to be treated, the optimal dose, and the optimal gestational age for starting and stopping the treatment.

Intrauterine Growth Restriction

Several definitions are used to define small–for–gestational age (SGA) or IUGR in the literature, but they usually refer to an infant born with a birth weight less than the 10th, 5th or the 3rd percentile for the gestational age, or to a fetus with an estimated weight below these percentiles.[30,31] Placental insufficiency is one of the major risk factors for IUGR, and it is typically seen in the most severe forms of the disease when there are no congenital or chromosomal anomalies. Placental insufficiency can result from deep placentation disorders, but also from other risk factors such as smoking and thrombophilia. Early placental smallness or placental dysfunction that can be detected in the first trimester can lead to IUGR and perinatal death related to IUGR.[32–34]

Low-Dose Aspirin for the Prevention of Intrauterine Growth Restriction

Meta-analyses of randomized trials without consideration for gestational age at initiation of LDA observed no impact of LDA on the risk of IUGR.[29,35] However, looking specifically at studies that evaluated LDA started before 16 weeks, LDA was associated with a significant reduction of IUGR and perinatal death.[20] **Fig. 2** reports the forest plot of the randomized trials that evaluated the impact of LDA started before 16 weeks on the prevention of IUGR. Similar to the results obtained for PE, LDA reduces by half the risk of IUGR (RR: 0.47; 95% CI: 0.36–0.62, $P<.01$). Roberge and colleagues[20] reported a mean birth weight increased by 209 g (95% CI: 100–319) with LDA started before 16 weeks in high-risk women.

Few studies evaluated the impact of LDA on placental function (or dysfunction) and placental pathology. However, 2 randomized trials reported an improvement of mid-trimester uterine artery pulsatility index in women who started LDA in early pregnancy.[36]

Who Should Receive Low-Dose Aspirin in Early Gestation?

Most randomized trials that evaluated the benefits of LDA before 16 weeks' gestation included women at high-risk for PE based on women's medical history (eg, chronic hypertension or prior PE) or based on abnormal uterine artery Doppler, but other risk factors such as nulliparity, multiple gestation, advanced maternal age, maternal obesity, and other chronic diseases (eg, diabetes, connective tissue disease) have been

Table 1
Characteristics of randomized trials that evaluated low-dose aspirin in early pregnancy for the prevention of preeclampsia

Authors, Year	N	Inclusion Criteria	Intervention	Aspirin Controls	Onset (Wk)
August et al,[57] 1994	54	History, risk factors[a]	100 mg	Placebo	13–15
Azar & Turpin,[58] 1990	91	History, risk factors[a]	100 mg[b]	No treatment	16
Beaufils et al,[28] 1985	102	History, risk factors[a]	150 mg[b]	No treatment	14
Benigni et al,[59] 1989	33	History, risk factors[a]	60 mg	Placebo	12
Bakhti & Vaiman,[60] 2011	84	Nulliparity	100 mg	No treatment	8–10
Caritis et al,[61] 1998 (Moore et al,[62] 2015)	523	High risk[b]	60 mg	Placebo	≤16
Chiaffarino et al,[63] 2004	40	Chronic hypertension with or without history risk factors[a]	100 mg	No treatment	<14
Dasari et al,[64] 1998	50	Nulliparity	100 mg	Placebo	12
Ebrashy et al,[65] 2005	139	Abnormal uterine artery Doppler plus history, risk factors[a]	75 mg	No treatment	14–16
Hermida et al,[66] 1997	107	History, risk factors[a]	100 mg	Placebo	12–16
Hermida et al,[67,68]1999	350	History, risk factors[a]	100 mg	Placebo	12–16
Jamal et al,[69] 2012	70	PCOS before pregnancy, 18–40 y, singleton, no history of diabetes or hypertension	80 mg	No treatment	6–12
Mesdaghinia et al,[70] 2011	80	Abnormal uterine artery Doppler	80 mg	No treatment	12–16
Michael & Walters,[71] 1992	110	Hypertension with history, risk factors[a]	100 mg	Placebo	16
Odibo et al,[72] 2015	90	Nulliparity plus multiple gestation	81 mg	Placebo	≤16
Porreco et al,[73] 1993	23	Any risk factors for PE	81 mg	Placebo	11–13
Tulppala et al,[74] 1997	66	Consecutive miscarriage	50 mg	Placebo	~7
Vainio et al,[75] 2002	90	Abnormal uterine artery Doppler plus history, risk factors[a]	0.5 mg/kg	Placebo	12–14
Villa et al,[76] 2013	121	Abnormal uterine artery Doppler plus history, risk factors[a]	100 mg	Placebo	12–14
Zhao et al,[77] 2012	237	High risk (hypertension, history, risk factors[a])	75 mg	Placebo	13–16

[a] Includes history of chronic hypertension, cardiovascular or endocrine disease, previous pregnancy hypertension or fetal growth restriction.
[b] Insulin treated diabetes, chronic hypertension, multiple pregnancy or PE in a previous pregnancy.
Data from Refs.[28,57–77]

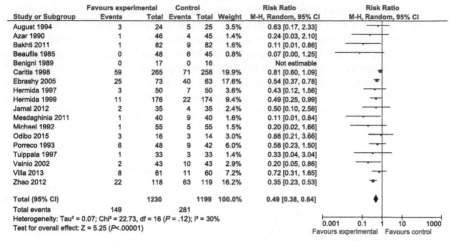

Study or Subgroup	Favours experimental Events	Total	Control Events	Total	Weight	Risk Ratio M-H, Random, 95% CI
August 1994	3	24	5	25	3.5%	0.63 [0.17, 2.33]
Azar 1990	1	46	4	45	1.4%	0.24 [0.03, 2.10]
Bakhti 2011	1	82	9	82	1.6%	0.11 [0.01, 0.86]
Beaufils 1985	0	48	6	45	0.8%	0.07 [0.00, 1.25]
Benigni 1989	0	17	0	16		Not estimable
Caritis 1998	59	265	71	258	19.9%	0.81 [0.60, 1.09]
Ebrashy 2005	25	73	40	63	17.6%	0.54 [0.37, 0.78]
Hermida 1997	3	50	7	50	3.6%	0.43 [0.12, 1.56]
Hermida 1999	11	176	22	174	9.4%	0.49 [0.25, 0.99]
Jamal 2012	2	35	4	35	2.4%	0.50 [0.10, 2.56]
Mesdaghinia 2011	1	40	9	40	1.6%	0.11 [0.01, 0.84]
Michael 1992	1	55	5	55	1.5%	0.20 [0.02, 1.66]
Odibo 2015	3	16	3	14	3.0%	0.88 [0.21, 3.66]
Porreco 1993	6	48	9	42	6.0%	0.58 [0.23, 1.50]
Tuippala 1997	1	33	3	33	1.4%	0.33 [0.04, 3.04]
Vainio 2002	2	43	10	43	2.9%	0.20 [0.05, 0.86]
Villa 2013	8	61	11	60	7.2%	0.72 [0.31, 1.65]
Zhao 2012	22	118	63	119	16.2%	0.35 [0.23, 0.53]
Total (95% CI)		1230		1199	100.0%	0.49 [0.38, 0.64]
Total events	149		281			

Heterogeneity: Tau² = 0.07; Chi² = 22.73, df = 16 (P = .12); I² = 30%
Test for overall effect: Z = 5.25 (P<.00001)

Fig. 1. Forest plot of randomized trials that evaluated the administration of LDA ≤16 weeks of gestation for the prevention of preeclampsia. (*Data from* Refs.[28,57–59,61,65–76])

considered.[13,14,37] Numerous factors can be used to screen women at high risk for PE, including medical history, biophysical factors, multiple gestation, and uterine artery Doppler. However, because LDA seems to be mainly effective for the prevention of preterm and severe PE that occurred in less than 1% to 2% of the population, no single factor, perhaps with the exception of a prior history of PE and chronic hypertension, has an adequate positive predictive value to be used alone. Actually, ACOG recommends that women with a prior early onset PE or those with 2 or more pregnancies with PE should receive aspirin, while guidelines from many national societies suggest that LDA should be started in early pregnancy in women presenting with 1 major factor or 2 minor risk factors for PE.[10,38] However, it remains controversial as to

Study or Subgroup	Experimental Events	Total	Control Events	Total	Weight	Risk Ratio M-H, Random, 95% CI
August 1994	0	24	1	25	0.7%	0.35 [0.01, 8.12]
Bakhti 2011	0	82	1	82	0.7%	0.33 [0.01, 8.06]
Beaufils 1985	4	48	13	45	6.6%	0.29 [0.10, 0.82]
Benigni 1989	2	17	6	16	3.5%	0.31 [0.07, 1.33]
Caritis 1998	15	265	23	258	18.4%	0.63 [0.34, 1.19]
Chiaffarino 2004	2	16	5	19	3.2%	0.47 [0.11, 2.13]
Dasari 1998	1	25	5	25	1.7%	0.20 [0.03, 1.59]
Ebrashy 2005	13	73	21	63	19.8%	0.53 [0.29, 0.98]
Hermida 1997	1	50	2	50	1.3%	0.50 [0.05, 5.34]
Hermida 1999	6	124	14	116	8.5%	0.40 [0.16, 1.01]
Jamal 2012	1	35	2	35	1.3%	0.50 [0.05, 5.27]
Mesdaghinia 2010	0	40	0	40		Not estimable
Odibo 2015	1	16	1	14	1.0%	0.88 [0.06, 12.73]
Tuippala 1997	3	33	3	33	3.1%	1.00 [0.22, 4.60]
Vainio 2002	1	43	3	43	1.5%	0.33 [0.04, 3.08]
Villa 2013	2	61	6	60	3.0%	0.33 [0.07, 1.56]
Zhao 2012	16	118	36	119	25.7%	0.45 [0.26, 0.76]
Total (95% CI)		1070		1043	100.0%	0.47 [0.36, 0.62]
Total events	68		142			

Heterogeneity: Tau² = 0.00; Chi² = 4.53, df = 15 (P = 1.00); I² = 0%
Test for overall effect: Z = 5.46 (P<.00001)

Fig. 2. Forest plot of randomized trials that evaluated the administration of low-dose aspirin ≤16 weeks of gestation for the prevention of intrauterine growth restriction. (*Data from* Refs.[28,57,59–76])

whether such an approach is efficient to predict women at high risk for preterm or severe PE.[39] A recent cost–benefit analysis by Werner and colleagues[40] demonstrated that such screening would be more cost-effective than the ACOG guidelines.

Uterine artery Doppler has been used in the first trimester to identify women at high risk for PE.[32] However, the predictive values are unclear and varied between studies.[41] Although an increased pulsatility index in the first trimester is associated with a higher risk of PE, the beneficial effect of adding uterine artery Doppler to maternal factors seems to be clinically limited to the prediction of the early onset forms of PE.[42] Serum markers, such as PAPP-A and PlGF are also useful for the prediction of PE, and also the early onset PE.[43]

There is an increasing body of evidence that the combination of biophysical, biochemical, and uterine artery Doppler in the first trimester could be used to predict most early onset PE (>80%) and most preterm PE, with a false-positive rate below 10%.[44,45] Such a screening strategy could also be used in high-risk women based on clinical factors.[46] In a recent prospective study of 35,948 pregnant women with singleton pregnancies screened in the first trimester, including 1058 (2.9%) of them who experienced PE, O'Gorman and colleagues[47] demonstrated that combination of those markers could identify 75% of preterm PE cases and 47% of term PE cases compared with 49% and 38% of cases, respectively, using maternal factors alone. Hypothetically, in a population with a prevalence of preterm or severe PE of 1%, the number needed to treat (NNT) would be approximately 20 to prevent 1 case. Park and colleagues[48] showed that screening women for early onset PE and treating those at high risk with 150 mg of aspirin led to a significant decrease in early onset PE (from 0.4% to 0.04%) in their population. The same strategy is being evaluated in a multicenter randomized trial (http://www.aspre.eu).

Low-Dose Aspirin Posology

LDA refers to a daily dose below 325 mg, but dosage of 160 mg or less daily is usually recommended during pregnancy, as it has been shown to be safe for the fetus.[49–51] The range of dosage used in randomized trials varied from 50 to 150 mg daily, with some trials adding dipyridamole. Most randomized trials that recruited participants in early pregnancy used a dosage of 100 mg.[13] At 75 to 81 mg, about 30% of pregnant women show evidence of aspirin resistance, and using higher dosage of aspirin in those women is associated with better pregnancy outcomes and less severe PE.[52,53] Based on available literature, the authors believe that a minimum of 80 mg should be used, and a dosage of 100 to 150 mg daily, started from the 12 weeks' or pregnancy should be considered in high-risk women. There are insufficient data to recommend a specific time to stop the prophylactic measures, because most studies stopped it at 36 to 37 weeks or at delivery. The authors, however, believe that it should be continued until at least the third trimester of pregnancy.

Low Molecular Weight Heparin

Placental vascular thrombosis is a frequent finding in early onset PE, and most thrombophilias increase the risk of the disease. Therefore, there has been a growing interest for the use of anticoagulants such as unfractionated heparin and LMWH in the prevention of PE and placenta-mediated adverse outcomes. However, most trials that used LMWH alone showed no improvement of pregnancy outcomes with LMWH compared with no treatment.[54,55] Still, recent data based on a few trials suggest that LMWH combined with LDA could be beneficial in the reduction of early onset PE and IUGR in women with prior history of early onset PE.[56] Interestingly, a large multicenter randomized trial observed a nonsignificant increase of adverse perinatal outcomes with

LMWH in women who were not taking concomitant LDA (RR: 1.20; 95% CI 0.7–2.2), while they observed a nonsignificant decrease of the similar outcomes with LMWH in those who were taking LDA (RR: 0.30; 95% CI 0.1–1.1).[54] Therefore, the authors believe that there is a potential benefit of adding LMWH to LDA in very high-risk women, but further studies are required.

SUMMARY

Studies have demonstrated that LDA administered in early gestation is efficient in reducing the risk of PE, IUGR, preterm birth, and perinatal death in high-risk women, especially those at high risk for deep placentation disorders, preterm PE, and severe IUGR. First-trimester screening programs for such adverse pregnancy outcomes are increasingly promising, and recent studies combining a first-trimester screening strategy with prophylactic LDA demonstrated a significant decrease of early onset PE. Although most national societies recommend the use of 60 to 80 mg of aspirin for the prevention of PE in high-risk women, most randomized trials that evaluated LDA started in early pregnancy used higher dosages. Future studies should evaluate the optimal dosage of LDA and the potential benefits of adding LMWH in women identified at high risk for early onset PE specifically.

REFERENCES

1. Report of the national high blood pressure education program working group on high blood pressure in pregnancy. Am J Obstet Gynecol 2000;183(1):S1–22.
2. Geographic variation in the incidence of hypertension in pregnancy. World Health Organization International Collaborative Study of hypertensive disorders of pregnancy. Am J Obstet Gynecol 1988;158(1):80–3.
3. Walker JJ. Pre-eclampsia. Lancet 2000;356(9237):1260–5.
4. Brosens I, Pijnenborg R, Vercruysse L, et al. The "Great Obstetrical Syndromes" are associated with disorders of deep placentation. Am J Obstet Gynecol 2011; 204(3):193–201.
5. Steegers EA, von Dadelszen P, Duvekot JJ, et al. Pre-eclampsia. Lancet 2010; 376(9741):631–44.
6. Ogge G, Chaiworapongsa T, Romero R, et al. Placental lesions associated with maternal underperfusion are more frequent in early-onset than in late-onset pre-eclampsia. J Perinat Med 2011;39(6):641–52.
7. Pijnenborg R, Dixon G, Robertson WB, et al. Trophoblastic invasion of human decidua from 8 to 18 weeks of pregnancy. Placenta 1980;1(1):3–19.
8. De Wolf F, De Wolf-Peeters C, Brosens I, et al. The human placental bed: electron microscopic study of trophoblastic invasion of spiral arteries. Am J Obstet Gynecol 1980;137(1):58–70.
9. Bujold E, Romero R, Chaiworapongsa T, et al. Evidence supporting that the excess of the sVEGFR-1 concentration in maternal plasma in preeclampsia has a uterine origin. J Matern Fetal Neonatal Med 2005;18(1):9–16.
10. Magee LA, Pels A, Helewa M, et al, Canadian Hypertensive Disorders of Pregnancy Working Group. Diagnosis, evaluation, and management of the hypertensive disorders of pregnancy: executive summary. J Obstet Gynaecol Can 2014; 36(5):416–41.
11. Patrelli TS, Dall'asta A, Gizzo S, et al. Calcium supplementation and prevention of preeclampsia: a meta-analysis. J Matern Fetal Neonatal Med 2012;25(12): 2570–4.

12. de Vries JI, van Pampus MG, Hague WM, et al. Low-molecular-weight heparin added to aspirin in the prevention of recurrent early-onset pre-eclampsia in women with inheritable thrombophilia: the FRUIT-RCT. J Thromb Haemost 2012; 10(1):64–72.

13. Bujold E, Roberge S, Lacasse Y, et al. Prevention of preeclampsia and intrauterine growth restriction with aspirin started in early pregnancy: a meta-analysis. Obstet Gynecol 2010;116(2 Pt 1):402–14.

14. Bujold E, Morency AM, Roberge S, et al. Acetylsalicylic acid for the prevention of preeclampsia and intra-uterine growth restriction in women with abnormal uterine artery Doppler: a systematic review and meta-analysis. J Obstet Gynaecol Can 2009;31(9):818–26.

15. Roberge S, Giguere Y, Villa P, et al. Early administration of low-dose aspirin for the prevention of severe and mild preeclampsia: a systematic review and meta-analysis. Am J Perinatol 2012;29(7):551–6.

16. Roberge S, Villa P, Nicolaides K, et al. Early administration of low-dose aspirin for the prevention of preterm and term preeclampsia: a systematic review and meta-analysis. Fetal Diagn Ther 2012;31(3):141–6.

17. Rumbold A, Duley L, Crowther CA, et al. Antioxidants for preventing pre-eclampsia. Cochrane Database Syst Rev 2008;(1):CD004227.

18. Meher S, Duley L. Progesterone for preventing pre-eclampsia and its complications. Cochrane Database Syst Rev 2006;(4):CD006175.

19. Meher S, Duley L. Exercise or other physical activity for preventing pre-eclampsia and its complications. Cochrane Database Syst Rev 2006;(2):CD005942.

20. Roberge S, Nicolaides KH, Demers S, et al. Prevention of perinatal death and adverse perinatal outcome using low-dose aspirin: a meta-analysis. Ultrasound Obstet Gynecol 2013;41(5):491–9.

21. ACOG Committee on Obstetric Practice. Diagnosis and management of preeclampsia and eclampsia. Int J Gynaecol Obstet 2002;77(1):67–75.

22. Moldenhauer JS, Stanek J, Warshak C, et al. The frequency and severity of placental findings in women with preeclampsia are gestational age dependent. Am J Obstet Gynecol 2003;189(4):1173–7.

23. Kim YM, Bujold E, Chaiworapongsa T, et al. Failure of physiologic transformation of the spiral arteries in patients with preterm labor and intact membranes. Am J Obstet Gynecol 2003;189(4):1063–9.

24. Kim YM, Chaiworapongsa T, Gomez R, et al. Failure of physiologic transformation of the spiral arteries in the placental bed in preterm premature rupture of membranes. Am J Obstet Gynecol 2002;187(5):1137–42.

25. Goodlin RC, Haesslein HO, Fleming J. Aspirin for the treatment of recurrent toxaemia. Lancet 1978;2(8079):51.

26. Crandon AJ, Isherwood DM. Effect of aspirin on incidence of pre-eclampsia. Lancet 1979;1(8130):1356.

27. Masotti G, Galanti G, Poggesi L, et al. Differential inhibition of prostacyclin production and platelet aggregation by aspirin. Lancet 1979;2(8154):1213–7.

28. Beaufils M, Uzan S, Donsimoni R, et al. Prevention of pre-eclampsia by early antiplatelet therapy. Lancet 1985;1(8433):840–2.

29. Askie LM, Duley L, Henderson-Smart DJ, et al. Antiplatelet agents for prevention of pre-eclampsia: a meta-analysis of individual patient data. Lancet 2007; 369(9575):1791–8.

30. Robson SC, Martin WL, Morris RK, et al. The investigation and management of the small-for-gestational-age fetus. Royal College of Obstetricians & Gynaecologists; 2014. p. 1–34.

31. Lausman A, Kingdom J, Maternal Fetal Medicine Committe, et al. Intrauterine growth restriction: screening, diagnosis, and management. J Obstet Gynaecol Can 2013;35(8):741–57.
32. Cnossen JS, Morris RK, ter Riet G, et al. Use of uterine artery Doppler ultrasonography to predict pre-eclampsia and intrauterine growth restriction: a systematic review and bivariable meta-analysis. CMAJ 2008;178(6):701–11.
33. Effendi M, Demers S, Giguere Y, et al. Association between first-trimester placental volume and birth weight. Placenta 2014;35(2):99–102.
34. Poon LC, Volpe N, Muto B, et al. Second-trimester uterine artery Doppler in the prediction of stillbirths. Fetal Diagn Ther 2013;33(1):28–35.
35. Duley L, Henderson-Smart DJ, Meher S, et al. Antiplatelet agents for preventing pre-eclampsia and its complications. Cochrane Database Syst Rev 2007;(2):CD004659.
36. Roberge S, Carpentier C, Demers S, et al. The impact of low-dose aspirin on utero-placental circulation: a systematic review. Ultrasound Obstet Gynecol 2014; 24th World Congress on Ultrasound in Obstetrics and Gynecology. September 14–17, 2014. Barcelona, Spain. p. 269.
37. Jeyabalan A. Epidemiology of preeclampsia: impact of obesity. Nutr Rev 2013; 71(Suppl 1):S18–25.
38. ACOG. Hypertension in pregnancy: practice guidelines, American College of Obstetrician and Gynecologist. Washington, DC: Library of Congress; 2013. Available at: http://www.acog.org/Resources-And-Publications/Task-Force-and-Work-Group-Reports/Hypertension-in-Pregnancy. Accessed January 19, 2016.
39. Verghese L, Alam S, Beski S, et al. Antenatal screening for pre-eclampsia: evaluation of the NICE and pre-eclampsia community guidelines. J Obstet Gynaecol 2012;32(2):128–31.
40. Werner EF, Hauspurg AK, Rouse DJ. A cost-benefit analysis of low-dose aspirin prophylaxis for the prevention of preeclampsia in the United States. Obstet Gynecol 2015;126(6):1242–50.
41. Audibert F, Boucoiran I, An N, et al. Screening for preeclampsia using first-trimester serum markers and uterine artery Doppler in nulliparous women. Am J Obstet Gynecol 2010;203(4):383.e1–8.
42. Poon LC, Staboulidou I, Maiz N, et al. Hypertensive disorders in pregnancy: screening by uterine artery Doppler at 11-13 weeks. Ultrasound Obstet Gynecol 2009;34(2):142–8.
43. Tsiakkas A, Cazacu R, Wright A, et al. Serum placental growth factor at 12, 22, 32 and 36 weeks' gestation in screening for preeclampsia. Ultrasound Obstet Gynecol 2015. [Epub ahead of print].
44. Bahado-Singh RO, Syngelaki A, Akolekar R, et al. Validation of metabolomic models for prediction of early-onset preeclampsia. Am J Obstet Gynecol 2015; 213(4):530.e1–10.
45. Wright D, Syngelaki A, Akolekar R, et al. Competing risks model in screening for preeclampsia by maternal characteristics and medical history. Am J Obstet Gynecol 2015;213(1):62.e1–10.
46. Demers S, Bujold E, Arenas E, et al. Prediction of recurrent preeclampsia using first-trimester uterine artery Doppler. Am J Perinatol 2014;31(2):99–104.
47. O'Gorman N, Wright D, Syngelaki A, et al. Competing risks model in screening for preeclampsia by maternal factors and biomarkers at 11-13 weeks gestation. Am J Obstet Gynecol 2015;214(1):103.e1–12.

48. Park F, Russo K, Williams P, et al. Prediction and prevention of early-onset pre-eclampsia: impact of aspirin after first-trimester screening. Ultrasound Obstet Gynecol 2015;46(4):419–23.

49. Rumack CM, Guggenheim MA, Rumack BH, et al. Neonatal intracranial hemorrhage and maternal use of aspirin. Obstet Gynecol 1981;58(5 Suppl):52S–6S.

50. Bloor M, Paech M. Nonsteroidal anti-inflammatory drugs during pregnancy and the initiation of lactation. Anesth Anal 2013;116(5):1063–75.

51. Ostensen ME, Skomsvoll JF. Anti-inflammatory pharmacotherapy during pregnancy. Expert Opin Pharmacother 2004;5(3):571–80.

52. Caron N, Rivard GE, Michon N, et al. Low-dose ASA response using the PFA-100 in women with high-risk pregnancy. J Obstet Gynaecol Can 2009;31(11):1022–7.

53. Wojtowicz A, Undas A, Huras H, et al. Aspirin resistance may be associated with adverse pregnancy outcomes. Neuro Endocrinol Lett 2011;32(3):334–9.

54. Rodger MA, Hague WM, Kingdom J, et al. Antepartum dalteparin versus no antepartum dalteparin for the prevention of pregnancy complications in pregnant women with thrombophilia (TIPPS): a multinational open-label randomised trial. Lancet 2014;384(9955):1673–83.

55. Martinelli I, Ruggenenti P, Cetin I, et al. Heparin in pregnant women with previous placenta-mediated pregnancy complications: a prospective, randomized, multicenter, controlled clinical trial. Blood 2012;119(14):3269–75.

56. Roberge S, Demers S, Nicolaides KH, et al. Prevention of pre-eclampsia by low-molecular weight heparin in addition to aspirin: a meta-analysis. Ultrasound Obstet Gynecol 2015. [Epub ahead of print].

57. August P, Helseth G, Edersheim T, et al. Sustained relase, low-dose aspirin ameliorates but does not prevent preeclampsia (PE) in a high risk population. In: Proceedings of 9th International Congress, International Society for the Study of Hypertension. Hypertension in Pregnancy. Sydney, Australia, March 15–18, 1994. p. 72.

58. Azar R, Turpin D. Effect of antiplatelet therapy in women at high risk for pregnancy-induced hypertension. In: Proceedings of 7th World Congress of Hypertension in Pregnancy. Perugia, Italy, October, 1990. p. 257.

59. Benigni A, Gregorini G, Frusca T, et al. Effect of low-dose aspirin on fetal and maternal generation of thromboxane by platelets in women at risk for pregnancy-induced hypertension. N Engl J Med 1989;321(6):357–62.

60. Bakhti A, Vaiman D. Prevention of gravidic endothelial hypertension by aspirin treatment administered from the 8th week of gestation. Hypertension Research 2011;34(10):1116–20. Corrigendum: Hypertension Research 2012;35(2) 244.

61. Caritis S, Sibai B, Hauth J, et al. Low-dose aspirin to prevent preeclampsia in women at high risk. National Institute of Child Health and Human Development Network of Maternal-Fetal Medicine Units. N Engl J Med 1998;338(11):701–5.

62. Moore GS, Allshouse AA, Post AL, et al. Early initiation of low-dose aspirin for reduction in preeclampsia risk in high-risk women: a secondary analysis of the MFMU High-Risk Aspirin Study. J Perinatol 2015;35(5):328–31.

63. Chiaffarino F, Parazzini F, Paladini D, et al. A small randomised trial of low-dose aspirin in women at high risk of pre-eclampsia. Eur J Obstet Gynecol Reprod Biol 2004;112(2):142–4.

64. Dasari R, Narang A, Vasishta K, et al. Effect of maternal low dose aspirin on neonatal platelet function. Indian Pediatr 1998;35(6):507–11.

65. Ebrashy A, Ibrahim M, Marzook A, et al. Usefulness of aspirin therapy in high-risk pregnant women with abnormal uterine artery Doppler ultrasound at 14-16 weeks pregnancy: randomized controlled clinical trial. Croat Med J 2005;46(5):826–31.

66. Hermida RC, Ayala DE, Iglesias M, et al. Time-dependent effects of low-dose aspirin administration on blood pressure in pregnant women. Hypertension 1997;30(3 Pt 2):589–95.

67. Ayala DE, Ucieda R, Hermida RC. Chronotherapy with low-dose aspirin for prevention of complications in pregnancy. Chronobiol Int 2013;30(1–2):260–79.

68. Hermida RC, Ayala DE, Fernandez JR, et al. Administration time-dependent effects of aspirin in women at differing risk for preeclampsia. Hypertension 1999; 34(4 Pt 2):1016–23.

69. Jamal A, Milani F, Al-Yasin A. Evaluation of the effect of metformin and aspirin on utero placental circulation of pregnant women with PCOS. Iran J Reprod Med 2012;10(3):265–70.

70. Mesdaghinia E, Talari H, Abedzadeh-Kalahroudi M. Effect of aspirin for prevention of preeclampsia in women with abnormal ultrasonic findings in uterine artery. Feyz 2011;15(2):98–104. Available at: http://applications.emro.who.int/imemrf/J_Kashan_Univ_Med_Sci/J_Kashan_Univ_Med_Sci_2011_15_2_98_104.pdf.

71. Michael C, Walters B, editors. Low-dose aspirin in the prevention of pre-eclampsia: current evaluation. Carnforth (United Kingdom): Parthenon Publishing Group Limited; 1992.

72. Odibo AO, Goetzinger KR, Odibo L, et al. Early prediction and aspirin for prevention of pre-eclampsia (EPAPP) study: a randomized controlled trial. Ultrasound Obstet Gynecol 2015;46(4):414–8.

73. Porreco RP, Hickok DE, Williams MA, et al. Low-dose aspirin and hypertension in pregnancy. Lancet 1993;341(8840):312.

74. Tulppala M, Marttunen M, Soderstrom-Anttila V, et al. Low-dose aspirin in prevention of miscarriage in women with unexplained or autoimmune related recurrent miscarriage: effect on prostacyclin and thromboxane A2 production. Hum Reprod 1997;12(7):1567–72.

75. Vainio M, Kujansuu E, Iso-Mustajarvi M, et al. Low dose acetylsalicylic acid in prevention of pregnancy-induced hypertension and intrauterine growth retardation in women with bilateral uterine artery notches. BJOG 2002;109(2):161–7.

76. Villa PM, Kajantie E, Raikkonen K, et al. Aspirin in the prevention of pre-eclampsia in high-risk women: a randomised placebo-controlled PREDO Trial and a meta-analysis of randomised trials. BJOG 2013;120(1):64–74.

77. Zhao YM, Xiao LP, Hu H, et al. Low-dose aspirin prescribed at bed time for the prevention of pre-eclampsia in high-risk pregnant women. Reprod Contracept 2012;32:355–9.

First-, Second-, and Third-Trimester Screening for Preeclampsia and Intrauterine Growth Restriction

Alejandro Rodriguez, MD[a],*, Methodius G. Tuuli, MD, MPH[b],
Anthony O. Odibo, MD, MSCE[a]

KEYWORDS

- Preeclampsia • Intrauterine growth restriction • Screening

KEY POINTS

- Preeclampsia and intrauterine growth restriction may result in adverse perinatal outcome; therefore, early detection and management could improve the outcome.
- Clinical characteristics, ultrasonography and Doppler parameters, and biochemical markers individually have been used in an attempt to predict these conditions with poor results.
- Predictive models combining different biochemical markers and uterine artery Doppler in every trimester have shown mixed results, although some show promise as potential screening tools.

INTRODUCTION

Preeclampsia and intrauterine growth restriction (IUGR) are major contributors to perinatal mortality and morbidity.[1] Although there is an increasing understanding of the pathophysiology of these conditions, their prevention remains a considerable challenge in obstetrics. It is now well-understood that, although the symptoms of preeclampsia and IUGR generally manifest in the second to third trimesters of pregnancy, their underlying pathology largely takes place in the first trimester.[2] This phenomenon has sparked great interest in the search for tests to predicting them early in pregnancy before these complications occur.

Funding Support: None.
[a] Division of Maternal-Fetal Medicine, Department of Obstetrics and Gynecology, University of South Florida Morsani College of Medicine, 2 Tampa General Circle, Tampa, FL 33606, USA;
[b] Division of Maternal-Fetal Medicine, Department of Obstetrics and Gynecology, Washington University School of Medicine, 4911 Barnes Jewish Hospital Plaza, Maternity Tower 6th floor, St Louis, MO 63110, USA
* Corresponding author.
E-mail address: Arodri24@health.usf.edu

Clin Lab Med 36 (2016) 331–351
http://dx.doi.org/10.1016/j.cll.2016.01.007
0272-2712/16/$ – see front matter © 2016 Elsevier Inc. All rights reserved.

labmed.theclinics.com

Several individual clinical factors, Doppler ultrasound parameters, and serum analytes have been evaluated for prediction of preeclampsia and/or IUGR. On their own, these tests generally have poor predictive value. This result may reflect the multifactorial nature of the preeclampsia syndrome. However, a combination of selected parameters and results of recent novel measures seem to be promising. The aim of this paper is to review the first-, second-, and third-trimester screening tests for preeclampsia and IUGR.

PATHOPHYSIOLOGY

Although the precise origin of preeclampsia remains elusive, it is believed to be multifactorial, with the placenta playing a central role. During the last several years, a clearer picture of the pathophysiology has begun to emerge.[3] A 2-stage model has been proposed in which poor placentation, the central initiating event, is thought to occur early. This first stage results from failure of the normal physiologic process in early pregnancy where endovascular trophoblast invades the maternal vasculature and replaces the smooth muscle normally present in the spiral arterioles with a noncontractile matrix material. The result of this normal but seemingly destructive event is a high flow, low resistance vascular conduit that perfuses the intervillous space.[4] This is reflected by a decrease in the uterine artery resistance with increasing gestation. Failure of the trophoblast invasion leaves a high resistance vasculature with persistent smooth muscle histology of the maternal blood vessels. This lack of transformation predisposes to hypoperfusion, hypoxia reperfusion injury, oxidative stress, and signs of placental maldevelopment in the second trimester.[5] Recent evidence suggests that a significant part of placental injury is mechanical damage resulting from intermittent perfusion as a result of persistence of smooth muscle in the spiral arterioles.[6]

The second stage of preeclampsia pathogenesis is the maternal response to abnormal placentation, which is initially adaptive, but subsequently results in widespread systemic injury. Key features of this second phase are systemic endothelial dysfunction[3,7] and an imbalance of circulating vasoactive factors.[8–10] Of note, many of the resulting features can be detected before clinical signs of pathology (preeclampsia or IUGR) appear, creating an opportunity for potential predictive tests.

There is emerging evidence that the pathophysiology described is more consistent with preterm preeclampsia with coexisting IUGR than term preeclampsia.[11] For example, placental pathologic studies indicate that preeclampsia or IUGR resulting in preterm delivery before 34 weeks has high rates of thrombotic placental pathologic findings of the villous trees.[12] In contrast, term preeclampsia and/or IUGR was associated with either normal or minimal pathologic findings.[13] Doppler studies also suggest that preterm preeclampsia/IUGR is associated with defective invasion of the spiral arteries, whereas the spiral artery defect plays a much smaller role in the cases nearer term.[14] Thus, term preeclampsia and IUGR seem to be associated with normal trophoblast transformation in the first trimester and late atherosclerotic changes in spiral arterioles. Such late changes may be the consequence of increased placental mass as occurs in diabetic and twin pregnancies, senescence of the placenta as in prolonged pregnancy or placental edema, and necrosis as in fetal hydrops.[15]

SCREENING TESTS FOR PREECLAMPSIA AND INTRAUTERINE GROWTH RESTRICTION

Screening tests are commonly used in clinical practice, yet the underlying principles of screening are widely misunderstood.[16] This overview assumes some basic understanding of the principles of screening, including use of receiver operating characteristic curves and likelihood ratios, the details of which can be reviewed in the following references.[17–21] Proposed screening tests for preeclampsia are grouped according to the type as well as the presumed pathophysiologic basis for the test (**Box 1**). We provide a brief discussion of each test or groups of tests and summarize results of studies evaluating their performance in screening for preeclampsia. For brevity, results of recent systematic reviews and metaanalysis are used when available and emphasis is placed on the more recent screening modalities. Where tests are uniquely used in any trimester, the designation is specified.

Clinical Factors

A number of prepregnancy and pregnancy-related factors have been associated with increased risk of preeclampsia and IUGR (**Box 2**). These factors may increase the likelihood of preeclampsia through placental mechanisms or predisposition to maternal cardiovascular disease. The use of clinical risk factors has the advantage of being free of cost, noninvasive, and routinely collected. However, clinical factors have not been found to be an effective screening tool for preeclampsia and IUGR in the general obstetric population owing to their poor sensitivity and specificity.[22] The role of risk

---

Box 1
Candidate screening tests for preeclampsia and intrauterine growth restriction

   i. Clinical risk factor screening

  ii. Placenta perfusion dysfunction related tests
      Uterine artery Doppler ultrasonography
      Two-dimensional placenta imaging
      Three-dimensional placenta imaging
         Placental volume
         Placenta quotient
         Placenta vascular indices

 iii. Maternal serum analytes
      Down syndrome markers
         Alpha fetoprotein
         Human chorionic gonadotropin
         Estriol
         Inhibin A
      A disintegrin and metalloproteases
      Placental protein 13

  iv. Endothelial dysfunction-related tests
      Circulated angiogenic factors
         Placental growth factor
         Soluble fms-like tyrosine kinase 1
         Vascular endothelial growth factor
         Soluble endoglin
      Endothelial cell adhesion molecules
         Selectin

   v. Markers of insulin resistance
      Tumor necrosis factor
      Sex hormone binding globulin
      Adiponectin
      Leptin

  vi. Genomics and proteomics

 vii. Maternal serum analytes

Box 2
Risk factors for preeclampsia and intrauterine growth restriction

A. Preeclampsia
  i. Prepregnancy factors
     Chronic hypertension
     Renal disease
     Diabetes mellitus
     Connective tissue disease
     Thrombophilia
     Uncontrolled hyperthyroidism
     Polycystic ovarian syndrome
     Age older than 40 years and younger than 20 years
     Obesity/insulin resistance
     Preeclampsia in a previous pregnancy
     Primiparity
     Limited sperm exposure
     Pregnancies from artificial reproductive technology
     Partner who fathered preeclamptic pregnancy with another woman
     Smoking (reduced risk)
     Family history of preeclampsia
  ii. Pregnancy-related factors
     Multifetal gestation
     Chromosomal abnormality (triploidy, trisomy 13)

B. Intrauterine growth restriction
  i. Prepregnancy factors
     Chronic hypertension
     Renal disease
     Diabetes with vasculopathy
     Autoimmune syndromes—antiphospholipid syndrome, lupus
     Thrombophilia
     Maternal hypoxemia (cyanotic heart disease, severe chronic anemia, chronic pulmonary disease)
     Uterine anomalies—large submucous myomas, septate uterus, synechiae
     Smoking
     Substance abuse—Alcohol, heroin, methadone, cocaine, therapeutic agents
     Malnutrition
     Family history of intrauterine growth restriction
  ii. Pregnancy-related factors
     Fetal chromosomal abnormality (trisomy 13, 18, and 21, triploidy, uniparental disomy)
     Fetal malformations (gastroschisis, omphalocele, diaphragmatic hernia, congenital heart defect)
     Maternal infection—malaria, rubella, cytomegalovirus, herpes, toxoplasmosis
     Multiple gestation

---

factor assessment may be in the identification of individuals at greater risk for preeclampsia and IUGR than baseline, in whom other screening test may be applied.[23] The combination of risk factors with other screening tests may improve their screening efficiency for preeclampsia and IUGR.[24]

Placenta Perfusion Dysfunction Related

Uterine artery Doppler velocimetry

Enhanced uterine artery resistance reflects a failure of trophoblastic invasion of the spiral arteries and is associated with the development of preeclampsia and IUGR.[15,25] Increased resistance to vascular flow can be measured noninvasively by Doppler flow studies of the myometrial segments of the arteries supplying the spiral arterioles. Increased uterine artery resistance as measured by pulsatility index (PI) or resistive index above a chosen value and/or percentile or the presence of unilateral or bilateral diastolic notches has been investigated for the prediction of preeclampsia and IUGR. The use of different criteria for defining abnormal uterine artery flow is one of the limitations to comparing results across different studies.

Abnormal uterine artery Doppler studies in the both the first and second trimesters have been shown to be associated with preeclampsia and IUGR. A recent update of a metaanalysis of studies using uterine artery Doppler indices to predict preeclampsia produced a number of important conclusions.[19,23] First, irrespective of the Doppler artery indices used, predictive accuracy in low-risk populations was moderate to minimal, whereas that in high-risk populations was minimal. The sensitivities and specificities of uterine artery Doppler in low-risk populations varied from 34% to 76% and 83% to 93%, respectively. Second, the best predictor indices were increased PI and the presence of bilateral notching, with positive likelihood ratio of 5. In high-risk populations, all uterine artery Doppler indices had poor predictive ability with positive and negative likelihood ratios of 2.5 to 3.3 and 0.4 to 0.8, respectively. Third, the predictive accuracy for early onset preeclampsia is moderate to good, irrespective of the index or combination of indices used.

Another recent systematic review and metaanalysis concluded that, for both preeclampsia and IUGR, Doppler testing was more accurate in the second than the first trimester (see below for role of uterine artery in the third trimester). Increased PI with notching in the second trimester emerged as the best predictor of preeclampsia. The authors strongly recommended their routine use in clinical practice.[26] That review has been strongly criticized and the recommendation labeled premature, as it is based on only 2 studies (one of which included 1757 low-risk women and the other 351 high-risk women) and the tests (increased PI with notching) produced insufficiently high positive likelihood ratios of positive (7.5) and poor negative likelihood ratios for both populations (0.59 and 0.82, respectively).[27] A number of methodologic concerns were appropriately raised, including absence of formal tests for heterogeneity, publication bias, and the inappropriate pooling of sensitivities and specificities.[27]

In conclusion, although uterine artery Doppler velocimetry shows promise, especially for the prediction of early onset preeclampsia and IUGR, standards are lacking for the gestational age of screening and criteria for an abnormal test. Thus, current evidence does not support routine screening with uterine artery Doppler imaging in low- or high-risk populations.

Three-dimensional placenta imaging

The size of the placenta and the vascular flow patterns within the placental villous tree in early pregnancy may predict adverse pregnancy outcomes, including preeclampsia and IUGR. Small placental volume results from shallow invasive activity of the extravillous trophoblast. This may be secondary to a reduction in oxygen tension in the intervillous space and/or the activation of inhibitors of trophoblast differentiation and proliferation.[4] Improvements in ultrasonographic imaging provide a tool for estimating placental volume and villous blood flow using 3- and 4-dimensional scanning techniques.[28,29] Parameters evaluated for predicting preeclampsia and IUGR include the placental volume itself, placental quotient and vascular indices.

Placental quotient The placental quotient, defined as the ratio of the placental volume to the fetal crown–rump length, quantifies the size of the placenta in relation to the fetus in the first trimester. Decreased placental volume at 11 to 14 weeks of gestation has been implicated in the subsequent development of preeclampsia and IUGR, with a predictive value similar to and independent of uterine artery Doppler.[30,31] Hafner and colleagues[30] reported a high negative predictive value of the placental quotient, enabling it to define a subgroup at low risk for perinatal complications. The placental quotient performed better in predicting severe preeclampsia with IUGR requiring delivery before 34 weeks' gestation. However, it was not particularly useful for screening in a low-risk population with sensitivity of 38.5% for preeclampsia and 27.1% for small for gestational age (SGA) fetuses. Combining the assessment of placental volume with the first trimester uterine artery Doppler screening may improve the detection rate of preeclampsia to values similar to that of late second trimester screening, with the added advantage of early screening.

Placental vascular indices Vascular indices within the placenta are calculated from 3-dimensional data formed by the voxels (the basic information units of volume) for vascularization assessment of organs and structures. These indices represent the total and relative amounts of power Doppler information within the volume of interest. The vascularization index (VI) quantifies the number of color-coded voxels to all voxels within the volume expressed as a percentage, flow index (FI) represents the power Doppler signal intensity from all color-coded voxels and vascularization FI (VFI) is the mathematical relationship derived from multiplying the VI by the FI. These indices are thought to reflect the number of blood vessels within the volume (VI), the intensity of flow at the time of the 3-dimensional sweep (FI), and both blood flow and vascularization (VFI). After acquisition of the 3-dimensional image, machine-specific software is used to calculate the placental indices. Three-dimensional ultrasonography with power Doppler has been demonstrated to be particularly useful and superior to 2-dimensional (2-D) ultrasonography in the determination of the distal vascular branches of the fetal placental blood vessels.[32] When the entire image of the placenta cannot be obtained in a single sweep, 'vascular biopsy' or 'sonobiopsy' has been proposed to obtain a representative sample of the placenta.[33] A recent study noted that 2 of the indices obtained from sonobiopsy (VI and VFI) are similar to those from whole placenta evaluation.[34]

Placental flow indices obtained by these techniques have been correlated with gestational age, alterations in fetal growth, amniotic fluid volume, and Doppler biometric parameters of fetoplacental circulation.[35–37] A reduction in these indices may be an early marker of placental dysfunction. A study in normal and growth-restricted pregnancies revealed that the FI, which identifies the most severe cases of placental impairment, was the most reliable index.[37] After assessing placental vascularization in 208 normal fetuses between 12 and 40 weeks of gestation and 13 pregnancies with IUGR at 22 to 39 weeks' gestation, Noguchi and colleagues[36] found that VI values in 8 of 13 fetal growth restricted pregnancies (61.5%), FI value in 1 IUGR pregnancy (7.7%), and VFI values of 6 IUGR pregnancies (46.2%) were below -1.5 standard deviations of the reference ranges for VI, FI, and VFI, respectively.

Although this technology shows promise, no large-scale studies have been performed to validate its use. In addition, technical and methodologic issues must be addressed before its general application.[38–41] First and second trimester studies using standardized techniques are underway to clarify the usefulness of this tool in predicting adverse pregnancy outcomes including preeclampsia and IUGR.

Two-dimensional placenta imaging

Examination of the placenta is a normal part of routine obstetric ultrasound examinations. In the standard B-mode, the normal placenta is relatively homogeneous with areas of differing echogenicity as pregnancy progresses secondary to varying degrees of calcification. Abnormalities in the placenta in 2-D imaging, including decreased length and thickness, infarcts, abnormal texture, and the presence of echogenic cystic lesions have been associated with adverse pregnancy outcomes including preeclampsia and IUGR. A method for systematic 2-D placental ultrasound examination has been described and used, often in combination with other parameters for screening.[42] Abnormal placental morphology is defined by shape, texture or both and determined by measurement of the maximal placental length and thickness with placental thickness greater than 4 cm or greater than 50% of placental length, defining an abnormal shape; categorizing placental texture as normal (homogeneously granular), heterogeneous (echogenic patches alternating with normal texture), or abnormal when the placenta contains either multiple echogenic cystic lesions or assumes a jellylike appearance with turbulent uteroplacental flow visible because of lack of normal villous development; and defining placental cord insertion as normal (>2 cm from the placental disc margin), lateral (within 2 cm of the margin), marginal (on the margin), or velamentous (inserting into the surrounding membranes).[42]

Using this method of placenta examination, Toal and colleagues[25] in a cohort of 60 high-risk women with abnormal uterine artery Doppler ultrasound examinations, found a higher odds of IUGR in patients with abnormally shaped placentas when compared with those with normally shaped placentas. The same group used placental morphology from 2-D imaging in combination with maternal serum screening and uterine artery Doppler to define a 'placenta function profile,' which was then used to screen for placenta-related adverse pregnancy outcomes, including IUGR and preeclampsia in 212 high-risk pregnancies.[43] Although the combined test proved useful in predicting women who would and would not have adverse pregnancy outcomes, there were no data reported on the predictive performance of the placental morphology from 2-D imaging of the placenta alone.

To date, no large-scale prospective studies have validated the use of 2-D placenta imaging in the prediction of preeclampsia or IUGR. This modality has significant limitations, including poor resolution, difficulty assessing nonanteriorly located placentas, and a wide variability in the morphology of normal placentas. Three- and 4-dimensional scanning techniques are significant improvements that are likely to prove more useful than 2-D imaging in delineating placental structure.

Maternal Serum Analytes

Maternal serum analytes provide minimally invasive tests of fetal and placental endocrine function as well as endothelial dysfunction. The current understanding of the pathophysiology of preeclampsia and IUGR provide the basis for these screening tests. The failure of trophoblastic invasion may be related to dysregulated secretory activity of the trophoblasts, whereas alteration in the surface layer of the syncytiotrophoblast may contribute to 'leakage' of human chorionic gonadotropin (hCG) and alpha-fetoprotein (AFP) into the maternal circulation.[44,45] Reduced placental size or defective syncytiotrophoblast formation may result in reduced production of placenta-derived proteins, such as pregnancy-associated protein A (PAPP-A).[46] Hypoxia–reoxygenation may be responsible for the increased secretion of proinflammatory cytokines, such as tumor necrosis factor (TNF)-α and interleukin (IL)-1ß, and antiangiogenic factors, such as the soluble receptor for vascular endothelial growth factor (sFLT-1).[47–49] Hypoxia–reoxygenation may also result in increased apoptosis in trophoblasts, leading to the release of free fetal DNA into maternal circulation.[49] Endothelial cell damage, platelet activation dysfunction, and disturbances in coagulation may be responsible for increased P-selectin and markers of insulin resistance.[7,50,51]

Many of the tests of fetal and placental endocrine function are measured in the first and/or second trimesters as part of routine prenatal care. The use of these analytes is attractive because the results are available routinely. However, they have generally yielded poor predictive characteristics, increasing interest in the development and testing of novel markers.

Fetal and placental endocrine dysfunction-related tests

Down syndrome markers Second trimester serum screening for Down syndrome is routinely offered to women, either as the triple test (AFP, hCG, and unconjugated estriol) or with the addition of inhibin A as the quadruple test. More recently, first trimester screening with fetal nuchal translucency, hCG, and PAPP-A is in use. Owing to their origin and sites of metabolism, these biochemical markers may be useful in the prediction of preeclampsia and IUGR. Several studies have investigated their role as predictive tests for preeclampsia and IUGR.

A recent metaanalysis summarized results of relevant studies to determine the accuracy of the 5 serum analytes used in Down serum screening (hCG, AFP, unconjugated estriol, PAPP-A, and inhibin A) for prediction of preeclampsia and/or SGA.[52] A total of 44 studies, including 169,637 pregnant women (4376 preeclampsia cases) and 86 studies, including 382,005 women (20,339 fetal growth restriction cases) met the selection criteria. The results showed low predictive accuracy overall. For preeclampsia, the best predictor was inhibin A of greater than 2.79 multiples of the median (MoM) with positive likelihood ratio of 19.5 (95% CI, 8.3–45.8) and negative likelihood ratio of 0.3 (95% CI, 0.1–0.7). For SGA infants, the best predictor was an AFP of greater than 2.0 MoM with a positive likelihood ratio of 28.0 (95% CI, 8.0–97.5) and a negative likelihood ratio of 0.8 (95% CI, 0.6–1.1). The authors acknowledged methodologic and reporting limitations in the included studies as well as heterogeneity, which resulted in wide CIs of the pooled estimates.

In conclusion, although an attractive screening modality owing to its wide spread availability, Down syndrome serum screening analytes by themselves have a low predictive accuracy for preeclampsia and SGA. However, they may be a useful means of risk assessment or used in combination with other screening tests.

A disintegrin and metalloproteases A disintegrin and metalloproteases (ADAM12) is a placenta-derived multidomain glycoprotein involved in controlling fetal and placental growth and development. ADAM12-S (the short isoform) is the secreted form and can bind to adhesion receptors and mediate shedding of oxytocinase, which may be associated with progressive growth of the placenta.[53,54] Reduced ADAM12 has been shown to be a potential marker of preeclampsia and IUGR in the first trimester.[55–57] Of note, concentration of ADAM12 in normal pregnancies varies with gestational age, African American race, and maternal weight, necessitating adjustment for these variables before comparing results with pathologic pregnancies.[58]

The screening performance of first trimester ADAM12 alone is poor. For a 5% false-positive rate, it can only detect 26.6% of the preeclampsia pregnancies and 7% to 20% of the SGA pregnancies.[56–58] After adjusting for maternal weight and race in a case control study, Poon and colleagues[58] noted that maternal serum ADAM12 concentration at 11 to 13 + 6 weeks of gestation in pregnancies developing preeclampsia or gestational hypertension was neither significantly different from normotensive pregnancies nor associated with the severity of preeclampsia. The authors concluded that the development of preeclampsia associated with low levels of ADAM12 may be a reflection of the association between the development of preeclampsia and increasing maternal weight.

In conclusion, studies to date suggest that ADAM12 may have a limited or no role as a predictive test for preeclampsia and IUGR. Results of ongoing studies may further clarify these observations.

Placental protein 13 Placental protein 13 (PP13), a member of the galectin family, is produced by syncytiotrophoblast. It binds to proteins on the extracellular matrix between the placenta and the endometrium and is thought to be involved in placental implantation and maternal vascular remodeling.[59,60] A decrease in the PP13 messenger RNA expression noted in trophoblasts obtained from women at 11 weeks' gestation who subsequently develop preeclampsia suggests that alteration in PP13 expression may be involved in the pathogenesis of preeclampsia.[61]

A number of studies have evaluated serum PP13 levels as a predictive test for preeclampsia and IUGR with conflicting results.[62–65] In a prospective nested case control study, Chafetz and colleagues[60] demonstrated that when serum PP13 at 9 to 12 weeks was expressed as MoM, sensitivities for preeclampsia and IUGR were 79% and 33%, respectively, at a 90% specificity rate. In another study, a sensitivity of 100% was obtained for early-onset preeclampsia at 80% specificity.[63] In addition, 2 prospective studies suggest a potential role for first trimester PP13 levels in combination with the slope between the first and second trimesters for predicting preeclampsia.[64,65] In a prospective cohort, Schneuer and colleagues[66] found that standardized levels by gestational age, smoking status, and maternal weight were inadequate for screening purposes when using a 5% fix rate for false positives, it showed a low sensitivity of 20.4% (95% CI, 14.9–26.8) and low positive predictive ratio 24.2% for prediction of SGA, with an area under the curve (AUC) of 0.73 (95% CI, 0.69–0.77). its ability to predict preeclampsia was also low with a sensitivity of 31.7% (95% CI, 18.1–48.1) and an AUC of 0.83 (95% CI, 0.78–.0.88). In contrast, a case-control study by Akolekar and colleagues[67] found that the addition of serum PP13 did not significantly improve the prediction of early preeclampsia provided by a combination of maternal factors, uterine artery PI, and PAPP-A. Other studies also found no association between low levels of PP13 and subsequent development of preeclampsia and IUGR.[62]

In conclusion, PP13 shows promise as a predictor of preeclampsia and IUGR, but results of preliminary studies are conflicting and limited by their case-control design and small sample sizes. It is expected that results of larger prospective studies currently underway will resolve these conflicting results and clarify its potential role in the prediction of preeclampsia and IUGR.

Endothelial dysfunction-related tests
Circulating angiogenic factors Growing evidence suggest that an imbalance between proangiogenic factors (such as vascular endothelial growth factor [VEGF] and placental growth factor [PIGF]) and antiangiogenic factors (such as sFlt-1 and soluble endoglin [sEng]) is related to the development of preeclampsia.[68] Generally, levels of proangiogenic factor levels are lower and antiangiogenic factors are increased in the maternal circulation before the onset of and during active disease.[68] Angiogenic factors are thought to contribute to normal trophoblastic proliferation and implantation. sFlt-1 blocks the effects of VEGF and PIGF by inhibiting interaction with their receptors.[69] This deprives maternal vascular endothelium of these essential proangiogenic factors and causes systemic endothelial dysfunction that may culminate in preeclampsia.[70,71]

Several studies suggest that PIGF concentration in the first trimester is decreased in women who go on to develop preeclampsia/IUGR and the levels inversely correlate with severity of the disease.[70,72–78] Kusanovic and colleagues[79] examined the role of maternal plasma PIGF, sEng, and sFlt-1 concentrations in early pregnancy

(6–15 weeks) and midtrimester (20–25 weeks) for predicting preeclampsia. They found that individual proangiogenic and antiangiogenic factors had a poor predictive value for preeclampsia. However, a combination of these analytes (PlGF to sEng ratio, its delta and slope) had great predictive performance with sensitivity of 100%, specificity of 98% to 99%, and positive likelihood ratios of 57.6, 55.6, and 89.6, respectively, for predicting early-onset preeclampsia.[79]

Urinary PlGF has also been explored as a possible screening test for preeclampsia with disappointing results. Savvidou and colleagues[80] demonstrated that first trimester urinary PlGF levels, were not different between pregnancies that developed preeclampsia and normotensive controls. Also, serum VEGF is unlikely to serve as a useful screening marker because it binds sFlt1 with a higher affinity than PlGF and free VEGF is extremely low in the sera, below the detection limit of currently available assays.[72,74]

Circulating sEng levels have been shown to increase earlier and more distinctly in pregnancies with subsequent preeclampsia compared with normal pregnancies.[81] This effect was particularly pronounced in gestations affected by early-onset pre-eclampsia.[82] Baumann and colleagues[83] reported that increased levels of sEng were paralleled by increased sFlt1/PlGF ratios and similar to sFlt1 levels. There are conflicting results among studies on sEng levels in the first trimester and subsequent development of preeclampsia.[81,83]

The current interest in angiogenic factors for the prediction of preeclampsia is promising, but most studies to date are limited by their retrospective design, nonstandardized assays, and small sample sizes. Results of an ongoing large, international, prospective study are expected to define the role for angiogenic factors in the prediction of preeclampsia.

Endothelial cell adhesion molecules P-selectin, a member of the selectin family of cell adhesion molecules expressed in platelets and endothelial cells, is involved in leukocyte–endothelial interactions.[84,85] Because preeclampsia is associated with increase in cytokine levels, endothelial cell damage and platelet activation, increased P-selectin expression is thought to play an important role in the pathophysiology of preeclampsia.[7,50,51]

P-selectin levels are significantly increased as early as 10 to 14 weeks in women destined to develop preeclampsia.[86] Banzola and colleagues[87] evaluated the performance of P-selectin, total activin A and VEGF receptor at 11 to 15 weeks' gestation in predicting preeclampsia. P-selectin was identified as the marker with the best discriminant ability between controls and preeclampsia. Bosio and colleagues[51] reported an area under the receiver operating characteristic curve of 0.93 at 10 to 14 weeks and a negative predictive value of close to 100% for P-selectin in predicting preeclampsia. These results are yet to be validated by a large study.

Markers of insulin resistance

Insulin resistance has long been implicated in the pathogenesis of preeclampsia. Possible mechanisms are endothelial dysfunction and disturbances in coagulation.[22] Fasting insulin levels have been shown to be increased before the onset of disease.[88] A number of investigators have attempted to use markers of insulin resistance (TNF-α, sex hormone-binding globulin, adiponectin, and leptin) to predict preeclampsia with mixed results.[88–94] Overall, none of them proved useful as a predictive test.

Genomics and Proteomics

Studies in recent years suggest that genetic polymorphisms may play a role in the development of preeclampsia. Maternal susceptibility loci for preeclampsia have been found on the short arm of chromosome 2 and the long arm of chromosome 4.[95,96] There is also evidence suggesting genetic or immunologic discordance between the mother and fetus as etiologic factors in preeclampsia.[22] Using villous sampling, Farina and colleagues[97] demonstrated altered gene expressions relating to angiogenesis and oxidative stress in first trimester trophoblasts of pregnancies that went on to develop preeclampsia. Founds and colleagues[98] reported 36 differentially expressed genes, providing promising potential biomarkers for preeclampsia and clues to pathogenesis. However, a genetic contribution to preeclampsia is likely complex and involves the interaction of multiple genes and 'environmental' factors.[19] Therefore, it is unlikely that any single genetic test will reliably predict preeclampsia.

Cell-free fetal DNA (cfDNA) has been reported as a potential noninvasive marker for placenta-related complications such as preeclampsia and IUGR.[99,100] A number of studies have reported increased numbers of fetal cells and cfDNA in pregnancies complicated by preeclampsia.[101,102] Although the exact mechanism for this observation is unclear, the leading hypothesis is the release of DNA fragments by apoptosis, which is known to be widespread in preeclampsia.[103] To date, studies evaluating the use of cfDNA for the prediction of preeclampsia have yielded largely disappointing results, with some studies suggesting no difference in the amount of cfDNA in preeclamptics as compared with normotensive controls.[104,105]

These preliminary findings suggest that genomic studies can improve our understanding of the early pathophysiology of preeclampsia/IUGR at the molecular level and provide potential targets for the development of clinical biomarkers in maternal blood. However, small sample sizes and differences in methodology limit their generalizability. Importantly, the current use of cfDNA in maternal blood is limited to pregnancies with male fetuses, because only male fragments of DNA can be clearly detected with certainty.[19] Large prospective studies using improved techniques are needed to investigate the role of cfDNA in the prediction of pregnancy complications including preeclampsia and IUGR.[106]

Combination of Tests

Because no single screening test is sufficiently predictive of preeclampsia and IUGR to permit routine clinical use, many investigators have attempted to improve the predictive value of tests by combining them.[56,59,83,87,107,108] The use of multiple parameters attempts to increase the specificity and sensitivity by exploring the different possible pathways to preeclampsia and IUGR. Generally, abnormal uterine artery Doppler, a reflection of inadequate trophoblastic invasion of the maternal spiral arteries is combined with abnormal biomarkers presumably resulting from dysregulated secretory activity of trophoblasts.[78,109] We review representative studies incorporating multiple tests, to illustrate the usefulness and limitations of the combined approached.

In a prospective cohort study including 3348 women, Espinoza and colleagues[110] noted that the combination of abnormal uterine artery Doppler and maternal plasma PlGF in the second trimester improved the specificity and positive likelihood ratio for prediction of any preeclampsia, early-onset preeclampsia, and severe preeclampsia, but similar negative likelihood ratios as the individual tests. Importantly, their results showed that among women with abnormal uterine artery Doppler ultrasonography, maternal plasma concentration of PlGF of less than 280 pg/mL identified most patients who would develop early-onset and/or severe preeclampsia.[110]

Poon and colleagues[111] showed that uterine artery PI combined with maternal factors, mean arterial pressure (MAP), serum PlGF, and PAPP-A improved detection rate of early preeclampsia to about 90% with a false-positive rate of 5%. Recently, the same group demonstrated that combination of the maternal factor–derived a priori risk, uterine artery PI, and MAP produced detection rates of 89% for early and 57% for late preeclampsia at a 10% false-positive rate.[112]

Plasencia and colleagues[108] reported that uterine artery PI at 11 to 13 + 6 weeks combined with the ratio of the PI at 21 to 24 + 6 weeks to the PI at 11 to 13 + 6 weeks reduced the false-positive rate from 15% to 5% for a 91% detection rate of early pre-eclampsia. Nicolaides and colleagues[59] showed that for a 10% false-positive rate with early preeclampsia, the detection rates were 80% for PP-13 (95% CI, 44%–98%), 40% for uterine artery PI (95% CI, 12%–74%), and 90% for the markers combined (95% CI, 55%–100%). Spencer and colleagues[56] reported that, when ADAM12-S was combined with mean uterine artery PI, the area under the receiver operating characteristic curve increased to 0.88, but addition of PAPP-A to ADAM12-S increased detection by only 1%.

Results of these combined screening studies have a number of features that provide useful insights for future research but are of limited clinical usefulness at present.

Third-Trimester Serum and Ultrasound Markers for Prediction of Preeclampsia and Intrauterine Growth Restriction

As mentioned, because the pathogenesis of early preeclampsia and IUGR seems to be different from late or term preeclampsia first- and second-trimester predictions tests have poorer performance in detecting late preeclampsia and IUGR. Consequently, different screening methods have been proposed.

Biochemical markers in the third trimester

Similar to how low PlGF and high sFlt-1 levels have been studied as markers in the first or second trimesters for the prediction of early preeclampsia, a recent prospective screening study by Valino and colleagues[113] found that, in the third trimester (specifically at 30–34 weeks), these markers individually have poor predictive values, but when combined with uterine artery PI and MAP, they showed a detection rate of 97.5% at a false-positive rate of 10% for prediction of preeclampsia before 37 weeks or 55.8% for preeclampsia after 37 weeks (AUC of 0.992). The same study reported that low PIFG, estimated fetal weight (EFW) and high sFlt-1 and uterine artery PI in the third trimester predicted SGA neonates with a sensitivity of 88.3% at a 10% false-positive rate before 37 weeks and 51% after 37 weeks (AUC of 0.954).[113] Another study from these authors found similarly that low sFlt-1 and increased MAP and PlGF were the best predictors of preeclampsia with a sensitivity of 73% at a false positive rate of 10% (AUC of 0.913). For SGA, the best predictors were EFW, PlGF, and uterine artery PI with a sensitivity of 62.8% at a 10% false-positive rate (AUC, 0.883).[114]

Chaiworapongsa and colleagues[115] in a prospective study recently reported the ratio between different angiogenic factors: PlGF, sEng, and sFlt-1 and its accuracy to predict late preeclampsia, severe late preeclampsia, SGA, and stillbirth. A PlGF/sEng ratio of less than 0.3 MoM was associated with late preeclampsia (adjusted odds ratio [aOR], 7.1; 95% CI, 3.6–13.8) and even higher for severe late preeclampsia (aOR, 16.1; 95% CI, 5.8–44.6) than subjects above that threshold. The same relationship was seen with the PlGF/sFlt-1 ratio of less than 0.3 MoM (the aOR for detection of late preeclampsia was 6.1 [95% CI, 3.1–11.8]) and for severe preeclampsia was 12.2 (95% CI, 4.6–32). Overall, it showed a sensitivity of 74% to 78%, respectively, and a specificity of 84% with an AUC of 0.88 and 0.86. These 2 ratios were not as good at predicting SGA with a sensitivity of 35.2% and 28.7% for an AUC of 0.62.[115]

Activin-A is a glycoprotein produced by the placenta, endothelium, and mononuclear cells that has been reported to be increased during preeclampsia. A study by Lai and colleagues[116] found that, in the third trimester, the detection rate for preeclampsia was 36% (95% CI, 22.9–50.8) and it increased to 50% when used in combination with maternal characteristics (95% CI, 35.5–64.5) for an AUC of 0.722 and 0.772, respectively.

Because it has been proposed that a potential mechanism for preeclampsia is via inflammatory mediators some of those have been studied as markers for the disease.[117] TNF-α and its receptor TNF-R1 are known to be increased in preeclampsia.[118] A case-control study by Mosimann and colleagues[119] evaluated TNF-R1 levels at 30 to 33 weeks as a predictor for preeclampsia. It revealed poor predictive capabilities with a detection rate of 28% (95% CI, 16.2–44.6) when measured with a false-positive rate of 10% (AUC, 0.645; 95% CI, 0588–0.7). When combined with maternal characteristics its detection rate increased to 40% (95% CI, 26.4–54.8) with an AUC of 0.777 (95% CI, 0.726–0.823).[119]

The same authors also published the result of other cytokines including macrophage inflammatory protein 1-alpha (MIP-1α), IL-8, IP10 (Interferon gamma-induced protein 10), MIP-1β, IL-18, were lower in preeclampsia than in control group, but in most cases they were either not detectable in the control or preeclampsia groups, or it was detected in less than 10% of each group, the only markers that were consistently detected were IL-1β, IL-1ra, IL-10, and MIP-1β (among others), but there were no differences in levels between the groups. They concluded that the cytokines did not provide prediction for preeclampsia.[120]

In a recent paper, Bakalis and colleagues[121] studied the use of different biomarkers for the screening of SGA at 30 to 34 weeks; the study included 490 subjects delivered with SGA and 9360 controls. They analyzed the prediction characteristics of PIGF, SFlt-1, PAPP-A, free βhCG, and AFP within 5 weeks of the testing and after 5 weeks. The MoM of PIGF and AFP were lower in the group affected with SGA of less than the fifth percentile and delivered within 5 weeks, whereas in the group delivered more than 5 weeks after the same biomarkers plus PAPP-A were lower. The values of sFlt-1 and β-hCG were higher in the group affected with SGA. The best performance for detection was by using a combination of maternal factors, EFW and PIGF, with a detection rate for a 10% false positive of 85% to 92% for SGA a less that the 10th or 3rd percentiles, respectively, when delivered within 5 weeks (AUC for SGA <10th of 0.953 [95% CI, 0.948–0.957] and of 0.98 [95% CI, 0.977–0.983] for SGA <3rd). For the subjects who delivered after 5 weeks the detection rate of this combination of markers was 57% at SGA less than 10% and 70.5% at SGA less than 3%, with an AUC of 0.844 (95% CI, 0.836–0.851) and 0.895 (95% CI, 0.889–0.901), respectively.[121]

Use of Doppler Ultrasonography for the Prediction of Preeclampsia and Intrauterine Growth Restriction in the Third Trimester

Uterine artery Doppler ultrasonography has been investigated and used as a marker of or surrogate for uteroplacental blood flow and its changes can predict groups at high risk of developing fetal growth restriction and preeclampsia.[122,123] As mentioned, it has been used widely in the first and second trimesters for the prediction of these conditions. More recently, Shwarzman and colleagues[124] in a prospective study found that patients with unilateral abnormal uterine artery Doppler waveforms have a higher risk of having a SGA neonate, lower APGAR scores, cesarean delivery, or a preterm delivery; when both uterine arteries had abnormal Doppler waveforms, the risk for IUGR and preeclampsia was also increased ($P = .01$).

A combination of maternal characteristics and uterine artery Doppler waveforms after 30 weeks has been reported to increase the ability to identify women at risk for development of preeclampsia. Bakalis and colleagues[125] in 2015 found that use of maternal characteristics plus EFW, uterine artery Doppler waveforms at a 10% false-positive rate they could predict 81.6% (95% CI, 77.6–85.2) of the SGA fetus who delivered within 5 weeks from the tests. Lai and colleagues[126] found that, for combination of maternal characteristics and uterine artery PI, the detection rate for intermediate preeclampsia (34–37 weeks) and late preeclampsia (after 38 weeks) were 70.3% and 54.6% respectively, for a 10% fixed false-positive rate. Conversely, Fadigas and associates[127] found no improvement in detection rates for SGA when uterine artery PI was a combined with maternal factor, fetal biometry, and MAP when compared with maternal factors and EFW alone.

In patients with an EFW at less than the 10th percentile screened at 30 to 40 weeks gestation, Lobmaier and colleagues[128] found that patients who developed preeclampsia had an higher uterine artery PI, low cerebroplacental Doppler ratio (uterine artery PI/middle cerebral artery PI), low PIGF, and high sFlt-1, but that the AUC for detecting preeclampsia was similar to that of uterine artery PI at 0.852 (95% CI, 0.792–0.918) and sFlt-1 at 0.839 (95% CI, 0.759–0.918), alone or in combination 0.86 (95% CI, 0.802–0.917).

SUMMARY AND FUTURE PERSPECTIVES

Accurate prediction of preeclampsia and IUGR is important for identifying those women who require more intensive monitoring, permit earlier recognition and intervention, allow targeting of potential preventive measures to those at risk, and timing interventions before the underlying condition is established. The ideal screening test for preeclampsia and IUGR must have high positive and low negative likelihood ratios to overcome their relatively low incidence rates, and be simple, acceptable, rapid, noninvasive, inexpensive, and feasible early in pregnancy with widely available technology. Currently, none of the screening tests meets these criteria. Although different measures of placental dysfunction have been associated with increased risk of adverse pregnancy outcomes, the ability of any single measure to accurately predict these outcomes is poor. Attempts to use predictive models combining analytes and measurements of placental structure and blood flow have so far produced mixed results, but provide useful insights for future research. The use of first-, second-, and third-trimester biochemical markers in combination with uterine artery Doppler screening may have the greatest potential as a screening tool. Finally, improvement in our knowledge of the pathogenesis of preeclampsia and IUGR will facilitate the development of novel modalities for prediction and intervention.

REFERENCES

1. McIntire DD, Bloom SL, Casey BM, et al. Birth weight in relation to morbidity and mortality among newborn infants. N Engl J Med 1999;340(16):1234–8.
2. Kaufmann P, Black S, Huppertz B. Endovascular trophoblast invasion: implications for the pathogenesis of intrauterine growth retardation and preeclampsia. Biol Reprod 2003;69(1):1–7.
3. Roberts JM, Cooper DW. Pathogenesis and genetics of pre-eclampsia. Lancet 2001;357(9249):53–6.
4. Caniggia I, Winter J, Lye SJ, et al. Oxygen and placental development during the first trimester: implications for the pathophysiology of pre-eclampsia. Placenta 2000;21(Suppl A):S25–30.
5. Scifres CM, Nelson DM. Intrauterine growth restriction, human placental development and trophoblast cell death. J Physiol 2009;587(Pt 14):3453–8.

6. Burton GJ, Woods AW, Jauniaux E, et al. Rheological and physiological consequences of conversion of the maternal spiral arteries for uteroplacental blood flow during human pregnancy. Placenta 2009;30(6):473–82.

7. Roberts JM, Taylor RN, Musci TJ, et al. Preeclampsia: an endothelial cell disorder. Am J Obstet Gynecol 1989;161(5):1200–4.

8. Hsu CD, Iriye B, Johnson TR, et al. Elevated circulating thrombomodulin in severe preeclampsia. Am J Obstet Gynecol 1993;169(1):148–9.

9. Mills JL, DerSimonian R, Raymond E, et al. Prostacyclin and thromboxane changes predating clinical onset of preeclampsia: a multicenter prospective study. JAMA 1999;282(4):356–62.

10. Taylor RN, Crombleholme WR, Friedman SA, et al. High plasma cellular fibronectin levels correlate with biochemical and clinical features of preeclampsia but cannot be attributed to hypertension alone. Am J Obstet Gynecol 1991; 165(4 Pt 1):895–901.

11. Vatten LJ, Skjaerven R. Is pre-eclampsia more than one disease? BJOG 2004; 111(4):298–302.

12. Moldenhauer JS, Stanek J, Warshak C, et al. The frequency and severity of placental findings in women with preeclampsia are gestational age dependent. Am J Obstet Gynecol 2003;189(4):1173–7.

13. Egbor M, Ansari T, Morris N, et al. Morphometric placental villous and vascular abnormalities in early- and late-onset pre-eclampsia with and without fetal growth restriction. BJOG 2006;113(5):580–9.

14. Melchiorre K, Wormald B, Leslie K, et al. First-trimester uterine artery Doppler indices in term and preterm pre-eclampsia. Ultrasound Obstet Gynecol 2008; 32(2):133–7.

15. von Dadelszen P, Magee LA, Roberts JM. Subclassification of preeclampsia. Hypertens Pregnancy 2003;22(2):143–8.

16. Schulz KF, Grimes DA, editors. The lancet handbook of essential concepts in clinical research. New York: Elsevier; 2006.

17. Jaeschke R, Guyatt GH, Sackett DL. Users' guides to the medical literature. III. How to use an article about a diagnostic test. B. What are the results and will they help me in caring for my patients? The Evidence-Based Medicine Working Group. JAMA 1994;271(9):703–7.

18. Lang TA, Secic M. How to report statistics in medicine. Philadelphia: American College of Physicians; 1997.

19. Lindheimer MD, Roberts J, Cunningham FG, editors. Chesley's hypertensive disorders in pregnancy. 3rd edition. Oxford: Elsevier Inc; 2009.

20. Riegelman RK, Rinke H, editors. Studying a study and testing a test. 2nd edition. Boston: Little, Brown and Co.; 1987.

21. Villar J, Say L, Shennan A, et al. Methodological and technical issues related to the diagnosis, screening, prevention, and treatment of pre-eclampsia and eclampsia. Int J Gynaecol Obstet 2004;85(Suppl 1):S28–41.

22. Farag K, Hassan I, Ledger WL. Prediction of preeclampsia: can it be achieved? Obstet Gynecol Surv 2004;59(6):464–82 [quiz: 485].

23. Conde-Agudelo A, Villar J, Lindheimer M. World Health Organization systematic review of screening tests for preeclampsia. Obstet Gynecol 2004;104(6): 1367–91.

24. Pilalis A, Souka AP, Antsaklis P, et al. Screening for pre-eclampsia and fetal growth restriction by uterine artery Doppler and PAPP-A at 11–14 weeks' gestation. Ultrasound Obstet Gynecol 2007;29(2):135–40.

25. Toal M, Keating S, Machin G, et al. Determinants of adverse perinatal outcome in high-risk women with abnormal uterine artery Doppler images. Am J Obstet Gynecol 2008;198(3):330.e1–7.

26. Cnossen JS, Morris RK, ter Riet G, et al. Use of uterine artery Doppler ultrasonography to predict pre-eclampsia and intrauterine growth restriction: a systematic review and bivariable meta-analysis. CMAJ 2008;178(6):701–11.

27. Conde-Agudelo A, Lindheimer M. Use of Doppler ultrasonography to predict pre-eclampsia. CMAJ 2008;179(1):53 [author reply: 53–4].

28. Pretorius DH, Nelson TR, Baergen RN, et al. Imaging of placental vasculature using three-dimensional ultrasound and color power Doppler: a preliminary study. Ultrasound Obstet Gynecol 1998;12(1):45–9.

29. Konje JC, Huppertz B, Bell SC, et al. 3-dimensional colour power angiography for staging human placental development. Lancet 2003;362(9391):1199–201.

30. Hafner E, Metzenbauer M, Höfinger D, et al. Comparison between three-dimensional placental volume at 12 weeks and uterine artery impedance/notching at 22 weeks in screening for pregnancy-induced hypertension, pre-eclampsia and fetal growth restriction in a low-risk population. Ultrasound Obstet Gynecol 2006;27(6):652–7.

31. Rizzo G, Capponi A, Pietrolucci ME, et al. Effects of maternal cigarette smoking on placental volume and vascularization measured by 3-dimensional power Doppler ultrasonography at 11+0 to 13+6 weeks of gestation. Am J Obstet Gynecol 2009;200(4):415.e1–5.

32. Matijevic R, Kurjak A. The assessment of placental blood vessels by three-dimensional power Doppler ultrasound. J Perinat Med 2002;30(1):26–32.

33. Merce LT, Barco MJ, Bau S. Reproducibility of the study of placental vascularization by three-dimensional power Doppler. J Perinat Med 2004;32(3):228–33.

34. Tuuli MG, Houser M, Odibo L, et al. Validation of placental vascular sonobiopsy for obtaining representative placental vascular indices by three-dimensional power Doppler ultrasonography. Placenta 2010;31(3):192–6.

35. Merce LT, Barco MJ, Bau S, et al. Assessment of placental vascularization by three-dimensional power Doppler "vascular biopsy" in normal pregnancies. Croat Med J 2005;46(5):765–71.

36. Noguchi J, Hata K, Tanaka H, et al. Placental vascular sonobiopsy using three-dimensional power Doppler ultrasound in normal and growth restricted fetuses. Placenta 2009;30(5):391–7.

37. Guiot C, Gaglioti P, Oberto M, et al. Is three-dimensional power Doppler ultrasound useful in the assessment of placental perfusion in normal and growth-restricted pregnancies? Ultrasound Obstet Gynecol 2008;31(2):171–6.

38. Raine-Fenning NJ, Welsh AW, Jones NW, et al. Methodological considerations for the correct application of quantitative three-dimensional power Doppler angiography. Ultrasound Obstet Gynecol 2008;32(1):115–7 [author reply: 117–8].

39. Raine-Fenning NJ, Nordin NM, Ramnarine KV, et al. Determining the relationship between three-dimensional power Doppler data and true blood flow characteristics: an in-vitro flow phantom experiment. Ultrasound Obstet Gynecol 2008;32(4):540–50.

40. Raine-Fenning NJ, Nordin NM, Ramnarine KV, et al. Evaluation of the effect of machine settings on quantitative three-dimensional power Doppler angiography: an in-vitro flow phantom experiment. Ultrasound Obstet Gynecol 2008;32(4):551–9.

41. Schulten-Wijman MJ, Struijk PC, Brezinka C, et al. Evaluation of volume vascularization index and flow index: a phantom study. Ultrasound Obstet Gynecol 2008;32(4):560–4.
42. Viero S, Chaddha V, Alkazaleh F, et al. Prognostic value of placental ultrasound in pregnancies complicated by absent end-diastolic flow velocity in the umbilical arteries. Placenta 2004;25(8–9):735–41.
43. Toal M, Chan C, Fallah S, et al. Usefulness of a placental profile in high-risk pregnancies. Am J Obstet Gynecol 2007;196(4):363.e1–7.
44. Redman CW. Current topic: pre-eclampsia and the placenta. Placenta 1991; 12(4):301–8.
45. Thomas RL, Blakemore KJ. Evaluation of elevations in maternal serum alpha-fetoprotein: a review. Obstet Gynecol Surv 1990;45(5):269–83.
46. Costa SL, Proctor L, Dodd JM, et al. Screening for placental insufficiency in high-risk pregnancies: is earlier better? Placenta 2008;29(12):1034–40.
47. Cindrova-Davies T, Spasic-Boskovic O, Jauniaux E, et al. Nuclear factor-kappa B, p38, and stress-activated protein kinase mitogen-activated protein kinase signaling pathways regulate proinflammatory cytokines and apoptosis in human placental explants in response to oxidative stress: effects of antioxidant vitamins. Am J Pathol 2007;170(5):1511–20.
48. Hung TH, Charnock-Jones DS, Skepper JN, et al. Secretion of tumor necrosis factor-alpha from human placental tissues induced by hypoxia-reoxygenation causes endothelial cell activation in vitro: a potential mediator of the inflammatory response in preeclampsia. Am J Pathol 2004;164(3):1049–61.
49. Tjoa ML, Cindrova-Davies T, Spasic-Boskovic O, et al. Trophoblastic oxidative stress and the release of cell-free feto-placental DNA. Am J Pathol 2006;169(2):400–4.
50. Redman CW. Platelets and the beginnings of preeclampsia. N Engl J Med 1990; 323(7):478–80.
51. Bosio PM, Cannon S, McKenna PJ, et al. Plasma P-selectin is elevated in the first trimester in women who subsequently develop pre-eclampsia. BJOG 2001;108(7):709–15.
52. Morris RK, Cnossen JS, Langejans M, et al. Serum screening with Down's syndrome markers to predict pre-eclampsia and small for gestational age: systematic review and meta-analysis. BMC Pregnancy Childbirth 2008;8:33.
53. Ito N, Nomura S, Iwase A, et al. ADAMs, a disintegrin and metalloproteinases, mediate shedding of oxytocinase. Biochem Biophys Res Commun 2004; 314(4):1008–13.
54. Iba K, Albrechtsen R, Gilpin B, et al. The cysteine-rich domain of human ADAM 12 supports cell adhesion through syndecans and triggers signaling events that lead to beta1 integrin-dependent cell spreading. J Cell Biol 2000;149(5): 1143–56.
55. Laigaard J, Sørensen T, Placing S, et al. Reduction of the disintegrin and metalloprotease ADAM12 in preeclampsia. Obstet Gynecol 2005;106(1):144–9.
56. Spencer K, Cowans NJ, Stamatopoulou A. ADAM12s in maternal serum as a potential marker of pre-eclampsia. Prenat Diagn 2008;28(3):212–6.
57. Cowans NJ, Spencer K. First-trimester ADAM12 and PAPP-A as markers for intrauterine fetal growth restriction through their roles in the insulin-like growth factor system. Prenat Diagn 2007;27(3):264–71.
58. Poon LC, Chelemen T, Granvillano O, et al. First-trimester maternal serum a disintegrin and metalloprotease 12 (ADAM12) and adverse pregnancy outcome. Obstet Gynecol 2008;112(5):1082–90.

59. Nicolaides KH, Bindra R, Turan OM, et al. A novel approach to first-trimester screening for early pre-eclampsia combining serum PP-13 and Doppler ultrasound. Ultrasound Obstet Gynecol 2006;27(1):13–7.

60. Chafetz I, Kuhnreich I, Sammar M, et al. First-trimester placental protein 13 screening for preeclampsia and intrauterine growth restriction. Am J Obstet Gynecol 2007;197(1):35.e1–7.

61. Sekizawa A, Purwosunu Y, Yoshimura S, et al. PP13 mRNA expression in trophoblasts from preeclamptic placentas. Reprod Sci 2009;16(4):408–13.

62. Cowans NJ, Spencer K, Meiri H. First-trimester maternal placental protein 13 levels in pregnancies resulting in adverse outcomes. Prenat Diagn 2008; 28(2):121–5.

63. Romero R, Kusanovic JP, Than NG, et al. First-trimester maternal serum PP13 in the risk assessment for preeclampsia. Am J Obstet Gynecol 2008;199(2): 122.e1–11.

64. Gonen R, Shahar R, Grimpel YI, et al. Placental protein 13 as an early marker for pre-eclampsia: a prospective longitudinal study. BJOG 2008;115(12):1465–72.

65. Huppertz B, Sammar M, Chefetz I, et al. Longitudinal determination of serum placental protein 13 during development of preeclampsia. Fetal Diagn Ther 2008;24(3):230–6.

66. Schneuer FJ, Nassar N, Khambalia AZ, et al. First trimester screening of maternal placental protein 13 for predicting preeclampsia and small for gestational age: in-house study and systematic review. Placenta 2012;33(9):735–40.

67. Akolekar R, Syngelaki A, Beta J, et al. Maternal serum placental protein 13 at 11-13 weeks of gestation in preeclampsia. Prenat Diagn 2009;29(12):1103–8.

68. Maynard S, Epstein FH, Karumanchi SA. Preeclampsia and angiogenic imbalance. Annu Rev Med 2008;59:61–78.

69. Powers RW, Roberts JM, Cooper KM, et al. Maternal serum soluble fms-like tyrosine kinase 1 concentrations are not increased in early pregnancy and decrease more slowly postpartum in women who develop preeclampsia. Am J Obstet Gynecol 2005;193(1):185–91.

70. Maynard SE, Min JY, Merchan J, et al. Excess placental soluble fms-like tyrosine kinase 1 (sFlt1) may contribute to endothelial dysfunction, hypertension, and proteinuria in preeclampsia. J Clin Invest 2003;111(5):649–58.

71. Sugimoto H, Hamano Y, Charytan D, et al. Neutralization of circulating vascular endothelial growth factor (VEGF) by anti-VEGF antibodies and soluble VEGF receptor 1 (sFlt-1) induces proteinuria. J Biol Chem 2003;278(15):12605–8.

72. Taylor RN, Grimwood J, Taylor RS, et al. Longitudinal serum concentrations of placental growth factor: evidence for abnormal placental angiogenesis in pathologic pregnancies. Am J Obstet Gynecol 2003;188(1):177–82.

73. Crispi F, Llurba E, Domínguez C, et al. Predictive value of angiogenic factors and uterine artery Doppler for early- versus late-onset pre-eclampsia and intrauterine growth restriction. Ultrasound Obstet Gynecol 2008;31(3):303–9.

74. Thadhani R, Mutter WP, Wolf M, et al. First trimester placental growth factor and soluble fms-like tyrosine kinase 1 and risk for preeclampsia. J Clin Endocrinol Metab 2004;89(2):770–5.

75. Teixeira PG, Cabral AC, Andrade SP, et al. Placental growth factor (PlGF) is a surrogate marker in preeclamptic hypertension. Hypertens Pregnancy 2008; 27(1):65–73.

76. Lam C, Lim KH, Karumanchi SA. Circulating angiogenic factors in the pathogenesis and prediction of preeclampsia. Hypertension 2005;46(5):1077–85.

77. Moore Simas TA, Crawford SL, Solitro MJ, et al. Angiogenic factors for the prediction of preeclampsia in high-risk women. Am J Obstet Gynecol 2007;197(3): 244.e1–8.
78. Akolekar R, Zaragoza E, Poon LC, et al. Maternal serum placental growth factor at 11 + 0 to 13 + 6 weeks of gestation in the prediction of pre-eclampsia. Ultrasound Obstet Gynecol 2008;32(6):732–9.
79. Kusanovic JP, Romero R, Chaiworapongsa T, et al. A prospective cohort study of the value of maternal plasma concentrations of angiogenic and anti-angiogenic factors in early pregnancy and midtrimester in the identification of patients destined to develop preeclampsia. J Matern Fetal Neonatal Med 2009;22(11):1021–38.
80. Savvidou MD, Akolekar R, Zaragoza E, et al. First trimester urinary placental growth factor and development of pre-eclampsia. BJOG 2009;116(5):643–7.
81. Rana S, Karumanchi SA, Levine RJ, et al. Sequential changes in antiangiogenic factors in early pregnancy and risk of developing preeclampsia. Hypertension 2007;50(1):137–42.
82. Signore C, Mills JL, Qian C, et al. Circulating soluble endoglin and placental abruption. Prenat Diagn 2008;28(9):852–8.
83. Baumann MU, Bersinger NA, Mohaupt MG, et al. First-trimester serum levels of soluble endoglin and soluble fms-like tyrosine kinase-1 as first-trimester markers for late-onset preeclampsia. Am J Obstet Gynecol 2008;199(3):266.e1–6.
84. Hsu-Lin S, Berman CL, Furie BC, et al. A platelet membrane protein expressed during platelet activation and secretion. Studies using a monoclonal antibody specific for thrombin-activated platelets. J Biol Chem 1984;259(14):9121–6.
85. Larsen E, Celi A, Gilbert GE, et al. PADGEM protein: a receptor that mediates the interaction of activated platelets with neutrophils and monocytes. Cell 1989;59(2):305–12.
86. Halim A, Kanayama N, el Maradny E, et al. Plasma P selectin (GMP-140) and glycocalicin are elevated in preeclampsia and eclampsia: their significances. Am J Obstet Gynecol 1996;174(1 Pt 1):272–7.
87. Banzola I, Farina A, Concu M, et al. Performance of a panel of maternal serum markers in predicting preeclampsia at 11-15 weeks' gestation. Prenat Diagn 2007;27(11):1005–10.
88. Spencer K, Yu CK, Rembouskos G, et al. First trimester sex hormone-binding globulin and subsequent development of preeclampsia or other adverse pregnancy outcomes. Hypertens Pregnancy 2005;24(3):303–11.
89. Williams MA, Farrand A, Mittendorf R, et al. Maternal second trimester serum tumor necrosis factor-alpha-soluble receptor p55 (sTNFp55) and subsequent risk of preeclampsia. Am J Epidemiol 1999;149(4):323–9.
90. Serin IS, Ozçelik B, Basbug M, et al. Predictive value of tumor necrosis factor alpha (TNF-alpha) in preeclampsia. Eur J Obstet Gynecol Reprod Biol 2002; 100(2):143–5.
91. Schipper EJ, Bolte AC, Schalkwijk CG, et al. TNF-receptor levels in preeclampsia–results of a longitudinal study in high-risk women. J Matern Fetal Neonatal Med 2005;18(5):283–7.
92. Leal AM, Poon LC, Frisova V, et al. First-trimester maternal serum tumor necrosis factor receptor-1 and pre-eclampsia. Ultrasound Obstet Gynecol 2009;33(2): 135–41.
93. Wolf M, Sandler L, Muñoz K, et al. First trimester insulin resistance and subsequent preeclampsia: a prospective study. J Clin Endocrinol Metab 2002;87(4): 1563–8.

94. D'Anna R, Baviera G, Corrado F, et al. Adiponectin and insulin resistance in early- and late-onset pre-eclampsia. BJOG 2006;113(11):1264–9.

95. Moses EK, Lade JA, Guo G, et al. A genome scan in families from Australia and New Zealand confirms the presence of a maternal susceptibility locus for pre-eclampsia, on chromosome 2. Am J Hum Genet 2000;67(6):1581–5.

96. Harrison GA, Humphrey KE, Jones N, et al. A genomewide linkage study of pre-eclampsia/eclampsia reveals evidence for a candidate region on 4q. Am J Hum Genet 1997;60(5):1158–67.

97. Farina A, Sekizawa A, De Sanctis P, et al. Gene expression in chorionic villous samples at 11 weeks' gestation from women destined to develop preeclampsia. Prenat Diagn 2008;28(10):956–61.

98. Founds SA, Conley YP, Lyons-Weiler JF, et al. Altered global gene expression in first trimester placentas of women destined to develop preeclampsia. Placenta 2009;30(1):15–24.

99. Alberry MS, Maddocks DG, Hadi MA, et al. Quantification of cell free fetal DNA in maternal plasma in normal pregnancies and in pregnancies with placental dysfunction. Am J Obstet Gynecol 2009;200(1):98.e1–6.

100. Caramelli E, Rizzo N, Concu M, et al. Cell-free fetal DNA concentration in plasma of patients with abnormal uterine artery Doppler waveform and intrauterine growth restriction–a pilot study. Prenat Diagn 2003;23(5):367–71.

101. Holzgreve W, Ghezzi F, Di Naro E, et al. Disturbed feto-maternal cell traffic in preeclampsia. Obstet Gynecol 1998;91(5 Pt 1):669–72.

102. Lo YM, Leung TN, Tein MS, et al. Quantitative abnormalities of fetal DNA in maternal serum in preeclampsia. Clin Chem 1999;45(2):184–8.

103. DiFederico E, Genbacev O, Fisher SJ. Preeclampsia is associated with widespread apoptosis of placental cytotrophoblasts within the uterine wall. Am J Pathol 1999;155(1):293–301.

104. Cotter AM, Martin CM, O'leary JJ, et al. Increased fetal DNA in the maternal circulation in early pregnancy is associated with an increased risk of preeclampsia. Am J Obstet Gynecol 2004;191(2):515–20.

105. Crowley A, Martin C, Fitzpatrick P, et al. Free fetal DNA is not increased before 20 weeks in intrauterine growth restriction or pre-eclampsia. Prenat Diagn 2007; 27(2):174–9.

106. NCI-NHGRI Working Group on Replication in Association Studies, Chanock SJ, Manolio T, et al. Replicating genotype-phenotype associations. Nature 2007; 447(7145):655–60.

107. Poon LC, Maiz N, Valencia C, et al. First-trimester maternal serum pregnancy-associated plasma protein-A and pre-eclampsia. Ultrasound Obstet Gynecol 2009;33(1):23–33.

108. Plasencia W, Maiz N, Poon L, et al. Uterine artery Doppler at 11 + 0 to 13 + 6 weeks and 21 + 0 to 24 + 6 weeks in the prediction of pre-eclampsia. Ultrasound Obstet Gynecol 2008;32(2):138–46.

109. Sibai B, Dekker G, Kupferminc M. Pre-eclampsia. Lancet 2005;365(9461): 785–99.

110. Espinoza J, Romero R, Nien JK, et al. Identification of patients at risk for early onset and/or severe preeclampsia with the use of uterine artery Doppler velocimetry and placental growth factor. Am J Obstet Gynecol 2007;196(4): 326.e1–13.

111. Poon LC, Kametas NA, Maiz N, et al. First-trimester prediction of hypertensive disorders in pregnancy. Hypertension 2009;53(5):812–8.

112. Poon LC, Karagiannis G, Leal A, et al. Hypertensive disorders in pregnancy: screening by uterine artery Doppler imaging and blood pressure at 11-13 weeks. Ultrasound Obstet Gynecol 2009;34(5):497–502.

113. Valino N, Giunta G, Gallo DM, et al. Biophysical and biochemical markers at 30-34 weeks' gestation in the prediction of adverse perinatal outcome. Ultrasound Obstet Gynecol 2015;47(2):194–202.

114. Valino N, Giunta G, Gallo DM, et al. Biophysical and biochemical markers at 35-37 weeks' gestation in the prediction of adverse perinatal outcome. Ultrasound Obstet Gynecol 2016;47:203–9.

115. Chaiworapongsa T, Romero R, Korzeniewski SJ, et al. Maternal plasma concentrations of angiogenic/antiangiogenic factors in the third trimester of pregnancy to identify the patient at risk for stillbirth at or near term and severe late preeclampsia. Am J Obstet Gynecol 2013;208(4):287.e1–15.

116. Lai J, Pinas A, Syngelaki A, et al. Maternal serum activin-A at 30-33 weeks in the prediction of preeclampsia. J Matern Fetal Neonatal Med 2013;26(8):733–7.

117. Conrad KP, Benyo DF. Placental cytokines and the pathogenesis of preeclampsia. Am J Reprod Immunol 1997;37(3):240–9.

118. Vince GS, Starkey PM, Austgulen R, et al. Interleukin-6, tumour necrosis factor and soluble tumour necrosis factor receptors in women with pre-eclampsia. Br J Obstet Gynaecol 1995;102(1):20–5.

119. Mosimann B, Wagner M, Birdir C, et al. Maternal serum tumour necrosis factor receptor 1 (TNF-R1) at 30-33 weeks in the prediction of preeclampsia. J Matern Fetal Neonatal Med 2013;26(8):763–7.

120. Mosimann B, Wagner M, Poon LC, et al. Maternal serum cytokines at 30-33 weeks in the prediction of preeclampsia. Prenat Diagn 2013;33(9):823–30.

121. Bakalis S, Gallo DM, Mendez O, et al. Prediction of small-for-gestational-age neonates: screening by maternal biochemical markers at 30-34 weeks. Ultrasound Obstet Gynecol 2015;46(2):208–15.

122. Campbell S, Diaz-Recasens J, Griffin DR, et al. New Doppler technique for assessing uteroplacental blood flow. Lancet 1983;1(8326 Pt 1):675–7.

123. Espinoza J, Romero R, Mee Kim Y, et al. Normal and abnormal transformation of the spiral arteries during pregnancy. J Perinat Med 2006;34(6):447–58.

124. Shwarzman P, Waintraub AY, Frieger M, et al. Third-trimester abnormal uterine artery Doppler findings are associated with adverse pregnancy outcomes. J Ultrasound Med 2013;32(12):2107–13.

125. Bakalis S, Stoilov B, Akolekar R, et al. Prediction of small-for-gestational-age neonates: screening by uterine artery Doppler and mean arterial pressure at 30-34 weeks. Ultrasound Obstet Gynecol 2015;45(6):707–14.

126. Lai J, Poon LC, Pinas A, et al. Uterine artery Doppler at 30-33 weeks' gestation in the prediction of preeclampsia. Fetal Diagn Ther 2013;33(3):156–63.

127. Fadigas C, Guerra L, Garcia-Tizon Larroca S, et al. Prediction of small-for-gestational-age neonates: screening by uterine artery Doppler and mean arterial pressure at 35-37 weeks. Ultrasound Obstet Gynecol 2015;45(6):715–21.

128. Lobmaier SM, Figueras F, Mercade I, et al. Angiogenic factors vs Doppler surveillance in the prediction of adverse outcome among late-pregnancy small-for-gestational-age fetuses. Ultrasound Obstet Gynecol 2014;43(5):533–40.

Maternal Serum Analytes as Predictors of Fetal Growth Restriction with Different Degrees of Placental Vascular Dysfunction

Matthew J. Blitz, MD, MBA*, Burton Rochelson, MD,
Nidhi Vohra, MD

KEYWORDS

- Serum analytes • Doppler velocimetry • Placental vascular dysfunction
- Placental pathology • Fetal growth restriction
- Absent or reverse end-diastolic velocity

KEY POINTS

- Abnormal levels of maternal serum analytes have been associated with perinatal complications such as fetal growth restriction (FGR) and preeclampsia secondary to placental vascular dysfunction.
- Placental vascular dysfunction can be assessed by direct and indirect methods, which include abnormal Doppler velocimetry and abnormal placental pathology.
- The ability to accurately predict adverse perinatal outcomes due to placental dysfunction remains elusive.
- A combination of abnormal analytes and absent or reversed end-diastolic velocity of the umbilical artery may identify FGR fetuses at highest risk of adverse outcomes.

INTRODUCTION

Fetal growth restriction (FGR), also referred to as intrauterine growth restriction (IUGR), is a significant cause of fetal and neonatal morbidity and mortality. The term generally describes a fetus that has not reached its growth potential because of fetal, placental, or maternal factors. Accurately identifying the FGR fetuses at highest risk for

Conflict of Interest: The authors declare no conflict of interest.
Division of Maternal-Fetal Medicine, Department of Obstetrics and Gynecology, Hofstra North Shore-LIJ School of Medicine, North Shore University Hospital, 300 Community Drive, Manhasset, NY 11030, USA
* Corresponding author.
E-mail address: mblitz@nshs.edu

Clin Lab Med 36 (2016) 353–367
http://dx.doi.org/10.1016/j.cll.2016.01.006
0272-2712/16/$ – see front matter © 2016 Elsevier Inc. All rights reserved.

adverse perinatal outcomes remains challenging and is of great importance in prenatal screening and antenatal fetal surveillance. The most common definition of FGR is an estimated fetal weight (EFW) less than the 10th percentile for gestational age. However, this description does not distinguish between fetuses that are constitutionally small and those that are pathologically small because of genetic or environmental factors.[1,2] Although multiple etiologic pathways may result in FGR, they often share a final common pathophysiologic mechanism: impaired uteroplacental blood flow.[3]

Invasion of extravillous trophoblasts into the maternal spiral arteries and decidual stroma is essential for successful placental development and function during pregnancy. Early placental development occurs in a hypoxic environment.[4] Endovascular plugs occlude the spiral arteries and prevent maternal blood flow from entering the intervillous space until 10 to 12 weeks of gestation.[5,6] At this time, the maternal intervillous circulation is established and the intraplacental oxygen concentration increases significantly.[7] Disruption and eventual replacement of the smooth muscle of the spiral arterioles with dilated, inelastic tubes devoid of maternal vasomotor control facilitates a high-flow, low-resistance vasculature.[8,9] In normal pregnancy, this corresponds to a decrease in uterine artery (UtA) resistance throughout gestation.[10]

Placental vascular dysfunction or maldevelopment results from deficient trophoblast invasion and spiral artery remodeling during early gestation. Placental vascular dysfunction leads to persistence of a high-resistance vasculature, impaired placental perfusion, oxidative stress, and ischemia-reperfusion injury.[11] The failure of transition of the UtA vascular bed from the normal high-resistance state to one of low resistance, which occurs in normal pregnancies, is associated with early-onset third-trimester complications of pregnancy and may be evaluated using UtA Doppler.

The degree of placental functional impairment can be described by various methods, including abnormal Doppler velocimetry and abnormal placental pathology. Abnormal umbilical artery (UmbA) Doppler, as indicated by absent or reversed end-diastolic velocity (A/REDV), can identify pathologically small fetuses with a severely compromised placental vasculature.[12,13] Placental pathology specimens from affected pregnancies demonstrate abundant fibrin deposition, dysregulated apoptosis, and sparsely branched, abnormally thin, and elongated vessels within the terminal villi representative of impaired angiogenesis.[14,15] Several pregnancy complications and adverse outcomes are associated with these findings, including FGR, preeclampsia, preterm birth, and pregnancy loss, including intrauterine fetal death (IUFD).[16]

Maternal serum biomarkers are widely used to screen for aneuploidy and open neural tube defects (NTD). Abnormal levels of these analytes have also been associated with placental dysfunction and its associated perinatal complications, as described above, in pregnancies with chromosomally normal fetuses.[17–20] However, no single biomarker or combination of biomarkers currently in use has yet been identified as adequate as a screening tool to predict adverse pregnancy outcomes in a low-risk or unselected population.[21,22] The predictive value of these analytes when used in a high-risk population, or in conjunction with other independent physiologic measures such as Doppler analysis, may prove to be higher. Maternal biochemical markers fundamentally reflect fetoplacental function, including endocrine as well as endothelial dysfunction. Reduced placental size and functional capacity may result in decreased production of pregnancy-associated plasma protein-A (PAPP-A) and unconjugated estriol (uE3). Leakage of other proteins, such as human chorionic gonadotropin (hCG), inhibin A, and α-fetoprotein (AFP), into the maternal circulation in increased quantities may occur secondary to placental hypoxia and apoptosis.

The aim of this article is to review the current understanding of the role of maternal serum analytes in predicting FGR secondary to placental vascular dysfunction, primarily as defined by Doppler analysis of the maternal and fetal circulation. First, the heterogeneous nature of FGR is discussed. Next, an overview is provided of the first- and second-trimester maternal serum analytes collected as part of routine screening for aneuploidy and open NTDs. This overview is followed by a discussion of the various methods of evaluating impaired placental function. Although much of the current literature has concentrated on the use of these biomarkers to predict preeclampsia, the focus here is on their ability to predict the FGR fetuses at highest risk for poor perinatal outcome. "Smallness," as Harrington said, "is an observation not a diagnosis."[23] If small fetal size alone is used as an outcome parameter, the efficacy of any test will be limited unless the small size is related to physiologic compromise of the fetoplacental circulation. Similarly, if the end points are FGR and/or preeclampsia at any gestational age, the predictive value of biochemical markers will be lower than if early-onset FGR and preeclampsia are the outcome variables studied. Early-onset FGR and preeclampsia are more likely to be better predicted by either biochemical or physiologic markers than would late onset FGR or preeclampsia.

FETAL GROWTH RESTRICTION

FGR is a heterogeneous condition with a spectrum of severity often determined by the degree of placental vascular compromise.[2] Historically, comparisons between studies have been challenging because of inconsistent terminology that failed to effectively distinguish between pathologically and constitutionally small fetuses. Stricter criteria for FGR, such as EFW less than the 5th percentile or abnormal UmbA Doppler, have been more strongly associated with adverse pregnancy outcomes.[24] Furthermore, it is important to distinguish between early- and late-onset FGR because they represent 2 distinct phenotypes with differences in severity. Early-onset FGR is associated with an increased risk of preeclampsia and a characteristic sequence of fetal deterioration that increases the risk of an IUFD and other adverse perinatal outcomes.[25] Early delivery is frequently required.

The ability to accurately predict which FGR fetuses will experience adverse outcomes has remained elusive. Although the combination of multiple abnormal maternal serum analytes and abnormal Doppler findings is strongly associated with adverse outcomes, the predictive value remains too low to be used as a screening test in a low-risk population. However, by developing prognostic groups for FGR or classifying the stages of fetal deterioration, new understandings of how to approach early diagnosis and intervention may emerge. Stepwise risk stratification of cases based on the severity of UmbA Doppler, as per Roman and colleagues,[17] may improve the predictive value of maternal serum analytes, as discussed later in this review. Stage-based management protocols, which consider the severity of placental insufficiency and the level of suspicion for fetal acidosis, as proposed by Figueras and Gratacos,[26] may minimize variation in clinical practice and improve perinatal outcomes by identifying optimal follow-up intervals and timing of delivery.

MATERNAL SERUM ANALYTES
Overview

Maternal serum screening allows early identification of pregnancies at increased risk for Down syndrome and trisomy 18 and has become a routine component of standard prenatal care. First-trimester screening, performed between 11 and 14 weeks, includes the biochemical markers β-hCG and PAPP-A combined with sonographic measurement of fetal nuchal translucency. In the second trimester, a triple screen (AFP, hCG, uE3) or quadruple screen (AFP, hCG, uE3, inhibin A) is typically offered between 15 and 20 weeks.

The ability to use these analytes, routinely collected for aneuploidy screening, to also detect adverse pregnancy outcomes secondary to placental vascular dysfunction is very appealing. Although they have been associated with adverse pregnancy outcomes in chromosomally normal pregnancies, studies to date suggest suboptimal predictive value of these markers, both individually and in combination. Of these analytes, PAPP-A and inhibin A appear to be the most robust biomarkers for the prediction of adverse pregnancy outcome. The accurate prediction of adverse pregnancy outcomes, before the onset of clinical manifestations, will allow more intensive monitoring in those who might benefit from it and may provide opportunities for prophylactic or therapeutic interventions.

First- and Second-Trimester Biomarkers

Human chorionic gonadotropin

In the first trimester, low free β-hCG levels are associated with adverse pregnancy outcomes, some more consistently than others. Dugoff and colleagues,[27] using data on more than 30,000 women in the United States from the FASTER (First and Second Trimester Evaluation of Risk) trial, demonstrated that free β-hCG levels less than the first percentile at 11 to 14 weeks are associated with early pregnancy loss. However, the association between low levels of free β-hCG and other clinical measures of placental dysfunction is less consistent. Fewer studies have examined elevated free β-hCG in the first trimester, but they have also yielded inconsistent findings.[22]

In the second trimester, an elevated hCG has been associated with FGR and adverse pregnancy outcomes, including preterm birth, preeclampsia, and IUFD. Gonen and colleagues[28] found that women with a second-trimester hCG greater than 2.5 multiple of the median (MoM) had a greater than 4-fold increased risk for hypertensive disorders of pregnancy and a nearly 3-fold increased risk for FGR. Another study noted that in women with an hCG greater than 4.0 MoM, more than 20% had severe adverse outcomes compared with only 10% of matched controls.[29] Low hCG in the first trimester may be a result of impaired placentation and decreased functional capacity, whereas high levels in the second trimester may be an adaptive response to hypoperfusion.[30]

Pregnancy-associated plasma protein-A

Multiple studies have found an association between low first-trimester PAPP-A and pregnancy complications, including FGR, preeclampsia, preterm birth, IUFD, and early miscarriage. The aforementioned study by Dugoff and colleagues[27] found that levels of PAPP-A at or less than the 5th percentile had an increased risk of all of these complications. First-trimester PAPP-A correlates with birth weight, and consequently, low PAPP-A increases the likelihood of having an FGR fetus.[31] A large study in the United Kingdom by Spencer and colleagues,[32] which included more than 46,000 women, found that PAPP-A levels less than the 5th percentile in chromosomally normal pregnancies were associated with a more than 3-fold increased risk of FGR but an overall detection rate of only 14%. Low PAPP-A has been associated with both early- and late-onset preeclampsia, but its predictive value is low unless combined with other maternal factors, biophysical tests, and biochemical markers.[33–36] Similarly, low first-trimester PAPP-A is associated with an increased risk of pregnancy loss at any gestational age but even more so with early pregnancy loss.[37,38] Although consistently associated with adverse outcomes, PAPP-A functions poorly as a screening test for these various complications due to low sensitivity and positive predictive values.

α-Fetoprotein

Many pregnancy complications have been associated with unexplained elevations in maternal serum AFP (MSAFP), including FGR, preeclampsia, preterm birth, placental abruption, and IUFD.[39–41] Multiple large studies have evaluated MSAFP elevations and the risk of having a low birth weight fetus. Although different MoM cutoffs were used, an increased risk was consistently noted, ranging from 2- to 10-fold.[42–44] Waller and colleagues[39] found that women with the highest MSAFP levels have the highest risk of IUFD, with a MoM greater than 3.0 conferring a 10-fold increased risk, whereas a MoM between 2.0 and 2.9 is associated with a 2- to 3-fold increased risk. Despite these many associations, an isolated elevation in MSAFP remains poorly predictive of adverse outcomes as three-fourths of these women will ultimately have a normal pregnancy.[45]

Unconjugated estriol

Low levels of uE3 in the second trimester have been associated with adverse pregnancy outcomes, including FGR, preeclampsia, spontaneous miscarriage, and IUFD.[19,46,47] After controlling for other biomarkers and maternal characteristics, one study found that an uE3 level less than 0.75 MoM was significantly and independently associated with a greater than 6-fold increased risk of FGR.[47]

Inhibin A

Elevated inhibin A in the second trimester may result from premature accelerated differentiation of the villous cytotrophoblasts and has been associated with adverse pregnancy outcomes, including FGR, preeclampsia, preterm birth, and IUFD when greater than 2.0 MoM.[48–50] Overall, studies examining the association between isolated elevations of inhibin A in the maternal serum with FGR and preeclampsia have produced inconsistent results.[51,52] Therefore, like the other analytes discussed, inhibin A is not yet considered useful as a predictive test for adverse outcomes in low-risk, unselected populations.

Combinations of Biomarkers

The readily available maternal serum analytes used for routine prenatal aneuploidy screening, when used individually in isolation, have a low predictive value for adverse pregnancy outcomes. Efforts have been made to combine multiple biomarkers to increase predictive performance.[21,50,53,54] Having 2 or more abnormal markers does significantly increase the risk of adverse outcomes, but the sensitivity and positive predictive value are thought to be too low to be clinically useful in an unselected population.[50] A systematic review by Hui and colleagues[21] found that when AFP and hCG both exceeded 2.5 MoM, the positive likelihood ratios for predicting FGR and preeclampsia were 6.18 and 5.68, respectively, but the confidence intervals were rather wide. A combination of low PAPP-A and high hCG in the first trimester has been associated with increased risk for early-onset severe preeclampsia in one study,[55] but a more comprehensive predictive model by Crovetto and colleagues,[56] which incorporated maternal characteristics, biophysical parameters, and angiogenic factors, did not support this finding in their multivariate analysis.

Comparisons between studies are hindered by significant heterogeneity in terms of the specific combinations of analytes examined, the cutoff values used to define abnormal, and the various adverse outcomes evaluated.[21] Whether a different combination of markers, or use in a more selected population at risk, would enhance the performance of such tests remains to be seen. In addition, most of the studies that have examined analytes in combination have looked at extreme values with dichotomous thresholds. The use of multivariate analysis using continuous values of analytes may also improve test performance.

PLACENTAL VASCULAR DYSFUNCTION
Overview

The severity or extent of placental vascular dysfunction varies based on the degree of deficient trophoblast invasion and spiral artery remodeling in early gestation. The corresponding clinical consequences often manifest at different stages of pregnancy. Although a miscarriage may occur in the first trimester and FGR or preeclampsia may present in the second or third trimesters, all 3 conditions involve a similar underlying pathologic process. An ischemic placenta with a high-resistance vasculature predisposes to hypoperfusion, oxidative stress, and ischemia-reperfusion injury.[11]

Although no combination of currently used biomarkers can accurately predict pathologic FGR and other adverse outcomes resulting from placental dysfunction, tests that also incorporate other parameters, such as Doppler ultrasound findings, and are applied to selected high-risk populations may prove more clinically useful. Placental dysfunction can be assessed by direct and indirect methods, which include abnormal Doppler velocimetry and placental pathology. Abnormal Doppler velocimetry can noninvasively identify a severely compromised placental vasculature.[12,13] Placental pathology specimens from affected pregnancies frequently demonstrate characteristic findings such as abundant fibrin deposition, dysregulated apoptosis, villous infarction, and villous morphologic alterations.[14,15,57]

Doppler studies may allow prophylactic or therapeutic interventions that could improve perinatal outcomes for at-risk FGR fetuses. Identification of such fetuses early in pregnancy allows initiation of prophylactic low-dose aspirin, which has been associated with a reduced incidence of FGR and preeclampsia when started by 16 weeks of gestation.[58] In addition, correlation of abnormal analytes, Doppler blood flow analysis, and placental pathology review may assist in counseling and management of subsequent pregnancies.

Uterine Artery Doppler

Nutrient and oxygen transport across the uterine arteries is essential for fetal and placental growth. Increased resistance to UtA blood flow can be measured in a noninvasive manner by Doppler ultrasound. In normal pregnancy, there is a decrease in UtA resistance throughout gestation, initially from trophoblast invasion of the spiral arteries and later possibly from a continued hormonal effect on the elasticity of the arterial walls.[10] The indices used to measure UtA resistance include systolic to diastolic velocity ratio (S/D), pulsatility index (PI), resistance index (RI), and the presence of persistent diastolic notching. Severe placental dysfunction may be associated with absent or reverse diastolic blood flow, which represents an ominous finding that may precede an IUFD.

Several studies have investigated whether abnormal UtA Dopplers can be used to identify women at risk of developing complications of uteroplacental insufficiency, such as FGR, preeclampsia, and IUFD.[59–62] Results have been inconsistent. Recent systematic reviews and meta-analyses suggest that UtA Doppler alone, in low-risk populations, has an overall poor predictive ability for detecting adverse outcomes.[63–65] More recently, efforts have been made to combine the results of abnormal UtA Dopplers with abnormal serum markers and other maternal or fetal characteristics to improve the predictive value for adverse outcomes.[34,66–68] Roeder and colleagues[69] found that abnormal serum analytes in conjunction with abnormal UtA Dopplers improve the prediction of preeclampsia and FGR by 9- to 15-fold. Crovetto and colleagues[68] developed a first-trimester predictive model for early-onset FGR that incorporated PAPP-A, free β-hCG, maternal blood pressure, and UtA Doppler, that identified 73% of cases at a 15% false positive rate. Overall, such studies have also yielded mixed results and low predictive ability, and therefore, routine screening with UtA Doppler velocimetry is not recommended.

Identification of at-risk FGR fetuses by predictive models that incorporate abnormal UtA Doppler studies early in gestation may allow prophylactic or therapeutic interventions that could improve perinatal outcomes. Initiation of prophylactic low-dose aspirin by 16 weeks of gestation has been associated with a reduced incidence of FGR and preeclampsia.[58] This effect is thought to be related to inhibition of vasoconstriction and platelet aggregation and increased UtA perfusion, thereby optimizing the development of the placental vasculature. The indications, optimal dosing, and most efficacious time of initiation for aspirin administration to prevent adverse outcomes in early-onset FGR have yet to be determined.

Umbilical Artery Doppler

In current clinical practice, UmbA Doppler is most useful for predicting, identifying, and monitoring fetuses with suspected early-onset FGR due to severe placental dysfunction.[70] The indices used to measure UmbA resistance include S/D, PI, and RI. Whereas UtA Doppler assesses placental resistance on the maternal side, UmbA Doppler evaluates placental resistance on the fetal side. When applied to pregnancies suspected of FGR, these 2 methods are comparable for predicting adverse outcomes.[71] When both are abnormal, there may be increased predictive value.

In high-risk pregnancies, Doppler ultrasound may reduce the risk of perinatal deaths and result in less obstetric interventions.[72] However, in low-risk, unselected populations, a recent Cochrane Review reiterated that there is insufficient evidence to support the routine use of UmbA or UtA Doppler.[73]

The authors' group and others have evaluated the combined use of UmbA Doppler and maternal serum biomarkers to predict adverse outcomes. Prior studies have noted that when second-trimester MSAFP is elevated and UmbA Doppler velocimetry is abnormal, there is a strong association with preterm delivery and FGR.[74,75] An elevated inhibin A has also been associated with FGR with abnormal UmbA Doppler.[76]

More recently, at the authors' institution, Roman and colleagues[17] stratified FGR cases by UmbA Doppler (A/REDV, elevated S/D ratio, and normal). Pregnancies with more severe placental dysfunction, as indicated by A/REDV, were more strongly associated with abnormal maternal serum analytes than the FGR fetuses with less severely abnormal or normal UmbA Doppler waveforms and than fetuses that were appropriately grown for gestational age (**Fig. 1**). In addition, by combining first- and second-trimester maternal biomarkers, 73% of FGR-A/REDV cases were identified at a 5% false positive rate (**Table 1**). After including other maternal risk factors such as chronic hypertension and pregestational diabetes, 91% of cases could be detected.

Stratification of FGR cases by UmbA Doppler revealed significant differences in perinatal outcomes. Among the FGR fetuses with A/REDV (n = 90), the mean gestational age at diagnosis was 25.7 ± 5.1 weeks and 82.6% delivered before 34 weeks. In contrast, among the FGR cases with an elevated S/D ratio (n = 46) and those with a normal UmbA Doppler (n = 215), the mean gestational age at diagnosis was 33.8 ± 4.0 weeks and 34.6 ± 4.5 weeks, and 15.2% and 5.6% delivered before

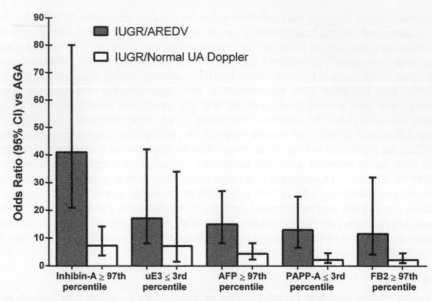

Fig. 1. Association with extreme levels of maternal first- and second-trimester analytes is stronger for IUGR/AREDV compared with IUGR/normal UA Doppler. Markers listed in decreasing order for the IUGR/AREDV group. Odds ratios compare each group to AGA and are adjusted for the existence of maternal risk factors. AGA, appropriately grown for gestational age; CI, confidence interval; FB2, free-β-human chorionic gonadotrophin second trimester; UA, umbilical artery. (*From* Roman A, Desai N, Krantz D, et al. Maternal serum analytes as predictors of IUGR with different degrees of placental vascular dysfunction. Prenat Diagn 2014;34(7):696; with permission.)

34 weeks, respectively. Furthermore, the incidence of preeclampsia was 35% in the FGR-A/REDV group, compared with 15.2% in the FGR-elevated S/D ratio group and 5% in the FGR-normal UmbA Doppler group. Similarly, the rate of fetal death was notably higher in the FGR-A/REDV group at 15.8% compared with 2.2% and 0.5% in the FGR-elevated S/D ratio group and the FGR-normal UmbA Doppler group, respectively.

Early-onset FGR with A/REDV on UmbA Doppler and extreme levels of maternal serum analytes likely represents the end of the spectrum in terms of placental dysfunction and its associated adverse outcomes. Most cases of FGR are likely secondary to more mild placental disease, which UmbA Doppler and serum analytes may fail to identify. Therefore, some have advocated for increased use of the cerebroplacental ratio (CPR), which has been said to correlate better with adverse outcomes than UmbA Doppler alone.[26] Further investigation is needed to determine if abnormal analytes can also predict an abnormal CPR.

Placental Pathology

The histopathological placental findings in FGR are varied, reflecting the heterogeneous nature of FGR. Although one-fourth of FGR cases have no abnormalities identified on routine placental examination, severe early-onset FGR cases are more consistently associated with macroscopic and histologic abnormalities.[57] The most common macroscopic abnormality in FGR placentas is patchy placental infarction,

Table 1
False-positive rate, detection rate, and positive predictive value of intrauterine growth restriction/absent or reversed end-diastolic velocity by biochemistry only or combined with maternal risk factors

	N	Biochemistry[a] Only	Biochemistry + Prior Risk
All patients			
False-positive rate	2590	5%	5%
DR IUGR/AREDV (95% CI)	33	73% (54%–87%)	91% (76%–98%)
DR IUGR/elevated S/D ratio (95% CI)	15	13% (2%–41%)	27% (8%–55%)
DR IUGR/normal Doppler (95% CI)	65	20% (11%–32%)	20% (11%–32%)
PPV[b]	—	1/30	1/24
Patients with no risk factors for IUGR			
False-positive rate	2556	5%	—
DR IUGR/AREDV (95% CI)	22	86% (65%–97%)	—
DR IUGR/elevated S/D ratio (95% CI)	13	15% (2%–45%)	—
DR IUGR/normal Doppler (95% CI)	65	20% (11%–32%)	—
PPV[b]	—	1/43	—

Risk factors for IUGR include chronic hypertension, pregestational diabetes, lupus, and inherited or acquired thrombophilia.

Abbreviations: AGA, appropriately grown for gestational age; CI, confidence interval; DR, detection rate; FPR, false-positive rate; N, number of cases with all 6 maternal serum markers; PPV, positive predictive value.

[a] Biochemistry includes a combination of first- and second-trimester analytes. Cutoff for biochemistry only was likelihood ratio of 2.3. Cutoff for biochemistry + prior risk was 1/280.

[b] PPV based on population incidence rates.

From Roman A, Desai N, Krantz D, et al. Maternal serum analytes as predictors of IUGR with different degrees of placental vascular dysfunction. Prenat Diagn 2014;34(7):696; with permission.

present in approximately one-quarter of cases, but this is also found in some non-FGR pregnancies. Common microscopic findings in FGR placentas include villous infarcts and villous morphologic alterations, such as syncytiotrophoblast "knots," excess cytotrophoblast cells, villous fibrosis, hypovascular terminal villi, reduced villous volume, reduced intervillous space, nonspecific inflammatory lesions, and fibrinoid necrosis.[57]

Abnormal Doppler studies in FGR pregnancies are associated with characteristic placental pathology, which reflects changes in the tertiary stem villi in response to chronic vasoconstriction. Specifically, an increased resistance of UmbA Doppler flow in FGR pregnancies is correlated with smaller placentas, increased vessel wall thickness of tertiary stem villi (due to hypertrophy), and reduced lumen circumference.[77,78] Interestingly, the nature of the placental lesions differ between cases of AEDV and REDV on UmbA Doppler. The AEDV cases have more occlusive lesions with luminal obliteration, and the REDV cases have more poorly vascularized terminal villi, abnormally thin-walled fetal stem vessels, villous stromal hemorrhage, and hemorrhagic endovasculitis.[79] Abnormal UtA Doppler is associated with impaired trophoblast migration in both early-onset FGR and preeclampsia.[57,80]

Studies have examined the association between abnormal levels of maternal serum analytes and abnormal placental pathology. Placental volume is reduced in pregnancies with low maternal serum PAPP-A concentrations, but this is not predictive of adverse pregnancy outcomes.[18,81] In addition, the volume and surface area of terminal villi are significantly decreased in pregnancies complicated by both FGR and low PAPP-A compared with pregnancies with FGR but with normal PAPP-A.[82] An elevated second-trimester hCG or MSAFP is more likely to have pathologic changes in the placenta in pregnancies complicated by FGR.[83]

Despite the association with abnormal Doppler studies and abnormal maternal serum analytes, abnormal placental pathology is a poor indicator of FGR severity, as regression analysis has shown that only 34% of variation in fetal growth is attributable to such lesions.[3] Further investigation is necessary to evaluate the association of specific clinical subgroups of FGR with abnormalities in serum analytes, Doppler studies, and placental pathology.

SUMMARY

The ability to accurately predict adverse perinatal outcomes due to placental dysfunction remains elusive. Combining first- and second-trimester maternal serum analytes with abnormal Doppler findings has increased the predictive value but currently used mathematical modeling techniques have not proven to be sufficient for this combination to be used as a screening test in a low-risk population. Additional studies on the appropriate patients for whom these tests may be more predictive, and on the development of prediction models using multivariate analysis of a combination of markers, may be helpful. More widespread use of cell-free fetal DNA (cffDNA) to predict aneuploidy may lead to a decline in conventional screening methods if that technique is eventually applied to the low-risk obstetric population. However, increased cffDNA in the maternal circulation has also been evaluated as a marker of placental dysfunction and may open new avenues for investigation, especially if combined with other biochemical and physiologic parameters. Nevertheless, at present, the authors recommend continued investigation into the use of first- and second-trimester markers in conjunction with maternal factors and biophysical tests to detect at-risk fetuses. Early identification of high-risk pregnancies with pathologic FGR, which may benefit from increased surveillance and prophylactic or therapeutic intervention, is one of the great goals of perinatology and efforts to develop progressively better predictive models will no doubt continue.

REFERENCES

1. Battaglia FC, Lubchenco LO. A practical classification of newborn infants by weight and gestational age. J Pediatr 1967;71(2):159–63.
2. Figueras F, Gratacos E. Update on the diagnosis and classification of fetal growth restriction and proposal of a stage-based management protocol. Fetal Diagn Ther 2014;36(2):86–98.
3. Salafia CM, Minior VK, Pezzullo JC, et al. Intrauterine growth restriction in infants of less than thirty-two weeks' gestation: associated placental pathologic features. Am J Obstet Gynecol 1995;173(4):1049–57.
4. James JL, Stone PR, Chamley LW. The regulation of trophoblast differentiation by oxygen in the first trimester of pregnancy. Hum Reprod Update 2006;12(2):137–44.
5. Jauniaux E, Gulbis B, Burton GJ. The human first trimester gestational sac limits rather than facilitates oxygen transfer to the foetus–a review. Placenta 2003;24(Suppl A):S86–93.
6. Burton GJ, Jauniaux E, Watson AL. Maternal arterial connections to the placental intervillous space during the first trimester of human pregnancy: the Boyd collection revisited. Am J Obstet Gynecol 1999;181(3):718–24.

7. Jauniaux E, Hempstock J, Greenwold N, et al. Trophoblastic oxidative stress in relation to temporal and regional differences in maternal placental blood flow in normal and abnormal early pregnancies. Am J Pathol 2003;162(1):115–25.

8. Harris LK, Aplin JD. Vascular remodeling and extracellular matrix breakdown in the uterine spiral arteries during pregnancy. Reprod Sci 2007;14(8 Suppl):28–34.

9. Whitley GS, Cartwright JE. Trophoblast-mediated spiral artery remodelling: a role for apoptosis. J Anat 2009;215(1):21–6.

10. Jurkovic D, Jauniaux E, Kurjak A, et al. Transvaginal color Doppler assessment of the uteroplacental circulation in early pregnancy. Obstet Gynecol 1991;77(3):365–9.

11. Prefumo F, Sebire NJ, Thilaganathan B. Decreased endovascular trophoblast invasion in first trimester pregnancies with high-resistance uterine artery Doppler indices. Hum Reprod 2004;19(1):206–9.

12. Morrow RJ, Adamson SL, Bull SB, et al. Effect of placental embolization on the umbilical arterial velocity waveform in fetal sheep. Am J Obstet Gynecol 1989;161(4):1055–60.

13. Spinillo A, Gardella B, Bariselli S, et al. Placental histopathological correlates of umbilical artery Doppler velocimetry in pregnancies complicated by fetal growth restriction. Prenat Diagn 2012;32(13):1263–72.

14. Scifres CM, Nelson DM. Intrauterine growth restriction, human placental development and trophoblast cell death. J Physiol 2009;587(Pt 14):3453–8.

15. Su EJ. Role of the fetoplacental endothelium in fetal growth restriction with abnormal umbilical artery Doppler velocimetry. Am J Obstet Gynecol 2015;213(4 Suppl):S123–30.

16. Burton GJ, Jauniaux E. Placental oxidative stress: from miscarriage to preeclampsia. J Soc Gynecol Investig 2004;11(6):342–52.

17. Roman A, Desai N, Krantz D, et al. Maternal serum analytes as predictors of IUGR with different degrees of placental vascular dysfunction. Prenat Diagn 2014;34(7):692–8.

18. Odibo AO, Patel KR, Spitalnik A, et al. Placental pathology, first-trimester biomarkers and adverse pregnancy outcomes. J Perinatol 2014;34(3):186–91.

19. Yaron Y, Cherry M, Kramer RL, et al. Second-trimester maternal serum marker screening: maternal serum alpha-fetoprotein, beta-human chorionic gonadotropin, estriol, and their various combinations as predictors of pregnancy outcome. Am J Obstet Gynecol 1999;181(4):968–74.

20. Dugoff L, Society for Maternal-Fetal Medicine. First- and second-trimester maternal serum markers for aneuploidy and adverse obstetric outcomes. Obstet Gynecol 2010;115(5):1052–61.

21. Hui D, Okun N, Murphy K, et al. Combinations of maternal serum markers to predict preeclampsia, small for gestational age, and stillbirth: a systematic review. J Obstet Gynaecol Can 2012;34(2):142–53.

22. Morris RK, Cnossen JS, Langejans M, et al. Serum screening with Down's syndrome markers to predict pre-eclampsia and small for gestational age: systematic review and meta-analysis. BMC Pregnancy Childbirth 2008;8:33.

23. Harrington K, Thompson MO, Carpenter RG, et al. Doppler fetal circulation in pregnancies complicated by pre-eclampsia or delivery of a small for gestational age baby: 2. Longitudinal analysis. Br J Obstet Gynaecol 1999;106(5):453–66.

24. Unterscheider J, Daly S, Geary MP, et al. Optimizing the definition of intrauterine growth restriction: the multicenter prospective PORTO Study. Am J Obstet Gynecol 2013;208(4):290.e1–6.

25. Savchev S, Figueras F, Sanz-Cortes M, et al. Evaluation of an optimal gestational age cut-off for the definition of early- and late-onset fetal growth restriction. Fetal Diagn Ther 2014;36(2):99–105.
26. Figueras F, Gratacos E. Stage-based approach to the management of fetal growth restriction. Prenat Diagn 2014;34(7):655–9.
27. Dugoff L, Hobbins JC, Malone FD, et al. First-trimester maternal serum PAPP-A and free-beta subunit human chorionic gonadotropin concentrations and nuchal translucency are associated with obstetric complications: a population-based screening study (the FASTER Trial). Am J Obstet Gynecol 2004;191(4):1446–51.
28. Gonen R, Perez R, David M, et al. The association between unexplained second-trimester maternal serum hCG elevation and pregnancy complications. Obstet Gynecol 1992;80(1):83–6.
29. Lepage N, Chitayat D, Kingdom J, et al. Association between second-trimester isolated high maternal serum maternal serum human chorionic gonadotropin levels and obstetric complications in singleton and twin pregnancies. Am J Obstet Gynecol 2003;188(5):1354–9.
30. Ong CY, Liao AW, Spencer K, et al. First trimester maternal serum free beta human chorionic gonadotrophin and pregnancy associated plasma protein A as predictors of pregnancy complications. BJOG 2000;107(10):1265–70.
31. Peterson SE, Simhan HN. First-trimester pregnancy-associated plasma protein A and subsequent abnormalities of fetal growth. Am J Obstet Gynecol 2008;198(5):e43–5.
32. Spencer K, Cowans NJ, Avgidou K, et al. First-trimester biochemical markers of aneuploidy and the prediction of small-for-gestational age fetuses. Ultrasound Obstet Gynecol 2008;31(1):15–9.
33. Poon LC, Stratieva V, Piras S, et al. Hypertensive disorders in pregnancy: combined screening by uterine artery Doppler, blood pressure and serum PAPP-A at 11-13 weeks. Prenat Diagn 2010;30(3):216–23.
34. Odibo AO, Zhong Y, Goetzinger KR, et al. First-trimester placental protein 13, PAPP-A, uterine artery Doppler and maternal characteristics in the prediction of pre-eclampsia. Placenta 2011;32(8):598–602.
35. Spencer K, Cowans NJ, Nicolaides KH. Low levels of maternal serum PAPP-A in the first trimester and the risk of pre-eclampsia. Prenat Diagn 2008;28(1):7–10.
36. Audibert F, Boucoiran I, An N, et al. Screening for preeclampsia using first-trimester serum markers and uterine artery Doppler in nulliparous women. Am J Obstet Gynecol 2010;203(4):383.e1–8.
37. Spencer K, Cowans NJ, Avgidou K, et al. First-trimester ultrasound and biochemical markers of aneuploidy and the prediction of impending fetal death. Ultrasound Obstet Gynecol 2006;28(5):637–43.
38. Goetzl L, Krantz D, Simpson JL, et al. Pregnancy-associated plasma protein A, free beta-hCG, nuchal translucency, and risk of pregnancy loss. Obstet Gynecol 2004;104(1):30–6.
39. Waller DK, Lustig LS, Cunningham GC, et al. Second-trimester maternal serum alpha-fetoprotein levels and the risk of subsequent fetal death. N Engl J Med 1991;325(1):6–10.
40. Williams MA, Hickok DE, Zingheim RW, et al. Elevated maternal serum alpha-fetoprotein levels and midtrimester placental abnormalities in relation to subsequent adverse pregnancy outcomes. Am J Obstet Gynecol 1992;167(4 Pt 1):1032–7.
41. Simpson JL, Elias S, Morgan CD, et al. Does unexplained second-trimester (15 to 20 weeks' gestation) maternal serum alpha-fetoprotein elevation presage

adverse perinatal outcome? Pitfalls and preliminary studies with late second- and third-trimester maternal serum alpha-fetoprotein. Am J Obstet Gynecol 1991; 164(3):829–36.

42. Milunsky A, Jick SS, Bruell CL, et al. Predictive values, relative risks, and overall benefits of high and low maternal serum alpha-fetoprotein screening in singleton pregnancies: new epidemiologic data. Am J Obstet Gynecol 1989;161(2):291–7.

43. Hamilton MP, Abdalla HI, Whitfield CR. Significance of raised maternal serum alpha-fetoprotein in singleton pregnancies with normally formed fetuses. Obstet Gynecol 1985;65(4):465–70.

44. Burton BK. Outcome of pregnancy in patients with unexplained elevated or low levels of maternal serum alpha-fetoprotein. Obstet Gynecol 1988;72(5):709–13.

45. Crandall BF, Robinson L, Grau P. Risks associated with an elevated maternal serum alpha-fetoprotein level. Am J Obstet Gynecol 1991;165(3):581–6.

46. Kim SY, Kim SK, Lee JS, et al. The prediction of adverse pregnancy outcome using low unconjugated estriol in the second trimester of pregnancy without risk of Down's syndrome. Yonsei Med J 2000;41(2):226–9.

47. Kowalczyk TD, Cabaniss ML, Cusmano L. Association of low unconjugated estriol in the second trimester and adverse pregnancy outcome. Obstet Gynecol 1998; 91(3):396–400.

48. Fitzgerald B, Levytska K, Kingdom J, et al. Villous trophoblast abnormalities in extremely preterm deliveries with elevated second trimester maternal serum hCG or inhibin-A. Placenta 2011;32(4):339–45.

49. Fraser RF 2nd, McAsey ME, Coney P. Inhibin-A and pro-alpha C are elevated in preeclamptic pregnancy and correlate with human chorionic gonadotropin. Am J Reprod Immunol 1998;40(1):37–42.

50. Dugoff L, Hobbins JC, Malone FD, et al. Quad screen as a predictor of adverse pregnancy outcome. Obstet Gynecol 2005;106(2):260–7.

51. Florio P, Ciarmela P, Luisi S, et al. Pre-eclampsia with fetal growth restriction: placental and serum activin A and inhibin A levels. Gynecol Endocrinol 2002; 16(5):365–72.

52. D'Anna R, Baviera G, Corrado F, et al. Is mid-trimester maternal serum inhibin-A a marker of preeclampsia or intrauterine growth restriction? Acta Obstet Gynecol Scand 2002;81(6):540–3.

53. Alkazaleh F, Chaddha V, Viero S, et al. Second-trimester prediction of severe placental complications in women with combined elevations in alpha-fetoprotein and human chorionic gonadotrophin. Am J Obstet Gynecol 2006; 194(3):821–7.

54. Wald NJ, Morris JK. Multiple marker second trimester serum screening for pre-eclampsia. J Med Screen 2001;8(2):65–8.

55. Jelliffe-Pawlowski LL, Baer RJ, Currier RJ, et al. Early-onset severe preeclampsia by first trimester pregnancy-associated plasma protein A and total human chorionic gonadotropin. Am J Perinatol 2015;32(7):703–12.

56. Crovetto F, Figueras F, Triunfo S, et al. First trimester screening for early and late preeclampsia based on maternal characteristics, biophysical parameters, and angiogenic factors. Prenat Diagn 2015;35(2):183–91.

57. Mifsud W, Sebire NJ. Placental pathology in early-onset and late-onset fetal growth restriction. Fetal Diagn Ther 2014;36(2):117–28.

58. Bujold E, Roberge S, Lacasse Y, et al. Prevention of preeclampsia and intrauterine growth restriction with aspirin started in early pregnancy: a meta-analysis. Obstet Gynecol 2010;116(2 Pt 1):402–14.

59. Papageorghiou AT, Yu CK, Bindra R, et al. Multicenter screening for pre-eclampsia and fetal growth restriction by transvaginal uterine artery Doppler at 23 weeks of gestation. Ultrasound Obstet Gynecol 2001;18(5):441–9.

60. Papageorghiou AT, Yu CK, Nicolaides KH. The role of uterine artery Doppler in predicting adverse pregnancy outcome. Best Pract Res Clin Obstet Gynaecol 2004;18(3):383–96.

61. Coleman MA, McCowan LM, North RA. Mid-trimester uterine artery Doppler screening as a predictor of adverse pregnancy outcome in high-risk women. Ultrasound Obstet Gynecol 2000;15(1):7–12.

62. Myatt L, Clifton RG, Roberts JM, et al. The utility of uterine artery Doppler velocimetry in prediction of preeclampsia in a low-risk population. Obstet Gynecol 2012;120(4):815–22.

63. Cnossen JS, Morris RK, ter Riet G, et al. Use of uterine artery Doppler ultrasonography to predict pre-eclampsia and intrauterine growth restriction: a systematic review and bivariable meta-analysis. CMAJ 2008;178(6):701–11.

64. Allen RE, Morlando M, Thilaganathan B, et al. Predictive accuracy of second trimester uterine artery Doppler indices for stillbirth: a systematic review and meta-analysis. Ultrasound Obstet Gynecol 2016;47(1):22–7.

65. Papageorghiou AT, Yu CK, Cicero S, et al. Second-trimester uterine artery Doppler screening in unselected populations: a review. J Matern Fetal Neonatal Med 2002;12(2):78–88.

66. Filippi E, Staughton J, Peregrine E, et al. Uterine artery Doppler and adverse pregnancy outcome in women with extreme levels of fetoplacental proteins used for Down syndrome screening. Ultrasound Obstet Gynecol 2011;37(5):520–7.

67. Di Lorenzo G, Ceccarello M, Cecotti V, et al. First trimester maternal serum PlGF, free beta-hCG, PAPP-A, PP-13, uterine artery Doppler and maternal history for the prediction of preeclampsia. Placenta 2012;33(6):495–501.

68. Crovetto F, Crispi F, Scazzocchio E, et al. First-trimester screening for early and late small-for-gestational-age neonates using maternal serum biochemistry, blood pressure and uterine artery Doppler. Ultrasound Obstet Gynecol 2014;43(1):34–40.

69. Roeder HA, Dejbakhsh SZ, Parast MM, et al. Abnormal uterine artery Doppler velocimetry predicts adverse outcomes in patients with abnormal analytes. Pregnancy Hypertens 2014;4(4):296–301.

70. Rochelson B, Schulman H, Farmakides G, et al. The significance of absent end-diastolic velocity in umbilical artery velocity waveforms. Am J Obstet Gynecol 1987;156(5):1213–8.

71. Ghosh GS, Gudmundsson S. Uterine and umbilical artery Doppler are comparable in predicting perinatal outcome of growth-restricted fetuses. BJOG 2009;116(3):424–30.

72. Alfirevic Z, Stampalija T, Gyte GM. Fetal and umbilical Doppler ultrasound in high-risk pregnancies. Cochrane Database Syst Rev 2013;(11):CD007529.

73. Alfirevic Z, Stampalija T, Medley N. Fetal and umbilical Doppler ultrasound in normal pregnancy. Cochrane Database Syst Rev 2015;(4):CD001450.

74. Weiner CP, Grant SS, Williamson RA. Relationship between second trimester maternal serum alpha-fetoprotein and umbilical artery Doppler velocimetry and their association with preterm delivery. Am J Perinatol 1991;8(4):263–8.

75. Jaffa A, Yaron Y, Har-Toov J, et al. Doppler velocimetry of the umbilical artery as a predictor of pregnancy outcome in pregnancies characterized by elevated

maternal serum alpha-fetoprotein and normal amniotic fluid alpha-fetoprotein. Fetal Diagn Ther 1997;12(2):85–8.

76. Bobrow CS, Holmes RP, Muttukrishna S, et al. Maternal serum activin A, inhibin A, and follistatin in pregnancies with appropriately grown and small-for-gestational-age fetuses classified by umbilical artery Doppler ultrasound. Am J Obstet Gynecol 2002;186(2):283–7.

77. Mitra SC, Seshan SV, Riachi LE. Placental vessel morphometry in growth retardation and increased resistance of the umbilical artery Doppler flow. J Matern Fetal Med 2000;9(5):282–6.

78. Giles WB, Trudinger BJ, Baird PJ. Fetal umbilical artery flow velocity waveforms and placental resistance: pathological correlation. Br J Obstet Gynaecol 1985; 92(1):31–8.

79. Salafia CM, Pezzullo JC, Minior VK, et al. Placental pathology of absent and reversed end-diastolic flow in growth-restricted fetuses. Obstet Gynecol 1997; 90(5):830–6.

80. Lin S, Shimizu I, Suehara N, et al. Uterine artery Doppler velocimetry in relation to trophoblast migration into the myometrium of the placental bed. Obstet Gynecol 1995;85(5 Pt 1):760–5.

81. Rizzo G, Capponi A, Pietrolucci ME, et al. First-trimester placental volume and vascularization measured by 3-dimensional power Doppler sonography in pregnancies with low serum pregnancy-associated plasma protein a levels. J Ultrasound Med 2009;28(12):1615–22.

82. Odibo AO, Zhong Y, Longtine M, et al. First-trimester serum analytes, biophysical tests and the association with pathological morphometry in the placenta of pregnancies with preeclampsia and fetal growth restriction. Placenta 2011;32(4): 333–8.

83. Morssink LP, de Wolf BT, Kornman LH, et al. The relation between serum markers in the second trimester and placental pathology. A study on extremely small for gestational age fetuses. Br J Obstet Gynaecol 1996;103(8):779–83.

Biophysical and Biochemical Screening for the Risk of Preterm Labor
An Update

Joseph R. Wax, MD*, Angelina Cartin, Michael G. Pinette, MD

KEYWORDS

- Cervical cerclage • Cervical length • Fetal fibronectin • Preterm birth
- Progesterone • Ultrasound

KEY POINTS

- Preterm birth, defined as delivery at less than 37 weeks' gestation, is the leading cause of perinatal morbidity and mortality in developed nations.
- The value of cervical lengths and fetal fibronectin (FFN) lies in their extremely high negative predictive values.
- Proper technique is critical for accurate and reproducible cervical length measurements.
- Supplemental progesterone administered to women carrying a singleton pregnancy after a previous spontaneous preterm birth significantly reduces the risk of recurrent spontaneous preterm birth.
- Vaginal progesterone is recommended in women with no prior spontaneous preterm birth and a cervical length less than 20 mm.

Preterm birth, defined as delivery at less than 37 weeks' gestation, is the leading cause of perinatal morbidity and mortality in developed nations. Twelve percent to 13% of US births are preterm, representing more than 500,000 births annually. In 2007, the preterm birth rate decreased to 12.7%, the first decrease in more than 2 decades (**Fig. 1**).[1] Medical costs for preterm newborns are more than 10 times those of term

This article is an update of an article previously published in *Clinics in Laboratory Medicine*, Volume 30, Issue 3, September 2010.

The authors report no conflict of interest.

Division of Maternal-Fetal Medicine, Department of Obstetrics and Gynecology, Maine Medical Center, Portland, ME 04102, USA

* Corresponding author. Maine Medical Partners Women's Health, 887 Congress Street, Suite 200, Portland, ME 04102.

E-mail address: waxj@mmc.org

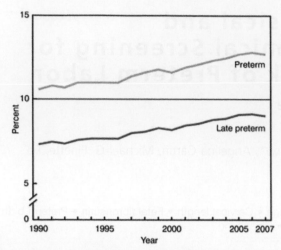

Fig. 1. Preterm birth rates: United States, final 1990 to 2006 and preliminary 2007. Preterm is less than 37 completed weeks of gestation. Late preterm is 34 to 36 completed weeks of gestation. (*Courtesy of* Centers for Disease Control and Prevention/National Center for Health Statistics, National Vital Statistics system.)

infants, and the average length of hospitalization is more than 6 times that of term infants.

Preterm deliveries may be categorized as *indicated* because of maternal or fetal complications or *spontaneous*, including births following preterm labor and preterm membrane rupture. The remainder of this discussion addresses only spontaneous preterm birth. Risk factors for spontaneous preterm birth are listed in **Box 1**. This lengthy catalog of heterogeneous associations of spontaneous preterm birth suggests etiologic heterogeneity as well. Although mechanisms of labor initiation are unknown, broad categories for these associations include inflammation, decidual hemorrhage, uterine overdistension, and early initiation of normal parturition.[2] Not surprisingly, long-standing goals identifying women destined to delivery preterm and offering effective preventive measures remain only partially fulfilled.

Proposed techniques for detecting at-risk pregnancies include risk factor–based scoring systems, home uterine activity monitoring, maternal serum chemistries, salivary estriol, cervicovaginal chemistries, and amniotic fluid analytes (**Box 2**). These modalities are characterized by inadequate screening efficiencies, invasiveness, expense, or lack of commercial availability. Moreover, their use does not demonstrate reduced spontaneous preterm birth rates. The remainder of this article discusses the respective biophysical and biochemical tests of sonographic cervical length measurement and cervicovaginal fetal fibronectin (FFN) that are widely evaluated and incorporated into the clinical care of patients at risk for spontaneous preterm birth.

CERVICAL LENGTH ASSESSMENT
Rationale

Labor is defined as regular uterine contractions resulting in progressive dilation and effacement of the cervix. Thus, the cervix provides the definitive window to diagnosing labor. Traditionally, the cervix has been viewed in dichotomous terms, as capable of maintaining pregnancy until term (competent) or not (incompetent). More recently, this paradigm has been challenged, with cervical function now viewed along a

Box 1		
Risk factors for spontaneous preterm birth		

Demographic

Age <18 y, >40 y

Lower socioeconomic status

Unmarried

Poor nutritional status

Psychosocial stressors

Inadequate prenatal care

Black race

Underweight

Smoker

Anemia

Interpregnancy interval <6 mo

Drug abuse

Prior preterm birth

Obstetric/Gynecologic

Uterus/cervix
  Fibroids
  Mullerian anomaly
  Conization/loop electrosurgical excise procedure
  Laceration
  Diethylstilbestrol exposure
  Overdistension
    Multiple gestation
    Polyhydramnios

Obstetric bleeding
  Abruption
  Threatened miscarriage

Inflammation
  Bacterial vaginosis
  Cystitis
  Systemic infection

continuum. Landmark research in the mid-1990s compared cervical lengths measured by transvaginal ultrasound (TVUS) in women with prior preterm births to cervical lengths in control subjects without previous preterm births. The investigators found that gestational age at delivery of the prior pregnancy correlated significantly with cervical length at 20 to 30 weeks in the subsequent gestation.[3]

These findings were expanded in a later multicenter study of 2915 women undergoing TVUS for cervix lengths at 24 weeks' gestation. The investigators observed that cervix lengths were normally distributed (**Fig. 2**) and that the risk of spontaneous preterm birth in the current pregnancy increased with decreasing cervical length (see **Fig. 2**; **Fig. 3**). A cervical length of 25 mm (10th percentile) seemed to be a clinically appropriate threshold of identifying preterm delivery risk, offering 37.3% sensitivity, 92.2% specificity, and a 97.4% negative predictive value.[4] Occasionally, echogenic material is noted within the amniotic fluid at the level of the cervix (**Fig. 4**). Initially

Box 2
Proposed biomarkers of preterm birth

Amniotic Fluid	Maternal Serum	Maternal Genital Tract
IL-6	IL-6	pH
Glucose	IL-8	FFN
Monocyte chemotactic protein-1	TNF-α	IL-6
Culture	ferritin	IL-8
Whole blood cell count	CRP	TNF-α
Gram stain	MSAFP	Bacterial vaginosis
CRP	uE3 (saliva)	—
PAPP-A	Corticotropin-releasing hormone	—
—	hCG	

Abbreviations: CRP, C-reactive protein; FFN, fetal fibronectin; IL, interleukin; MSAFP, maternal serum alpha fetoprotein; PAPP-A, pregnancy-associated placental protein A; TNF-α, tumor necrosis factor α; uE3, unconjugated estriol.

thought to represent blood clot, this debris is an inflammatory exudate consisting of fibrin, white blood cells, and bacteria.[5] Presence of this material known as sludge incurs a risk of preterm birth significantly increased greater than that incurred by the cervical length alone (**Fig. 5**).[6]

Sonographic Technique for Cervical Length Assessment

Proper technique is critical for accurate and reproducible cervical length measurements. Therefore, the Perinatal Quality Foundation developed the cervical length

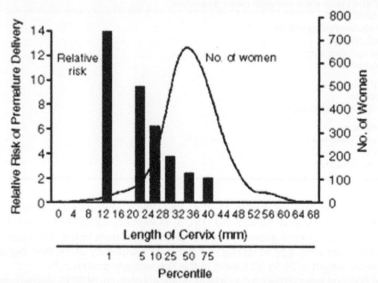

Fig. 2. Distribution of subjects among percentiles for cervical length measured by TVUS at 24 weeks of gestation (*solid line*) and relative risk of spontaneous preterm delivery before 35 weeks of gestation according to percentiles for cervical length (*bars*). The risks among women with values at or less than the 1st, 5th, 10th, 25th, 50th, and 75th percentiles for cervical length are compared with the risk among women with values greater than the 75th percentile. (*From* Iams JD, Goldenberg RL, Meis PJ, et al. The length of the cervix and the risk of spontaneous premature delivery. N Engl J Med 1996;334:567–72; with permission. Copyright ©1996 Massachusetts Medical Society. All rights reserved.)

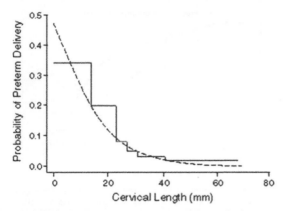

Fig. 3. Estimated probability of spontaneous preterm delivery before 35 weeks of gestation from the logistic-regression analysis (*dashed line*) and observed frequency of spontaneous preterm delivery (*solid line*) according to cervical length measured by TVUS at 24 weeks. (*From* Iams JD, Goldenberg RL, Meis PJ, et al. The length of the cervix and the risk of spontaneous premature delivery. N Engl J Med 1996;334:567–72; with permission. Copyright ©1996 Massachusetts Medical Society. All rights reserved.)

education and review (CLEAR) program composed of online continuing medical education lectures and voluntary image review (https://clear.perinatalquality.org/). Successful completion of the requirements leads to cervical length ultrasound certification. The CLEAR criteria for proper cervical length measurement are included in **Box 3**. Patients should be examined with an empty bladder to avoid dynamic cervical changes. The TVUS probe is introduced into the anterior vaginal fornix under real-time visualization. Use of TVUS limits measurement variation to 5% to 10%, a marked improvement over digital examination or transabdominal ultrasound. A midsagittal view of the cervix is obtained. The probe is then withdrawn just enough to allow the image to blur and then advanced just until the image comes back into focus. This sequence avoids excessive probe pressure on the cervix, which can result in falsely lengthened cervical measurements.

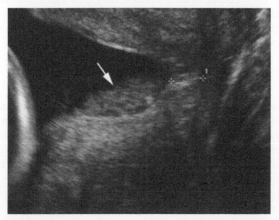

Fig. 4. Echogenic debris (*arrow*) at level of internal cervical os known as sludge. (*From* Wax JR, Cartin A, Pinette MG. Biophysical and biochemical screening for the risk of preterm labor. Clin Lab Med 2010;30(3):693–707; with permission.)

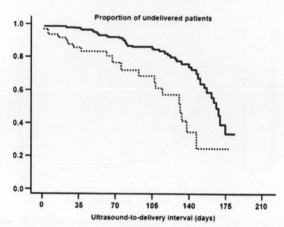

Fig. 5. Kaplan-Meier survival analysis of the ultrasound-to-delivery interval (days) according to the presence or absence of amniotic fluid sludge in asymptomatic high-risk patients for preterm delivery. Patients with sludge (*dotted line*) had a shorter ultrasound-to-delivery interval than those without AF sludge (*solid line*). (AF sludge positive, median: 127 [95% CI: 120–134] days vs AF sludge negative, median: 161 [95% CI: 153–169] days; log rank test, P<.001). (*From* Kusanovic JP, Espinoza J, Romero R, et al. Clinical significance of the presence of amniotic fluid 'sludge' in asymptomatic patients at high risk for spontaneous preterm delivery. Ultrasound Obstet Gynecol 2007;30:710. John Wiley & Sons, Inc; with permission.)

The on-screen electronic calipers are placed at the notches representing the internal and external cervical os, thereby identifying the bounds of the cervical length measurement (**Fig. 6**). Three such measurements are taken, and the shortest of the 3 is reported as the cervical length because the initial determination is often longer than the others.

Despite the aforementioned safeguards for ensuring proper cervical length assessments, several pitfalls may still impact this measurement. Before 20 weeks' gestation, the lower uterine segment is not particularly well developed, making it difficult to reliably determine the location of the internal os (**Fig. 7**). Commonly observed lower uterine segment focal myometrial contractions may give the false impression of either increased cervical length or dilation of the internal cervical os (**Fig. 8**). Finally, cervical dynamicism, or spontaneous cervical lengthening or shortening, may occur during the examination, precluding an accurate evaluation.[7]

FETAL FIBRONECTIN
Rationale

FFN, a glycoprotein, is a component of the amniochorionic extracellular matrix. Its function is thought to act as a glue, aiding in membrane adherence to the decidua. FFN may normally be detected in cervicovaginal secretions less than 20 weeks' and 37 weeks' or greater gestation (**Fig. 9**).[8] Between these gestational ages, cervicovaginal FFN is associated with an increased risk of spontaneous preterm birth, suggesting inappropriate release and leakage of FFN in response to inflammation or uterine activity. A recent meta-analysis of FFN testing among women symptomatic for preterm labor calculated a spontaneous preterm birth detection rate of 76.1% (95% confidence interval [CI] 69.1%–81.9%), positive predictive value 25.9%, and negative predictive value of 97.6% for delivery within 7 days of testing.[9] Among asymptomatic, generally low-risk patients, FFN testing at 24 to 30 weeks demonstrated test-positive

---

Box 3
Cervical length education and review cervical measurement criteria

Measurement is taken on a transvaginal image:
a. Transvaginal measurements are the gold standard for ultrasound cervix measurements.
b. Short cervix can be missed on transabdominal scans.

The transvaginal image is filled primarily with the cervix, and the field of view is optimized for measurement:
a. The cervix occupies approximately 75% of the image.
b. The bladder area is visible.

The anterior width of the cervix equals the posterior width:
a. The anterior cervical thickness is equal to the posterior cervical thickness.
b. The echogenicity is similar both anteriorly and posteriorly.
c. There is limited concavity created by the transducer.

The maternal bladder is empty:
a. The maternal bladder has a variable effect on the cervical length.

The internal os is seen:
a. The internal os is a small triangular area at the superior portion of the endocervical canal.
b. The internal os is adjacent to the uterine cavity.

The external os is seen:
a. The external os is a small triangular area at the inferior portion of the endocervical canal.
b. The anterior and posterior portions of the cervix come together at the external os.

The endocervical canal is visible throughout:
a. The endocervical canal is a linear echogenicity created by the interface between the anterior and posterior walls of the cervix.
b. The canal extends between the internal and external os.

Caliper placement is correct:
a. Calipers are placed where the anterior and posterior walls of the cervix touch at the internal and external os.
b. Calipers do not extend to the outer-most edge of the cervical tissue.
c. Calipers extend along the endocervical canal.
d. If the cervix is curved, 2 or more linear measurements are performed and the values added together to obtain the cervical length. Do not trace the cervical length.

Cervix mobility is considered:
a. Insert transvaginal probe to view the cervix; withdraw probe until the image blurs to reduce compression from the transducer, and then reapply just enough pressure to create the best image.
b. Apply mild suprapubic or fundal pressure to watch for funneling. Reduce probe pressure while fundal or suprapubic pressure is applied.
c. Visualize the cervix for 3 to 5 minutes and watch for shortening or funneling.

---

rates of 3.1% to 3.5%, detection rates of 17% to 19%, and positive predictive values of 13% to 24%, with 97% specificity.[10] Although intended for use in singleton pregnancies, a recent study evaluated FFN testing in symptomatic women carrying twins. The results demonstrated somewhat diminished sensitivity for delivery within 14 days of testing versus singletons (71% vs 82%) but similar negative predictive values (97% vs 99%).[11]

Technique

A specimen for FFN testing is obtained from patients during a vaginal speculum examination. The test is intended for use in women symptomatic for preterm labor with minimal (<3 cm) cervical dilation at 24 0/7 to 34 0/7 weeks' gestation or asymptomatic women from 22 0/7 to 30 6/7 weeks' gestation to provide additional information

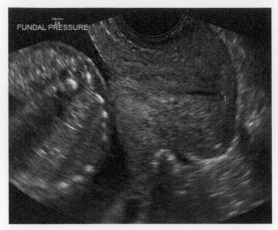

Fig. 6. Normal cervical length measurement.

regarding preterm delivery risk. The manufacturer-provided polyester swab is rotated across the posterior vaginal fornix for 10 seconds to absorb secretions and then placed in the provided tube of buffer. The specimen is labeled and transported to the laboratory for analysis. Validity of the test requires no antecedent cervical manipulation, such as sexual intercourse, digital examination, vaginal ultrasound, culturing, or Papanicolaou smear. Likewise, contamination of the collection swab with lubricants, soaps, or disinfectants may interfere with the test, invalidating results.

In order to improve patient acceptance and permit nonphysician personnel to obtain samples for FFN testing, investigators have evaluated blind collection techniques without a speculum examination. FFN test results following collection by speculum and blind methods were in agreement greater than 95% of the time, indicating excellent agreement as measured by the kappa statistic ($\kappa = 0.90$).[12] Another study found that blind collection offered similar detection rates and negative predictive values to those observed with the recommended speculum examination.[13]

FFN may be distinguished from other fibronectins by FDC-6 monoclonal antibodies directed against the unique III-CS region of FFN, forming the basis for the available

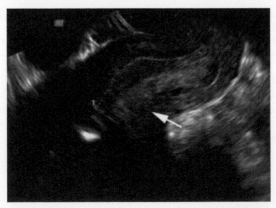

Fig. 7. Second trimester cervical ultrasound demonstrates undeveloped lower uterine segment (*arrow*). (*From* Wax JR, Cartin A, Pinette MG. Biophysical and biochemical screening for the risk of preterm labor. Clin Lab Med 2010;30(3):699; with permission.)

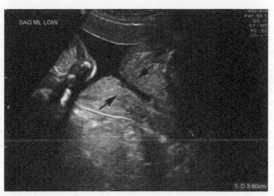

Fig. 8. Focal myometrial contraction of lower uterine segment (*arrows*). (*From* Wax JR, Cartin A, Pinette MG. Biophysical and biochemical screening for the risk of preterm labor. Clin Lab Med 2010;30(3):700; with permission.)

laboratory test. The assay is a solid-phase enzyme-linked immunosorbent assay. Specimen processing via an automatic analyzer requires approximately 20 minutes. If spectrophotometric evaluation at a wavelength of 550 nm notes a sample signal intensity greater than or equal to the calibrated value corresponding to the FFN concentration of 0.050 mcg/mL, the result is reported as positive. If the signal intensity is less than the calibrated value, the test result is negative. Internal controls are run with every sample and, if unmet, lead to an invalid test result.

GESTATIONAL AGE AND RISK-SPECIFIC APPROACH TO USING CERVICAL LENGTH AND FETAL FIBRONECTIN IN CLINICAL EVALUATION AND MANAGEMENT

From a clinical perspective, integrating cervical length and FFN into preterm birth risk assessment algorithms is best done in the context of gestational age at evaluation (<24 weeks, ≥24 weeks), history of previous spontaneous preterm birth (yes = high risk, no = low risk), and presence or absence of preterm labor symptoms. Thus, the following discussion is framed in the context of these variables. Importantly, the value

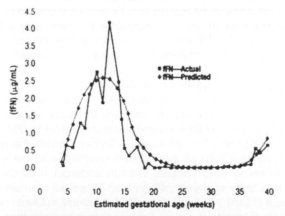

Fig. 9. FFN may normally be detected in cervicovaginal secretions less than 20 weeks' and 37 weeks' or greater gestation. (*From* Ascarelli MH, Morrison JC. Use of fetal fibronectin in clinical practice. Obstet Gynecol Surv 1997;52:1S-12. Lippincott Williams & Wilkins, Inc; with permission.)

of cervical lengths and FFN lies in their extremely high negative predictive values. FFN testing among symptomatic women in particular is associated with fewer hospital admissions for preterm labor, shorter lengths of stay, fewer medical interventions, and lower costs.[14–18]

Earlier than 24 Weeks' Gestation

Cervical length and cerclage

FFN is not usually performed during this time period, as previously noted. A shortened(<25 mm) cervix in high-risk patients at this gestational age raises the question of cervical insufficiency, classically referred to as incompetent cervix. No objective diagnostic criteria exist for this condition, and there is no uniformly agreed on definition. However, a reasonable description is "a clinical diagnosis characterized by recurrent painless dilation and spontaneous midtrimester birth, generally in the absence of predisposing conditions, such as spontaneous membrane rupture, bleeding, and infection, characteristics that shift the presumed underlying cause away from cervical incompetence and support other components of the preterm birth syndrome."[19]

At 20 to 24 weeks, the clinician should rule out uterine contractions, ruptured membranes, acute chorioamnionitis, and fetal death. If present, these conditions are managed according to existing guidelines.[20,21] If absent, cervical cerclage may be considered. If patients are less than 20 weeks pregnant, one may first consider repeating the cervical length after 3 to 7 days of restricted physical activity to ensure accuracy because cervical length sonography less than 20 weeks is technically difficult.[22] A recent meta-analysis of randomized trials of cerclage for preterm birth prevention in singleton high-risk pregnancies with a short cervix suggested that cerclage was associated with a significantly lower risk of delivery at less than 35 weeks, with a relative risk (RR) of 0.61 (95% CI 0.40–0.92). Among singletons with a shortened cervix and prior midtrimester loss, cerclage was also associated with a reduced likelihood of delivery at less than 35 weeks (39% vs 23.4%, number needed to treat = 8, RR = 0.57; 95% CI 0.33–0.99).[23] Similar findings were noted in a recent randomized trial of cerclage versus no cerclage in women with a history of spontaneous preterm birth.[24]

Current evidence does not support cerclage for the incidental finding of a shortened cervix in women without a prior spontaneous preterm birth or midtrimester loss.[25] Other groups known to be at increased risk for spontaneous preterm birth include twins and women who have undergone prior cervical cone biopsy or loop electrosurgical excision procedures.[25–31] In the former group, cerclage for a short cervix is associated with an increased rate of preterm birth at less than 35 weeks, RR = 2.15 (95% CI 1.15–4.01).[23] In the latter group, efficacy of cerclage for a shortened cervix has not been evaluated, leaving management speculative.[22]

Additional investigations evaluated the presence or absence of various biomarkers to improve identification of candidates for cerclage by midtrimester cervical sonography. Sakai and colleagues[32] performed cervical ultrasound on 16,508 women in a general obstetric population at 20 to 24 weeks. Clinicians made the decision to offer cerclage for a cervix less than 25 mm without knowledge of cervical interleukin 8 (IL-8) levels, a marker of inflammation. Women undergoing cerclage with normal IL-8 levels were less likely to deliver at less than 37 weeks than similar patients not receiving a cerclage (33.0% vs 54.5%, P = .01). In contrast, subjects undergoing cerclage with elevated IL-8 levels were more likely to deliver preterm than similar subjects not receiving a cerclage (78.0% vs 54.1%, P = .03).[32] Thus, IL-8 levels, though not commercially available for this purpose, may deserve further evaluation for identifying patients who may experience benefit or even harm from a cerclage.

In another study, Keeler and colleagues[33] stratified delivery outcomes by results of FFN testing obtained from 18 to 24 weeks at the time of TVUS cervical lengths. Subjects with cervical lengths less than 25 mm were randomized to cerclage or no cerclage, without clinician knowledge of the FFN result. Spontaneous preterm birth at less than 35 weeks occurred with similar frequency among FFN-positive women with (44.1%) or without (55.2%) cerclage (P = .45) as well as FFN-negative subjects with (17.8%) or without (17.0%) cerclage (P = .99). The investigators concluded that, although FFN does not aid cerclage candidate selection, it may aid counseling regarding pregnancy outcomes.[33]

Cervical length and progesterone

Supplemental progesterone administered to women carrying a singleton pregnancy after a previous spontaneous preterm birth significantly reduces the risk of recurrent spontaneous preterm birth.[34] Remarkably, the effect is most pronounced in patients with very preterm (<32 weeks) deliveries. Unfortunately, no such protective effect is observed in twin and triplet gestations.[35–37] The mechanism by which progesterone acts is unclear but may involve suppressing the fetal inflammatory response and inhibiting cervical ripening.[38–40] Supplemental progesterone is administered in one of several forms, intramuscularly or intravaginally, according to established protocols.[25] Regardless, not all women benefit from progesterone; among those who do, the benefit may vary. Several studies have, therefore, evaluated midtrimester cervical length to identify women potentially benefiting from progesterone therapy.

O'Brien and colleagues[41] randomized 659 women with a history of spontaneous preterm birth to receive daily treatment with either 90 mg vaginal progesterone gel or placebo from 16 to 22 6/7 weeks until 37 weeks or early delivery occurred. There was no difference between groups with regard to the primary outcome of delivery at 32 weeks or less, 10.0% and 11.3%, respectively.[41] Interestingly, a secondary analysis reevaluated the original results by cervical length at study enrollment. Outcomes of subjects with cervical lengths of 28 mm or less were compared by assignment with progesterone or placebo. Among women with a shortened cervix, progesterone therapy was associated with significantly less frequent delivery at 32 weeks or less, neonatal intensive care admissions, and shorter neonatal intensive care length of stay.[42]

Another multicenter trial evaluated TVUS cervical lengths at 20 to 25 weeks in a general obstetric population of singletons and twins. Women with cervical lengths of 15 mm or less were offered randomization to daily oral progesterone 200 mg or placebo from 24 to 33 6/7 weeks. The frequency of spontaneous preterm birth at less than 34 weeks was significantly lower in progesterone group (19.2% vs 34.4%). Although no differences were observed in perinatal morbidity or mortality, the study was not powered to evaluate these outcomes.[43] Subgroup analysis of another recent randomized placebo-controlled study of 90 mg vaginal progesterone daily demonstrated a reduction of preterm delivery among women with cervical lengths of 10.0 to 20.9 mm at 19 to 23 6/7 weeks and no prior spontaneous preterm birth.[44] Based on the 2 last reports, vaginal progesterone is recommended in women with no prior spontaneous preterm birth and a cervical length less than 20 mm.[25] Therefore, consideration may be given to a policy of universal cervical length screening.[25]

24 to 34 Weeks' Gestation

This period in pregnancy is beyond the window of classic cervical insufficiency and also marks the early phase of ex utero fetal viability. Thus, clinicians are now concerned with the prevention, diagnosis, and treatment of preterm labor. Unfortunately, our ability to predict and prevent preterm birth remains quite limited. Therefore, efforts have concentrated on the accurate diagnosis of preterm labor to allow selective and timely obstetric interventions for optimizing neonatal outcomes of fetuses destined for early delivery. Such measures include maternal administration of antibiotics to prevent invasive group B streptococcal infections, glucocorticoid administration to accelerate fetal lung maturity, and tocolysis to abate uterine contractions and permit maternal transport to a facility capable of providing specialized care of preterm infants. Equally important is the ability to reliably rule out preterm labor among symptomatic women in order to avoid the potential morbidity, expense, and inconvenience of such treatment.

At less than 37 weeks, clinical symptoms of at least 6 contractions per hour accompanied by cervical dilation by digital examination of at least 3 cm and 80% effacement, particularly in the presence of ruptured membranes or vaginal bleeding, comfortably allows one to diagnose preterm labor. Contractions without these associated findings are less clear, leaving the diagnosis uncertain. Therefore, in the authors' practice, they have adopted a guideline that incorporates both TVUS cervical length and FFN testing for evaluating patients presenting with suspected preterm labor.[2]

During the initial assessment, patients undergo a vaginal speculum examination. If the membranes are unruptured, a vaginal swab for FFN testing is obtained and held aside. A group B streptococcal culture is obtained as well. If a digital cervical examination and contraction frequency establishes a preterm labor diagnosis, treatment proceeds as outlined. If the diagnosis remains unclear, TVUS of the cervix is performed. A cervical length greater than 30 mm effectively rules out preterm labor; the FFN swab does not need to be sent; and patients can be managed expectantly. A cervical length less than 20 mm effectively confirms the diagnosis of preterm labor, allowing treatment to proceed. Again, the FFN swab may be discarded. A cervical length of 20 to 30 mm is considered inconclusive. The FFN swab is sent to the laboratory for processing. A positive FFN result leads to the presumptive diagnosis of preterm labor, whereas a negative result permits expectant care.

Finally, the authors recommend screening women presenting with preterm labor symptoms for asymptomatic bacteriuria. Identification and treatment of this condition significantly reduces the risk of preterm delivery, RR 0.56 (95% CI 0.43–0.73).[45] Likewise, diagnosis and treatment of bacterial vaginosis in symptomatic women with a prior spontaneous preterm birth can also reduce recurrent preterm delivery risk, RR 0.42 (95% CI 0.27–0.67).[46]

Understandably, not all obstetric care providers always have resources available for TVUS cervical lengths. In such cases, the authors think that FFN offers sufficiently high sensitivity and negative predictive value to assist in guiding initial clinical decision-making. Similarly, not all facilities offer FFN testing. Moreover, cervical manipulation may have occurred before deciding on FFN testing. In these cases, where available, incorporating TVUS cervical lengths with other available clinical information may assist clinical decision-making.

SUMMARY

Etiologic and physiologic heterogeneity confound the clinical prediction and prevention of spontaneous preterm birth. Research over the past 15 years demonstrates the remarkable progress made in these areas. Fruits of these labors include TVUS cervical length, cervicovaginal FFN, progesterone therapy, and more selective use of cervical cerclage. Future research is likely to evaluate other markers of preterm birth, maternal abdominal surface uterine electromyography, and proteomic evaluation of maternal and amniotic fluids.[47–50] Imaging and clinical and research laboratories will play central roles in the unfolding story of preterm birth prediction and prevention.

REFERENCES

1. Hamilton BE, Martin JA, Ventura SJ. Births: preliminary data for 2007. National vital statistics reports, March 18, 2009. Available at: http://www.cdc.gov/nchs/data/nvsr/nvsr57/nvsr57_12.pdf.
2. Iams JD. Prediction and early detection of preterm labor. Obstet Gynecol 2003; 101:402–12.
3. Iams JD, Johnson FF, Sonek J, et al. Cervical competence as a continuum: a study of ultrasonographic cervical length and obstetric performance. Am J Obstet Gynecol 1995;172(4 Pt 1):1097–106.
4. Iams JD, Goldenberg RL, Meis PJ, et al. The length of the cervix and the risk of spontaneous premature delivery. National Institute of Child Health and Human Development Maternal Fetal Medicine Unit Network. N Engl J Med 1996; 334(9):567–72.
5. Romero R, Kusanovic JP, Espinoza J, et al. What is amniotic fluid 'sludge'? Ultrasound Obstet Gynecol 2007;30(5):793–8.
6. Kusanovic JP, Espinoza J, Romero R, et al. Clinical significance of the presence of amniotic fluid 'sludge' in asymptomatic patients at high risk for spontaneous preterm delivery. Ultrasound Obstet Gynecol 2007;30(5):706–14.
7. Yost NP, Bloom SL, Twickler DM, et al. Pitfalls in ultrasonic cervical length measurement for predicting preterm birth. Obstet Gynecol 1999;93(4):510–6.
8. Ascarelli MH, Morrison JC. Use of fetal fibronectin in clinical practice. Obstet Gynecol Surv 1997;52(4 Suppl):S1–12.
9. Sanchez-Ramos L, Delke I, Zamora J, et al. Fetal fibronectin as a short-term predictor of preterm birth in symptomatic patients: a meta-analysis. Obstet Gynecol 2009;114(3):631–40.
10. Goldenberg RL, Mercer BM, Meis PJ, et al. The preterm prediction study: fetal fibronectin testing and spontaneous preterm birth. NICHD Maternal Fetal Medicine Units Network. Obstet Gynecol 1996;87(5 Pt 1):643–8.
11. Singer E, Pilpel S, Bsat F, et al. Accuracy of fetal fibronectin to predict preterm birth in twin gestations with symptoms of labor. Obstet Gynecol 2007;109(5): 1083–7.
12. Stafford IP, Garite TJ, Dildly GA, et al. A comparison of speculum and nonspeculum collection of cervicovaginal specimens for fetal fibronectin testing. Am J Obstet Gynecol 2008;199(2):131.e1–4.
13. Roman AS, Koklanaris N, Paidas MJ, et al. "Blind" vaginal fetal fibronectin as a predictor of spontaneous preterm delivery. Obstet Gynecol 2005;105(2):285–9.
14. Joffe GM, Jacques D, Bemis-Heys R, et al. Impact of the fetal fibronectin assay on admissions for preterm labor. Am J Obstet Gynecol 1999;180(3 Pt 1):581–6.
15. Incerti M, Ghidini A, Korker V, et al. Performance of cervicovaginal fetal fibronectin in a community hospital setting. Arch Gynecol Obstet 2007;275(5):347–51.
16. Abenhaim HA, Morin L, Benjamin A. Does availability of fetal fibronectin testing in the management of threatened preterm labor affect the utilization of hospital resources? J Obstet Gynaecol Can 2005;27(7):689–94.
17. Mozurkewich EL, Naglie G, Krahn MD, et al. Predicting preterm birth: a cost-effectiveness analysis. Am J Obstet Gynecol 2000;182(6):1589–98.
18. Lowe MP, Zimmerman B, Hansen W. Prospective randomized controlled trial of fetal fibronectin on preterm labor management in a tertiary care center. Am J Obstet Gynecol 2004;190(2):358–62.
19. Owen J, Iams JD, Hauth JC. Vaginal sonography and cervical incompetence. Am J Obstet Gynecol 2003;188(2):586–96.

20. ACOG practice bulletin No. 139. Premature rupture of membranes. Obstet Gynecol 2013;122:918–30.
21. ACOG practice bulletin No. 102. Management of stillbirth. Obstet Gynecol 2009; 113(3):748–61.
22. Harger JH. Cerclage and cervical insufficiency: an evidence-based analysis. Obstet Gynecol 2003;100(6):1313–27.
23. Berghella V, Odibo AO, To MS, et al. Cerclage for short cervix on ultrasonography: meta-analysis of trials using individual patient-level data. Obstet Gynecol 2005;106(1):181–9.
24. Owen J, Hankins G, Iams JD, et al. Multicenter randomized trial of cerclage for preterm birth prevention in high-risk women with shortened mid-trimester cervical length. Am J Obstet Gynecol 2009;201:375.e1–8.
25. Committee on Practice Bulletins—Obstetrics, The American College of Obstetricians and Gynecologists. Practice bulletin no. 130: prediction and prevention of preterm birth. Obstet Gynecol 2012;120:964–73.
26. Sjoborg KD, Vistad I, Myhr SS, et al. Pregnancy outcome after cervical cone excision: a case-control study. Acta Obstet Gynecol Scand 2007;86(4):423–8.
27. Berghella V, Pereira L, Gariepy A, et al. Prior cone biopsy: prediction of preterm birth by cervical ultrasound. Am J Obstet Gynecol 2004;191(4):1393–7.
28. Crane JM. Pregnancy outcome after loop electrosurgical excision procedure: a systematic review. Obstet Gynecol 2003;102(5 Pt 1):1058–62.
29. Samson SA, Bentley JR, Fahey TJ, et al. The effect of loop electrosurgical excision procedure on future pregnancy outcome. Obstet Gynecol 2005;105(2): 325–32.
30. Noehr B, Jensen A, Fredericksen K, et al. Loop electrosurgical excision of the cervix and risk for spontaneous preterm delivery in twin pregnancies. Obstet Gynecol 2009;114(3):511–5.
31. Jakobsson M, Gissler M, Paavonen J, et al. Loop electrosurgical excision procedure and the risk for preterm birth. Obstet Gynecol 2009;114(3):504–10.
32. Sakai M, Shiozaki A, Tabata M, et al. Evaluation of effectiveness of prophylactic cerclage of a short cervix according to interleukin-8 in cervical mucus. Am J Obstet Gynecol 2006;194(1):14–9.
33. Keeler SM, Roman AS, Coletta JM, et al. Fetal fibronectin testing in patients with short cervix in the midtrimester: can it identify optimal candidates for ultrasound-indicated cerclage? Am J Obstet Gynecol 2009;200(2):159.e1–6.
34. Meis PJ, Klebanoff M, Thom E, et al. Prevention of recurrent preterm birth by 17 alpha-hydroxyprogesterone caproate. N Engl J Med 2003;348(24):2379–85.
35. Norman JE, Mackenzie F, Owen P, et al. Progesterone for the prevention of preterm birth in twin pregnancy (STOPPIT): a randomized, double-blind, placebo controlled study and meta-analysis. Lancet 2009;373(9680):2034–40.
36. Rouse DJ, Caritis SN, Peaceman AM. A trial of 17 alpha-hydroxyprogesterone caproate to prevent prematurity in twins. N Engl J Med 2007;357(5):454–6.
37. Caritis SN, Rouse DJ, Peaceman AM, et al. Prevention of preterm birth in triplets using 17 alpha-hydroxyprogesterone caproate – a randomized controlled trial. Obstet Gynecol 2009;113(2 Pt 1):285–92.
38. Peltier MR, Berlin Y, Tee SC, et al. Does progesterone inhibit bacteria-stimulated interleukin-8 production by lower genital tract epithelial cells? J Perinat Med 2009; 37(4):328–33.
39. Yellon SM, Ebner CA, Elovitz MA. Medroxyprogesterone acetate modulates remodeling, immune cell census, and nerve fibers in the cervix of a mouse model for inflammation-induced preterm birth. Reprod Sci 2009;16(3):257–64.

40. Schwartz N, Xue X, Elovitz MA, et al. Progesterone suppresses the fetal inflammatory response ex vivo. Am J Obstet Gynecol 2009;201(2):211.e1–9.

41. O'Brien JM, Adair CD, Lewis DF, et al. Progesterone vaginal gel for the reduction of recurrent preterm birth: primary results from a randomized, double-blind, placebo-controlled trial. Ultrasound Obstet Gynecol 2007;30(5):687–96.

42. DeFranco EA, O'Brien JM, Adair CD, et al. Vaginal progesterone is associated with a decrease in risk for early preterm birth and improved neonatal outcome in women with a short cervix: a secondary analysis from a randomized, double-blind, placebo-controlled trial. Ultrasound Obstet Gynecol 2007;30(5):697–705.

43. Fonseca EB, Celik E, Parra M, et al. Progesterone and the risk of preterm birth among women with a short cervix. N Engl J Med 2007;357(5):462–9.

44. Hassan SS, Romero R, Vidyadhari D, et al. Vaginal progesterone reduces the rate of preterm birth in women with a sonographic short cervix: a multicenter, randomized, double-blind, placebo-controlled trial. PREGNANT Trial. Ultrasound Obstet Gynecol 2011;38:18–31.

45. Romero R, Oyarzun E, Mazor M, et al. Meta-analysis of the relationship between asymptomatic bacteriuria and preterm delivery/low birth weight. Obstet Gynecol 1989;73(4):576–82.

46. Leitich H, Brunbauer M, Bodnar-Aderl B, et al. Antibiotic treatment of bacterial vaginosis in pregnancy: a meta-analysis. Am J Obstet Gynecol 2003;188(3):752–8.

47. Verdenik I, Pajntar M, Leskosek B. Uterine electrical activity as predictor of preterm birth in women with preterm contractions. Eur J Obstet Gynecol Reprod Biol 2001;95(2):149–53.

48. Grgic O, Matijevic R. Uterine electrical activity and cervical shortening in the midtrimester of pregnancy. Int J Gynaecol Obstet 2008;102(3):246–8.

49. Garfield RE, Maner WL, Maul H, et al. Use of uterine EMG and cervical LIF in monitoring pregnant patient. BJOG 2005;112(Suppl 1):103–8.

50. Marque CK, Terrien J, Rihana S, et al. Preterm labour detection by use of a biophysical marker: the uterine electrical activity. BMC Pregnancy Childbirth 2007;7(Supple 1):S1–5.

The Past, Present, and Future of Preimplantation Genetic Testing

Anthony N. Imudia, MD*, Shayne Plosker, MD

KEYWORDS

- Aneuploidy • Embryo research • Preimplantation genetic diagnosis (PGD)
- Preimplantation genetic screening (PGS) • Preimplantation genetic testing (PGT)
- Single-gene disorder

KEY POINTS

- Preimplantation genetic screening (PGS) has helped many individuals prevent the birth of children with severe genetic diseases and also the need for selective abortion associated with postgravid antenatal screening techniques.
- Given the disadvantages associated with cleavage-stage biopsy for preimplantation genetic testing (PGT), most centers have adopted trophectoderm biopsy and cryopreservation of tested blastocysts for subsequent transfer as a new clinical paradigm.
- Utilization of newer genetic testing platform for PGS for aneuploidy is becoming an effective way to improve the chances of live birth, especially if elective single-embryo transfer is considered.
- Increasing knowledge of the human embryo and the genetic basis of human disease coupled with the development of these new genetic testing platforms will lead to increased application and use of PGT.

INTRODUCTION

Clinically applicable PGT was first accomplished in 1990, when it was announced that 2 women at risk for transmitting recessive X-linked diseases were pregnant with female fetuses as a result of in vitro fertilization (IVF) followed by embryo biopsy and sexing by polymerase chain reaction (PCR) for the Y chromosome.[1] At present, PGT has been used to identify more than 200 genetic disorders (https://genesisgenetics.org/pgd - What we test for). The indications of PGT include the identification of embryos harboring autosomomal recessive diseases, autosomal dominant diseases, sex chromosome–linked diseases, genetic mutations with important late-onset implications, chromosomal

Disclosure: None.
Division of Reproductive Endocrinology and Infertility, University of South Florida Morsani College of Medicine, 2 Tampa General Circle, Suite 6022, Tampa, FL 33606, USA
* Corresponding author. 2 Tampa General Circle, Suite 6022, Tampa, FL 33606.
E-mail address: aimudia@health.usf.edu

structural abnormalities (translocations), chromosomal numeric abnormalities (aneuploidies), and mitochondrial disorders. Additionally, PGT can be used for gender selection for medical (X-linked diseases or nonmendelian disorders with unequal gender distribution) or social (family balancing) reasons. PGT is necessary to identify HLA-matched embryos to permit the creation of a savior sibling whose umbilical cord blood could provide stem cells for a sibling in need of a stem cell transplant. If the sibling's condition is due to a single gene mutation, then concurrent preimplantation genetic diagnosis (PGD) for both HLA matching and absence of the mutation is required.[2]

The techniques and technologies used for PGT have evolved rapidly, providing greater promise for this treatment strategy. In the past, polar bodies from oocytes or 2-pronuclei (2PN) zygotes, or blastomeres from cleavage-stage embryos not older than 3 days post–egg retrieval, were analyzed. More recently, trophectoderm biopsy of day 5 or day 6 blastocyst embryos has replaced day 3 or earlier biopsy. Trophectoderm biopsy provides more genetic material, is less likely to delay embryo development, and is less likely to yield a false-positive result due to mosaicism.[3–10] Previously, fluorescence in situ hybridization (FISH) was used to screen embryos for aneuploidy or diagnose the presence of translocations. This technology was fraught with technical limitations, such as hybridization errors, interpretation error, and ability to test only a few chromosomes. Randomized controlled trials conducted using FISH technique, prior to the advent of trophectoderm biopsy, in women at risk for aneuploidy due to advanced reproductive age, found lower pregnancy rates after embryo biopsy.[11] Recently, several platforms have evolved that are capable of accurately evaluating all 23 chromosome pairs, including comparative genomic hybridization (CGH) microarray, single-nucleotide polymorphism (SNP) microarray, real-time PCR, and next-generation sequencing (NGS). The advent of trophectoderm biopsy and more accurate assays has resulted in a recent resurgence in the use of PGT for aneuploidy screening.[12]

There is no doubt that PGT has helped deliver remarkable gifts to many people; however, its use and application are not without risks or controversy. There is little or no medical or ethical debate about the benefit of PGD in diagnosing embryos at risk for inheriting lethal or significant, diseases, such as cystic fibrosis, Tay-Sachs disease, sickle cell anemia, or Huntington chorea. Medical debate has centered around the use of PGT for aneuploidy screening. Despite absence of medical benefit in improving live birth rates, PGS accounted for approximately 60% of all PGT procedures in Europe in 2009 to 2010.[13] PGT techniques are also used clinically to prevent transmission of genes associated with late-onset diseases, curable diseases, and increased, but not absolute, risk of disease. It is in these areas where many of the ethical concerns with PGT have been debated. The management of devastating late-onset conditions, such as Huntington chorea, poses challenges in disclosing, or hiding, the presence of the Huntington mutation when potentially affected parents choose not to know their status. Creation of a human being for the purpose of being a savior sibling is an area of intense ethical discussion. Another contentious application is the use of PGT to sex embryos for family balancing and to select for specific genetic traits.[14–17] With more and increasing knowledge of the human genome and stem cell biology, the full potential of PGT has yet to be realized. This review discusses the techniques and clinical application of PGT and the debate surrounding its associated uncertainty and expanded use in modern medicine.

HISTORIC PERSPECTIVE AND DEFINITION

In 1986, a group of experts met to discuss the feasibility of prenatal testing in the human preimplantation period to avoid the need for selective abortion associated with other antenatal screening techniques, like chorionic villus sampling (CVS) and amniocentesis.[18] This group of experts determined that 2 sets of people would be candidates: those with low risk of having a child affected by sporadic genetic disorders, like aneuploidy among older mothers, and those at persistent high risk of having a child with a genetic disease. The experts concluded that this second group of patients were most likely to benefit from PGD, and they predicted that "preimplantation genetic screening would not be widely applied to all IVF patients, but only in order to detect the specific disease or diseases for which a particular couple is at high risk." Shortly after this meeting, in 1988, it was reported that expression of the human genome occurs between the 4-cell and 8-cell stages of preimplantation development,[19] and in 1990 a group of researchers and clinicians in London announced the pregnancies of 2 women who conceived female twins after transfer of IVF-created embryos that were biopsied and sexed by PCR for the Y chromosome.[1] So began the clinical application of PGT.

In the first reported cases of PGT, 5 women at risk for transmitting recessive X-linked diseases underwent ovarian stimulation with exogenous gonadotropins, oocyte retrieval was performed, and the oocytes were fertilized in vitro. On day 3 of embryo culture, 1 to 2 cells were aspirated from the embryos after zona pellucida thinning, and Y-chromosome–specific DNA from the biopsied cells was amplified by PCR—a technique that had only recently been developed. Day 3 embryos identified as female were transferred back, and 2 of the women became pregnant with twins. Female gender of these fetuses was confirmed at 10 weeks by CVS. This application of PGT in which a specific genetic disease is being tested for is referred to officially as preimplantation genetic diagnosis (PGD) and it is defined in the International Committee Monitoring Assisted Reproductive Technology (ICMART) and the World Health Organization (WHO) revised glossary of assisted reproductive technology terminology as the "analysis of polar bodies, blastomeres, or trophectoderm from oocytes, zygotes, or embryos for the detection of specific genetic, structural, and/or chromosomal alterations."[20]

The application of PGT in IVF for improving IVF success rates or decreasing the chance of offspring with sporadic genetic disorders is referred to as PGS. PGS is defined in the ICMART/WHO glossary as the "analysis of polar bodies, blastomeres, or trophectoderm from oocytes, zygotes, or embryos for the detection of aneuploidy, mutation, and/or DNA rearrangement."[20] When experts convened in 1986, they predicted PGS as a means to increase live birth rates among women of advanced maternal age. After initial broad introduction of PGS into IVF for this indication, several randomized controlled trials not only failed to prove PGS's ability to improve live birth rates in women undergoing IVF but also suggested a lower birth rate in women of advanced reproductive age.[11] These findings resulted in a temporary decline in the use of PGS with IVF for several years. The concept has experienced a remarkable resurgence recently, relabeled as comprehensive chromosome screening, with the advent of embryo biopsy at a more advanced stage of development (trophectoderm biopsy of day 5 or day 6 blastocysts rather than polar body biopsy or blastomere biopsy no later than day 3) and replacement of the previously used FISH technique of a limited number of chromosomes with comprehensive chromosome screening of all 22 autosomes as well as the sex chromosomes.[12] Contrary to the experts' predictions in 1986, both PGD and PGS are offered to many patients in several settings.

INDICATIONS FOR PREIMPLANTATION GENETIC DIAGNOSIS

The frequency of use and the indications for PGD in the United States and worldwide is increasing. A 2006 survey reported that 74% of US IVF centers provided PGD to patients.[21] In the United States, 4% of 141,000 IVF cycles involved PGT in 2008, compared with 6% of 175,000 cycles in 2013 (SART.org).[22] Although some people consider PGD an early type of prenatal diagnostic testing performed on the embryo in vitro prior to transfer to the uterus, prospective parents often choose PGD to avoid traditional prenatal testing (CVS or amniocentesis) and subsequent termination of an affected fetus. In its original applications PGD was primarily used for mendelian disorders. Mendelian disorders are single-gene defects often defined by describing their basic pedigree patterns: autosomal dominant, autosomal recessive, X-linked (recessive or dominant), and Y-linked (rare). They require a particular genotype at a locus for expression of a character.[23] The widely used Online Mendelian Inheritance in Man (OMIM) (http://www.ncbi.nlm.nih.gov/omim/) is an on-line database created to describe the genes and phenotypes associated with all known mendelian disorders. Over the past 2 decades, the use of PGD in single-gene disorders has had tremendous expansion. Furthermore, more recently, PGD has shown promise in polygenic disorders, sometimes referred to as *nonmendelian*, where phenotypes or characters are dependent on multiple loci. These are conditions in which the pedigrees do not follow traditional monogenetic heritability. More complicated is that often in nonmendelian disorders variability outside the nuclear genetic loci has an etiologic or influential role on the phenotype, such as epigenetic modifications, mitochondrial (and mitochondrial DNA [mtDNA]) abnormalities, post-translational modifications, and the recognized contributions from the environment.

Common mendelian disorders that use PGD in many centers include cystic fibrosis, β-thalassemia, sickle cell disease, myotonic dystrophy, Huntington disease, fragile X syndrome, and spinal muscular atrophy among other disorders.[14,24–26] More recently, a portion of PGD cases includes HLA typing in addition to monogenic testing for a particular condition, which aids treatment strategies for a living sibling or other relative. One example of this is with Fanconi anemia.[27,28] As discussed previously, some of the first applications of PGD involved conditions with X-linked inheritance and amplification of a sequence on the Y chromosome to identify women who were presumably healthy for transfer.[1,26] Soon after, several monogenic disorders like cystic fibrosis followed as the most common indications for PGD as long as a probe containing the causative mutation could be created and used to amplify the DNA sequence in the genome of the embryonic cell. More than 200 single-gene disorders have been reportedly identified with PGD.[26]

Nonmendelian disorders are much more complex scientifically and ethically. Many common multifactorial disorders, such as congenital heart disease, cleft palate/lip, and some behavioral disorders, are currently not conducive to PGD because the polygenic, epigenetic, and environmental contributions to such a phenotype are not completely understood. One of the few situations where PGD may be helpful for nonmendelian or polygenic disorders is when there is unequal gender incidence.[29] For example, disorders, such as breast cancer, rheumatoid arthritis, and multiple sclerosis, have a significantly increased incidence in female offspring. On the other hand, a male sibling born to a family with an autistic child is more likely to have autism than a female sibling.[30] In these cases, PGD may be used simply for gender selection of embryos to diminish the risk to offspring. Gender selection, even for medical indications, is ethically debatable and likely will undergo continuous scrutiny.[31]

Another indication for PGD is in chromosomal disorders. Numeric and structural chromosomal abnormalities are both possible findings in spontaneous miscarriages and in an affected fetus, although overwhelmingly most are numeric.[32] Numeric chromosomal abnormalities include findings, such as polyploidy, monosomy, and trisomies. Although structural alterations represent a small number of miscarriages, they represent a majority of PGD cases done for chromosomal abnormalities.[14] Structural alterations include translocations, inversions, deletions, and other rearrangements in the chromosomes. A parent may harbor an unrecognized balanced translocation, which, when segregation occurs in gametogenesis and subsequent fertilization occurs, becomes an unbalanced abnormality in the offspring. Over the past several years, in the European PGD Consortium, reciprocal translocations have represented more PGD cases from chromosomal abnormalities than robertsonian translocations or other related structural/chromosomal findings.[14]

Finally, mitochondrial disorders are another growing indication for PGD, although more research in this area is needed. Several mitochondrial abnormalities are actually due to mutations in the nuclear DNA and, thus, a PGD process similar to that with a single-gene disorder can be carried out. When mitochondrial diseases are a result of a mutation in mtDNA, the phenotype or affected tissues do not become recognizable until the number of mutated mitochondria reaches an intolerable load within the cell. Many cells in identified mitochondrial diseases have heteroplasmy because a certain percentage of normal and mutated mitochondria exists within the same cell. Therefore, an individual is not affected unless a critical threshold of mutated mitochondria is reached. Often, because of primarily maternal inheritance of mtDNA from the ooplasm, the mother is a carrier of an unknown small percentage of mutated mtDNA that is propagated and expanded in her offspring. Such enhancement of the proportion of mutated mtDNA in the embryo/fetus is explained partially by the bottleneck theory, where at some point in early oogenesis the number of mitochondria per cell is rapidly depleted to very few and then subsequently rapidly expanded in the fetus.[33–37] Once a woman is identified as having an increased risk of transmitting mutated mitochondria to her offspring, her options are to take a chance at spontaneous conception, use donor oocytes, or try PGD to identify embryos with an acceptable ratio of normal to mutated mtDNA. PGD in this scenario is limited because the severity or penetrance of some mitochondrial diseases cannot be accurately predicted by the ratio of normal to abnormal mtDNA. In this scenario, PGD may not completely eliminate the risk of having an affected child but could dramatically lower it. In the future, nuclear transfer from the maternal oocyte into enucleated donor oocytes may prove a means of preventing mitochondrial disorders.[35,38,39] Embryos created using nuclear transfer would contain DNA from 3 sources – paternal nuclear DNA, maternal nuclear DNA, and donor mtDNA.

TECHNIQUES

PGT, either PGD or PGS, requires multiple steps and manipulations of the gametes and embryos to select unaffected embryos for transfer and subsequent potential pregnancy.

The steps involved in PGD are as follows:

1. For single-gene disorders, genotyping of the mutation from parental blood or cheek swab samples and creation of probes by a genetics laboratory, this process can take several weeks
2. Superovulation, oocyte retrieval, IVF with intracytoplasmic sperm injection (ICSI), and embryo culture. ICSI of a single sperm is preferred to standard insemination to avoid DNA contamination from sperm surrounding the embryo in the zona pellucida. Stripping surrounding cumulus cells from the oocyte, a requirement for ICSI, minimizes the risk of DNA contamination by these cells
3. Embryo, or more rarely oocyte polar body, are biopsied. PGT has been performed on the first polar body in unfertilized oocytes, the second polar body from

2PN zygotes,[40,41] blastomeres from day 2 or day 3 cleavage-stage embryos, and trophectoderm from blastocyst embryos. Current practice favors trophectoderm biopsy. Oocyte or embryo biopsy requires breaching the zona pellucida. In the past this was accomplished using acid Tyrode solution. Current technique uses a laser to create an opening in the zona pellucida through which trophectoderm cells are obtained

4. Transport of the biopsy specimen to the reference laboratory performing the evaluation

5. DNA amplification, almost always using PCR.[42] An alternative amplification strategy is whole-genome amplification

6. Testing the amplified DNA with the previously created probes for single-gene disorders

7. When trophectoderm biopsy is performed, cryopreservation of embryos immediately after biopsy is required. Embryo cryopreservation is required because the endometrium's window of implantation will have already closed by the time the genetic results are available

8. Frozen embryo transfer of an unaffected embryo or embryos is performed once the genetic analysis has determined the carrier status of the embryo

The steps involved in PGS are as follows:

1. Superovulation, oocyte retrieval, IVF with ICSI, and embryo culture

2. Biopsy of embryo, or more rarely oocyte polar body

3. Transport of the biopsy specimen to the genetics laboratory performing the evaluation

4. Amplification and testing of the specimen using CGH microarray, SNP microarray, real-time PCR, or NGS

5. When trophectoderm biopsy is performed, cryopreservation of embryos immediately after biopsy

6. Frozen embryo transfer of an embryo with a normal chromosome number in the case of PGS, or with absence of an unbalanced translocation, once the genetic analysis has determined the carrier status of the embryo

Compared with cleavage-stage biopsy, trophectoderm biopsy has the advantages of more cells yielding more DNA, decreased risk of delayed embryo development or destruction, and decreased prevalence of mosaicism compared with cleavage-stage embryos.[4,43–48] The trophectoderm gives rise to the placenta, and, as such, trophectoderm biopsy is analogous to CVS. Discordance in ploidy status between the trophectoderm and the inner cell mass (which gives rise to the fetus) occurs 3% to 5% of the time. A disadvantage of trophectoderm biopsy includes the need to cryopreserve the biopsied embryos and transfer at a later date, except in rare instances where the genetics laboratory is onsite at the IVF program to perform aneuploidy screening. Because many embryos do not progress from cleavage stage to blastocyst stage, patients need to be counseled that there may not be a specimen to biopsy, particularly when few oocytes are retrieved.

GENOMIC TESTING OF SINGLE GENE DISORDER

Genotyping and direct sequencing are the most common methods of identifying single-gene disorders. DNA amplification is required prior to testing, most commonly using PCR. Whole-genome amplification has also been used to perform simultaneous evaluation for single-gene disorders and assessment of all 23 chromosome pairs. Karyomapping using SNP haplotyping is another approach. Any approach that requires

DNA amplification risks allele dropout (ADO). ADO occurs when 1 of the 2 alleles fails to amplify. ADO can lead to misdiagnosis, for example, misinterpreting an embryo with 2 copies of a recessive gene as being a heterozygote or an embryo with only 1 copy of a recessive gene as being affected. Linkage analysis assays, which confirm equal amplification of both sperm-derived and oocyte-derived DNA, are used to identify ADO occurrence.

DIAGNOSTIC PLATFORMS FOR PREIMPLANTATION GENETIC SCREENING

A majority of US IVF centers that provide PGT continue to recommend subsequent prenatal testing (CVS or amniocentesis) to confirm the results due to the small frequency of errors that could occur during PGT.[21,49] Furthermore, genetic counseling of prospective parents prior to the start of a PGT cycle is essential due to the complexity of the multistep procedures, cost, alternatives, interpretation of testing, technical limitations, and outcomes.[49] Like much of technology, no single technique for PGT is perfect and they all carry a risk for misdiagnosis, an outcome that is often unacceptable for some couples.[50] Thus, technology is continually making strides for improved diagnostic accuracy while ensuring rapid and comprehensible results.

In the past, FISH and PCR were the 2 most used techniques for cellular analysis in IVF/PGD cycles.[28,51,52] FISH is a technique where fluorescent-labeled DNA probes are used to bind to specific regions of a chromosome to identify a particular section or presence of a chromosome. It is primarily used to test for chromosomal abnormalities, such as aneuploidy or translocations, but is also used for gender selection for X-linked disorders instead of using PCR. The number of probes used in FISH in each round of hybridization is limited in PGD, which limits the expansion of testing of all 23 chromosome pairs, yet FISH is technically easier than PCR with much less concern for contamination from other DNA material. PCR involves amplification of specific DNA fragments to produce enough material for subsequent analysis. Producing a large enough quantity of DNA from a single cell for mutation analyses is one of the main challenges with PCR. Improvements in PCR techniques have evolved over the past 1 to 2 decades to reduce the chance of erroneous results. The inclusion of additional processes, such as nested PCR, fluorescent PCR, genetic haplotyping, whole-genome amplification, array comparative genomic hybridization (CGH), NGS, and multiplex PCR (additional polymorphic linked markers are also amplified with the region of interest to assure correct allele amplification), among others, have improved accuracy.[28,51-62] Many genetics laboratories have recently shifted toward the use of microarrays with SNP or CGH to evaluate the ploidy status of all 23 chromosomes pairs when performing PGT.[63-67] Although these approaches do not identify balanced chromosomal errors, they do identify unbalanced errors and aneuploidy in all 23 chromosomes pairs.

DIAGNOSTIC ACCURACY

There are numerous decisions that must be made by a couple as they progress through an entire cycle of IVF/PGD. During the process, many complicated discussions ensue when an erroneous, inconsistent, or incomplete result is encountered. Precision in handling, manipulation, biopsy, and observation of the gametes and embryos is critical for reducing adverse outcomes. Numerous causes of misdiagnosis have been reported in the literature.[28,55] The most commonly discussed adverse outcomes are thought to be due to human error, ADO, contamination from other (usually maternal or paternal) DNA, and mosaicism. Human and/or laboratory error can occur at every step along the way and laboratory personnel have an obligation to follow stringent quality-control mechanisms throughout the process. Furthermore, training, not only in the laboratory techniques but also in the interpretation and delivery of reports and results, is crucial. As the technology used in PGD becomes more complicated, interpretation of the results is more challenging and often not as black and white as it may seem. Couples may be faced with a decision of whether or not to transfer an embryo based on a calculated estimate of risk, incomplete results, or limited to no information on the day of planned transfer rather than confirmation of an unaffected or euploid embryo. In addition, it is difficult to perform multiple testing mechanisms on a single embryonic cell. Just because an embryo may be negative for a particular single-gene mutation does not ensure an otherwise normal embryo void of other chromosomal or epigenetic abnormalities. Thus, there has been more recent adoption of microarray CGH platforms that allow for broadened specific and generalized genomic screening in an embryonic blastomere/trophectoderm—an application that is showing more technical promise.[26,61,63–72] It is vital that such information and potential outcomes be delivered to patients both preprocedurally and postprocedurally.

ADO is a commonly cited cause of misdiagnosis, especially with PCR.[28,55] Anytime a small amount of genetic material is utilized for testing, especially from a single cell, there is a chance that 1 of the 2 alleles will fail to hybridize to the probe and not be amplified or detected. The improvements in PCR techniques and adoption of different SNP and CGH microarray platforms, as discussed previously, show more promise in their abilities to detect ADO and provide optimal results.

Contamination is another problem that must always be considered. A majority of PGD cycles use ICSI to remove the 2 most common DNA contaminant sources: cumulus cells around the oocyte and remaining sperm surrounding the oocyte in conventional insemination. This is particularly true with PCR, because even a small amount of contaminant DNA can be dramatically amplified and the results difficult to interpret or erroneously reported. It seems that the issue of contamination is less of a concern with newer platforms for PGT that use whole-genome amplification but adherence to strict laboratory techniques is often encouraged to avoid any potential contamination because this can occur as carryover from either an operator or equipment used on a previous PGD case.[55]

Finally, mosaicism usually is a factor that affects diagnostic accuracy in PGD cases. Both germline and embryonic mosaicism can occur.[51] Inherent in any PGD case is that removal of 1 or a few blastomeres from the embryo assumes that those cells represent the DNA makeup of the embryo and are identical to the cells that remain after biopsy. Yet cells begin to differentiate into the inner cell mass and trophectoderm early in development. It is possible that the cells in the trophectoderm may not represent the cells in the inner cell mass, what is considered the developing fetus.[5–10] Furthermore, the ratio of normal to abnormal cells within the embryo itself could vary and alter the ultimate phenotype. Also, there is the potential for an oocyte or embryo to self-correct any chromosomal abnormality—terms coined *aneuploidy rescue* in meiosis II or *trisomy rescue* in embryonic mitotic divisions.[73] Such suggestions only complicate testing protocols surrounding PGD and may ultimately lead to more biopsy requirements for confirmatory testing. Although these issues are being addressed by performing more trophectoderm biopsy, it is currently not clear whether this approach will completely eliminate the issue of mosaicism.

CONTROVERSIES SURROUNDING PREIMPLANTATION GENETIC TESTING

For many people at risk for transmitting genetic disease, proceeding with PGD and PGS may be more palatable than prenatal diagnostic techniques, like CVS or amniocentesis, because PGD and PGS avoid the need for consideration of pregnancy termination. Because of this, along with the expanding knowledge of the human genome, some investigators have raised the concern that potentially controversial genetic manipulations may be available, including selection for optimization of characteristics that may be considered desirable, like intelligence or longevity.[74] Other investigators have argued that these possibilities are reasonable, allowing for "procreative beneficence" and setting a child up for the "best possible life."[75] On the other hand, the definition of the "best possible life" is debatable because characteristics considered disease by some may be desirable to others. One example of this is genetically inherited deafness—some patients have used PGD to prevent having a child with deafness, whereas some individuals within deaf communities would consider options to increase their chances of having a deaf child.[15]

As discussed previously, another issue that separates PGS and PGD from other antenatal diagnostic screening techniques is that PGS and PGD require the use of IVF. In standard IVF protocols, embryos in excess of what is needed for procreative needs are often created. With this excess, patients must decide (1) which embryos to put back and (2) what to do with those embryos that they do not want to use for procreative purposes. When choosing which embryos to transfer after IVF with PGS/PGD, issues clinicians need to address with patients include the potential inaccuracy of the PGS/PGD results, whether or not embryos carrying recessively inherited mutations or sex-linked disease are reasonable for transfer, and what other genetic information regarding the embryos should be revealed. It has been said that PGS/PGD should be used not as a program of eugenics, to try and wipe out genetic disease but rather to prevent disease, meaning that embryos that are merely carriers of disease should be used for transfer.[76] There is variation among clinicians, however, as to how much patient autonomy they allow in testing embryos.[77]

In addition to deciding which embryos to replace, patients must decide what to do with embryos created in excess of what they need for their reproductive use. Some patients struggle with this decision.[78] Traditional options that have existed for patients with excess embryos after IVF/ICSI have included cryopreservation for future reproductive use, discarding excess embryos, donating excess embryos to research, or donating embryos to other couples for reproductive uses. Some couples opt to not fertilize only a few oocytes to reduce the chances of having excess embryos; however, with PGD and PGS, excess embryos are desirable to increase the chances that good-quality embryos with the desired genetic makeup are available for transfer.

FUTURE OF PREIMPLANTATION GENETIC TESTING: POLICY AND ACCESS

Many investigators have advocated for increased monitoring of applications of PGT[14] and of the long-term health outcomes of the children born from these technologies,[79] but there is no consensus on how this monitoring ought to be done. Some investigators have advocated for government involvement and legislation.[80] In the United States, there is little legislation, restriction, or monitoring of PGD/PGS use and application; however, the American Society for Reproductive Medicine (ASRM) provides reasonable practice guidelines for the use of PGT.[49] The ASRM recommends thorough counseling of couples considering PGT, including genetic counseling, discussion of the risks associated with IVF, embryo biopsy, extended embryo culture, and discussion of the limitations of PGS/PGD, including the risk for misdiagnosis.

The ASRM also recommends a discussion of prenatal diagnostic testing options to confirm PGS/PGD results and the risks associated with the procedures, the possibility that all embryos may be affected, the disposition of embryos in which testing is inconclusive, the disposition of embryos not transferred, and a discussion of alternative options to avoid passing on genetic disease, including the use of donor gametes. Adhering to these recommendations will ensure transparency in the applications of these technologies and allow patients to make more informed decision in electing to use these techniques in their reproductive needs.

In the United States and many other countries, reproductive decisions like PGD/PGS and IVF ultimately are left to individuals and their physicians.[49] On the other hand, there are some countries where strict legislation and restrictions on PGD/PGS and IVF limit access to these treatments.[49,76,81] Some experts have warned that these restrictions may be contributing to the phenomenon of reproductive tourism, where patients travel to other countries for treatments that are not available in their own countries. This concern has raised further concern that a for-profit reproductive services market is being created in which patients without sufficient financial resources will be consigned to genetic fate.[82] In addition to legislation, reimbursement and financing for medical procedures may influence which procedures clinicians offer and, therefore, can limit access patients have to different medical treatments.[49] Although health care reimbursement in the United States may change dramatically in the future, it is unlikely that United States clinicians will stop offering techniques like PGD/PGS and IVF, given that many of these procedures are by and large privately financed.[82,83]

Although controversy in techniques, application, and policy guiding preimplantation screening exists, innovations stemming from current PGD technology may help alleviate some of these controversies. For example, in regard to the use of PGD for sibling HLA matching, recently, it was discovered that human embryonic stem cell lines could be derived from a single biopsied embryonic cell.[84] This could allow for the development of stem cell lines without the destruction of embryos. Furthermore, it could potentially allow for study of specific diseases in affected embryos[85] and for matched tissue generation for children from biopsied PGD embryos — thus avoiding the controversy sparked by the birth of Adam Nash, the first child born after PGD for sibling HLA matching.[84,86]

SUMMARY

As predicted, PGT has helped many individuals prevent the birth of children with severe genetic diseases and also the need for selective abortion associated with postgravid antenatal screening techniques.[18] Given the disadvantages associated with cleavage-stage biopsy for PGT,[4–7,48] most centers have adopted trophectoderm biopsy and cryopreservation of tested blastocysts for subsequent transfer as a new clinical paradigm. Utilization of newer genetic testing platform for PGS for aneuploidy is becoming an effective way to improve the chances of live birth, especially if elective single-embryo transfer is considered.[12,87,88] Increasing knowledge of the human embryo and the genetic basis of human disease coupled with the development of these new genetic testing platforms will lead to increased application and use of PGT. Collaborative efforts among clinicians of different disciplines, scientists, and policymakers are necessary to ensure that this increased application and use is done in a responsible fashion.

ACKNOWLEDGMENTS

The authors would like to acknowledge Amber R. Cooper, MD, and Emily S. Jungheim, MD, for their initial contributions to this topic.

REFERENCES

1. Handyside AH, Kontogianni EH, Hardy K, et al. Pregnancies from biopsied human preimplantation embryos sexed by Y-specific DNA amplification. Nature 1990;344(6268):768–70.
2. Brezina PR, Kutteh WH. Clinical applications of preimplantation genetic testing. BMJ 2015;350:g7611.
3. Carson SA, Gentry WL, Smith AL, et al. Trophectoderm microbiopsy in murine blastocysts: comparison of four methods. J Assist Reprod Genet 1993;10(6):427–33.
4. Scott RT Jr, Upham KM, Forman EJ, et al. Cleavage-stage biopsy significantly impairs human embryonic implantation potential while blastocyst biopsy does not: a randomized and paired clinical trial. Fertil Steril 2013;100(3):624–30.
5. Johnson DS, Cinnioglu C, Ross R, et al. Comprehensive analysis of karyotypic mosaicism between trophectoderm and inner cell mass. Mol Hum Reprod 2010;16(12):944–9.
6. Johnson DS, Gemelos G, Baner J, et al. Preclinical validation of a microarray method for full molecular karyotyping of blastomeres in a 24-h protocol. Hum Reprod 2010;25(4):1066–75.
7. Munne S, Sandalinas M, Escudero T, et al. Chromosome mosaicism in cleavage-stage human embryos: evidence of a maternal age effect. Reprod Biomed Online 2002;4(3):223–32.
8. Munne S, Weier HU, Grifo J, et al. Chromosome mosaicism in human embryos. Biol Reprod 1994;51(3):373–9.
9. Novik V, Moulton EB, Sisson ME, et al. The accuracy of chromosomal microarray testing for identification of embryonic mosaicism in human blastocysts. Mol Cytogenet 2014;7(1):18.
10. Vanneste E, Voet T, Le Caignec C, et al. Chromosome instability is common in human cleavage-stage embryos. Nat Med 2009;15(5):577–83.
11. Mastenbroek S, Twisk M, van der Veen F, et al. Preimplantation genetic screening: a systematic review and meta-analysis of RCTs. Hum Reprod Update 2011;17(4):454–66.
12. Scott RT Jr, Upham KM, Forman EJ, et al. Blastocyst biopsy with comprehensive chromosome screening and fresh embryo transfer significantly increases in vitro fertilization implantation and delivery rates: a randomized controlled trial. Fertil Steril 2013;100(3):697–703.
13. Moutou C, Goossens V, Coonen E, et al. ESHRE PGD Consortium data collection XII: cycles from January to December 2009 with pregnancy follow-up to October 2010. Hum Reprod 2014;29(5):880–903.
14. Goossens V, Harton G, Moutou C, et al. ESHRE PGD Consortium data collection IX: cycles from January to December 2006 with pregnancy follow-up to October 2007. Hum Reprod 2009;24(8):1786–810.
15. Dennis C. Genetics: deaf by design. Nature 2004;431(7011):894–6.
16. Verlinsky Y, Rechitsky S, Schoolcraft W, et al. Designer babies - are they a reality yet? Case report: simultaneous preimplantation genetic diagnosis for fanconi anaemia and HLA typing for cord blood transplantation. Reprod Biomed Online 2000;1(2):31.
17. Tajima H, Sueoka K, Moon SY, et al. The development of novel quantification assay for mitochondrial DNA heteroplasmy aimed at preimplantation genetic diagnosis of Leigh encephalopathy. J Assist Reprod Genet 2007;24(6):227–32.

18. Whittingham DG, Penketh R. Prenatal diagnosis in the human pre-implantation period. Meeting held at the Ciba Foundation on the 13th November 1986. Hum Reprod 1987;2(3):267–70.

19. Braude P, Bolton V, Moore S. Human gene expression first occurs between the four- and eight-cell stages of preimplantation development. Nature 1988; 332(6163):459–61.

20. Zegers-Hochschild F, Adamson GD, de Mouzon J, et al. International committee for monitoring assisted reproductive technology (ICMART) and the World Health Organization (WHO) revised glossary of ART terminology, 2009. Fertil Steril 2009; 92(5):1520–4.

21. Baruch S, Kaufman D, Hudson KL. Genetic testing of embryos: practices and perspectives of US in vitro fertilization clinics. Fertil Steril 2008;89(5):1053–8.

22. Available at: http://sart.org/. Accessed December 10, 2015.

23. Strachan T, Read A. Genes in pedigrees and populations. Human molecular genetics 3. 3rd edition. New York: Garland Science; 2004. p. 102–11.

24. Spits C, Sermon K. PGD for monogenic disorders: aspects of molecular biology. Prenat Diagn 2009;29(1):50–6.

25. Goossens V, Harton G, Moutou C, et al. ESHRE PGD Consortium data collection VIII: cycles from January to December 2005 with pregnancy follow-up to October 2006. Hum Reprod 2008;23(12):2629–45.

26. Fragouli E. Preimplantation genetic diagnosis: present and future. J Assist Reprod Genet 2007;24(6):201–7.

27. Verlinsky Y, Rechitsky S, Schoolcraft W, et al. Preimplantation diagnosis for Fanconi anemia combined with HLA matching. JAMA 2001;285(24):3130–3.

28. Yaron YGV, Gamzu R, Malcov M. Genetic analysis of the embryo. In: Gardner DWA, Howles C, Shoham Z, editors. Textbook of assisted reproductive technologies. 3rd edition. London: Informa; 2009. p. 403–16.

29. Amor DJ, Cameron C. PGD gender selection for non-mendelian disorders with unequal sex incidence. Hum Reprod 2008;23(4):729–34.

30. Yeargin-Allsopp M, Rice C, Karapurkar T, et al. Prevalence of autism in a US metropolitan area. JAMA 2003;289(1):49–55.

31. Pennings G. Personal desires of patients and social obligations of geneticists: applying preimplantation genetic diagnosis for non-medical sex selection. Prenat Diagn 2002;22(12):1123–9.

32. ESHRE Capri Workshop Group, Collins J, Diedrich K, Franks S, et al. Genetic aspects of female reproduction. Hum Reprod Update 2008;14(4):293–307.

33. Instability of the human genome: mutation and DNA repair. In: Strachan T, Read A, editors. Human molecular genetics 3. 3rd edition. New York: Garland Science; 2004. p. 316–49.

34. Anderson S, Bankier AT, Barrell BG, et al. Sequence and organization of the human mitochondrial genome. Nature 1981;290(5806):457–65.

35. Poulton J, Kennedy S, Oakeshott P, et al. Preventing transmission of maternally inherited mitochondrial DNA diseases. BMJ 2009;338:b94.

36. Marchington DR, Macaulay V, Hartshorne GM, et al. Evidence from human oocytes for a genetic bottleneck in an mtDNA disease. Am J Hum Genet 1998; 63(3):769–75.

37. Cree LM, Samuels DC, de Sousa Lopes SC, et al. A reduction of mitochondrial DNA molecules during embryogenesis explains the rapid segregation of genotypes. Nat Genet 2008;40(2):249–54.

38. Tachibana M, Sparman M, Sritanaudomchai H, et al. Mitochondrial gene replacement in primate offspring and embryonic stem cells. Nature 2009;461(7262): 367–72.
39. Cree L, Loi P. Mitochondrial replacement: from basic research to assisted reproductive technology portfolio tool-technicalities and possible risks. Mol Hum Reprod 2015;21(1):3–10.
40. Verlinsky Y, Cieslak J, Ivakhnenko V, et al. Preimplantation diagnosis of common aneuploidies by the first- and second-polar body FISH analysis. J Assist Reprod Genet 1998;15(5):285–9.
41. Verlinsky Y, Ginsberg N, Lifchez A, et al. Analysis of the first polar body: preconception genetic diagnosis. Hum Reprod 1990;5(7):826–9.
42. Hattori H, Kaneda T, Ohtsuka K. Preparative 2-dimensional electrophoresis–slab NEPHGE/SDS-PAGE. Seikagaku 1992;64(6):416–20 [in Japanese].
43. Goossens V, De Rycke M, De Vos A, et al. Diagnostic efficiency, embryonic development and clinical outcome after the biopsy of one or two blastomeres for preimplantation genetic diagnosis. Hum Reprod 2008;23(3):481–92.
44. McArthur SJ, Leigh D, Marshall JT, et al. Blastocyst trophectoderm biopsy and preimplantation genetic diagnosis for familial monogenic disorders and chromosomal translocations. Prenat Diagn 2008;28(5):434–42.
45. Michiels A, Van Assche E, Liebaers I, et al. The analysis of one or two blastomeres for PGD using fluorescence in-situ hybridization. Hum Reprod 2006; 21(9):2396–402.
46. Tarin JJ, Conaghan J, Winston RM, et al. Human embryo biopsy on the 2nd day after insemination for preimplantation diagnosis: removal of a quarter of embryo retards cleavage. Fertil Steril 1992;58(5):970–6.
47. van de Velde H, De Vos A, Sermon K, et al. Embryo implantation after biopsy of one or two cells from cleavage-stage embryos with a view to preimplantation genetic diagnosis. Prenat Diagn 2000;20(13):1030–7.
48. De Vos A, Staessen C, De Rycke M, et al. Impact of cleavage-stage embryo biopsy in view of PGD on human blastocyst implantation: a prospective cohort of single embryo transfers. Hum Reprod 2009;24(12):2988–96.
49. Practice Committee of Society for Assisted Reproductive Technology, Practice Committee of American Society for Reproductive Medicine. Preimplantation genetic testing: a practice committee opinion. Fertil Steril 2008;90:S136.
50. Rechitsky S, Verlinsky O, Amet T, et al. Reliability of preimplantation diagnosis for single gene disorders. Mol Cell Endocrinol 2001;183(Suppl 1):S65–8.
51. Kearns WG, Pen R, Graham J, et al. Preimplantation genetic diagnosis and screening. Semin Reprod Med 2005;23(4):336–47.
52. Sermon K, van Steirteghem A, Liebaers I. Preimplantation genetic diagnosis. Lancet 2004;363(9421):1633–41.
53. Hattori M, Yoshioka K, Sakaki Y. High-sensitive fluorescent DNA sequencing and its application for detection and mass-screening of point mutations. Electrophoresis 1992;13(8):560–5.
54. Moustafa H, Rizk B, Nagy Z. Preimplantation genetic diagnosis for single-gene disorders. In: Rizk B, Garcia-Velasco J, Sallam H, et al, editors. Infertility and assisted reproduction. New York: Cambridge University Press; 2008. p. 657–76.
55. Wilton L, Thornhill A, Traeger-Synodinos J, et al. The causes of misdiagnosis and adverse outcomes in PGD. Hum Reprod 2009;24(5):1221–8.
56. Thornhill AR, deDie-Smulders CE, Geraedts JP, et al. ESHRE PGD Consortium 'Best practice guidelines for clinical preimplantation genetic diagnosis (PGD) and preimplantation genetic screening (PGS)'. Hum Reprod 2005;20(1):35–48.

57. Renwick PJ, Trussler J, Ostad-Saffari E, et al. Proof of principle and first cases using preimplantation genetic haplotyping–a paradigm shift for embryo diagnosis. Reprod Biomed Online 2006;13(1):110–9.
58. Sherlock J, Cirigliano V, Petrou M, et al. Assessment of diagnostic quantitative fluorescent multiplex polymerase chain reaction assays performed on single cells. Ann Hum Genet 1998;62(Pt 1):9–23.
59. Fiorentino F, Magli MC, Podini D, et al. The minisequencing method: an alternative strategy for preimplantation genetic diagnosis of single gene disorders. Mol Hum Reprod 2003;9(7):399–410.
60. Zhang L, Cui X, Schmitt K, et al. Whole genome amplification from a single cell: implications for genetic analysis. Proc Natl Acad Sci U S A 1992;89(13):5847–51.
61. Wilton L. Preimplantation genetic diagnosis and chromosome analysis of blastomeres using comparative genomic hybridization. Hum Reprod Update 2005; 11(1):33–41.
62. Bejjani BA, Shaffer LG. Application of array-based comparative genomic hybridization to clinical diagnostics. J Mol Diagn 2006;8(5):528–33.
63. Bisignano A, Wells D, Harton G, et al. PGD and aneuploidy screening for 24 chromosomes: advantages and disadvantages of competing platforms. Reprod Biomed Online 2011;23(6):677–85.
64. Li G, Jin H, Xin Z, et al. Increased IVF pregnancy rates after microarray preimplantation genetic diagnosis due to parental translocations. Syst Biol Reprod Med 2014;60(2):119–24.
65. Treff NR, Northrop LE, Kasabwala K, et al. Single nucleotide polymorphism microarray-based concurrent screening of 24-chromosome aneuploidy and unbalanced translocations in preimplantation human embryos. Fertil Steril 2011; 95(5):1606.e1-2–12.e1-2.
66. Treff NR, Su J, Tao X, et al. Single-cell whole-genome amplification technique impacts the accuracy of SNP microarray-based genotyping and copy number analyses. Mol Hum Reprod 2011;17(6):335–43.
67. Treff NR, Tao X, Schillings WJ, et al. Use of single nucleotide polymorphism microarrays to distinguish between balanced and normal chromosomes in embryos from a translocation carrier. Fertil Steril 2011;96(1):e58–65.
68. Wells D, Sherlock JK, Handyside AH, et al. Detailed chromosomal and molecular genetic analysis of single cells by whole genome amplification and comparative genomic hybridisation. Nucleic Acids Res 1999;27(4):1214–8.
69. Hu DG, Webb G, Hussey N. Aneuploidy detection in single cells using DNA array-based comparative genomic hybridization. Mol Hum Reprod 2004; 10(4):283–9.
70. Le Caignec C, Spits C, Sermon K, et al. Single-cell chromosomal imbalances detection by array CGH. Nucleic Acids Res 2006;34(9):e68.
71. Spits C, Le Caignec C, De Rycke M, et al. Whole-genome multiple displacement amplification from single cells. Nat Protoc 2006;1(4):1965–70.
72. Spits C, Le Caignec C, De Rycke M, et al. Optimization and evaluation of single-cell whole-genome multiple displacement amplification. Hum Mutat 2006;27(5): 496–503.
73. Kuliev A, Verlinsky Y. Meiotic and mitotic nondisjunction: lessons from preimplantation genetic diagnosis. Hum Reprod Update 2004;10(5):401–7.
74. Committee on Ethics, American College of Obstetricians and Gynecologists, Committee on Genetics, American College of Obstetricians and Gynecologists. ACOG committee opinion No. 410: ethical issues in genetic testing. Obstet Gynecol 2008; 111(6):1495–502.

75. Savulescu J, Kahane G. The moral obligation to create children with the best chance of the best life. Bioethics 2009;23(5):274–90.
76. Aarden E, van Hoyweghen I, Vos R, et al. Providing preimplantation genetic diagnosis in the United Kingdom, The Netherlands and Germany: a comparative in-depth analysis of health-care access. Hum Reprod 2009;24(7):1542–7.
77. Wertz DC, Fletcher JC, Nippert I, et al. In focus. Has patient autonomy gone to far? Geneticists' views in 36 nations. Am J Bioeth 2002;2(4):W21.
78. Lyerly AD, Steinhauser K, Voils C, et al. Fertility patients' views about frozen embryo disposition: results of a multi-institutional U.S. survey. Fertil Steril 2008;93(2):499–509.
79. Reddy UM, Wapner RJ, Rebar RW, et al. Infertility, assisted reproductive technology, and adverse pregnancy outcomes: executive summary of a National Institute of Child Health and Human Development workshop. Obstet Gynecol 2007;109(4):967–77.
80. Simpson JL, Rebar RW, Carson SA. Professional self-regulation for preimplantation genetic diagnosis: experience of the American Society for Reproductive Medicine and other professional societies. Fertil Steril 2006;85(6):1653–60.
81. Jones HW Jr, Cohen J. IFFS surveillance 07. Fertil Steril 2007;87(4 Suppl 1):S1–67.
82. Spar D. Reproductive tourism and the regulatory map. N Engl J Med 2005;352(6):531–3.
83. Jain T, Harlow BL, Hornstein MD. Insurance coverage and outcomes of in vitro fertilization. N Engl J Med 2002;347(9):661–6.
84. Klimanskaya I, Chung Y, Becker S, et al. Human embryonic stem cell lines derived from single blastomeres. Nature 2006;444(7118):481–5.
85. Mateizel I, De Temmerman N, Ullmann U, et al. Derivation of human embryonic stem cell lines from embryos obtained after IVF and after PGD for monogenic disorders. Hum Reprod 2006;21(2):503–11.
86. Crockin S. Adam nash: legally speaking, a happy ending or slippery slope? Reprod Biomed Online 2001;2(1):6–7.
87. Forman EJ, Hong KH, Ferry KM, et al. In vitro fertilization with single euploid blastocyst transfer: a randomized controlled trial. Fertil Steril 2013;100(1):100–7.e101.
88. Forman EJ, Hong KH, Franasiak JM, et al. Obstetrical and neonatal outcomes from the BEST trial: single embryo transfer with aneuploidy screening improves outcomes after in vitro fertilization without compromising delivery rates. Am J Obstet Gynecol 2014;210(2):157.e1–6.

Screening for Open Neural Tube Defects

David A. Krantz, MA*, Terrence W. Hallahan, PhD,
Jonathan B. Carmichael, PhD

KEYWORDS

- Alpha fetoprotein • Maternal serum • Spina bifida • Anencephaly
- Adverse pregnancy outcome

KEY POINTS

- Biochemical prenatal screening was initiated with the use of maternal serum alpha feto-protein to screen for open neural tube defects.
- Screening has evolved to include multiple marker and sequential screening protocols involving serum and ultrasound markers to screen for aneuploidy.
- Most recently cell-free DNA screening for aneuploidy has been initiated and whether or not it becomes the primary form of screening for aneuploidy it is not effective in identifying neural tube defects.
- Although ultrasound is highly effective in identifying neural tube defects in high-risk populations, in decentralized health systems where screening of the general population takes place maternal serum screening still plays a significant role.
- Abnormal maternal serum alpha fetoprotein alone or in combination with other markers may indicate adverse pregnancy outcome in the absence of open neural tube defects.

Maternal serum screening for fetal congenital anomalies began in the early 1970s with the advent of alpha fetoprotein (AFP) screening for neural tube defects.[1,2] It was from this screening protocol that the initial observation that AFP is low in Down syndrome–affected pregnancies was made.[3] Today, screening for Down syndrome is highly complex with protocols that include various combinations of serum, ultrasound, and cell-free DNA markers across the first and second trimesters of pregnancy. Although, cell-free DNA testing shows great promise in high-risk populations conventional maternal serum screening remains the most appropriate screening approach in low-risk populations.[4] For those women who undergo second trimester conventional

---

This article is an update of an article previously published in Clinics in Laboratory Medicine, Volume 30, Issue 3, September 2010.
Disclosure Statement: The authors are employees of PerkinElmer.
Eurofins/NTD, 80 Ruland Road, Suite 1, Melville, NY 11747, USA
* Corresponding author.
E-mail address: DAVID.KRANTZ@PERKINELMER.COM

screening, risk assessment for open neural tube defects is an integral part of the process. However, in those instances where patients have undergone aneuploidy screening (first trimester conventional or cell-free DNA screening) it is important to offer these women screening for open neural tube defects in the second trimester. The most common approach to such screening is evaluation of AFP in maternal serum.

Maternal serum AFP (MSAFP) screening is conducted between 15 and 21 weeks of gestation. Blood specimens may be collected as liquid whole blood or dried blood spots.[5] Median MSAFP levels increase steadily by about 15% per week from a concentration of approximately 25 IU/mL at 15 weeks of gestation to a level of approximately 60 IU/mL at 21 weeks of gestation. To account for this upward trend in normal levels throughout pregnancy, values of AFP are converted into multiples of the gestational age–specific median (MoMs) by dividing the patient's analytical AFP concentration by the median concentration for that gestational age. The MoM values are then typically corrected for demographic factors, such as maternal weight, ethnicity, and diabetic status.

Patients with higher maternal weight tend to have on average lower MSAFP levels than those with lower maternal weight.[6] As a result, the MoM values for patients with higher maternal weight are adjusted downward, whereas patients with lower maternal weight are adjusted upward (**Fig. 1**).

MSAFP levels have been demonstrated to vary by ethnicity. The most significant shift is observed in African American patients who tend to have MoM values that are on average 16% greater than in white patients after weight adjustment.

Insulin-dependent diabetes mellitus affects open neural tube defect screening in two ways. First, the incidence of open neural tube defects is three- to four-fold higher in patients with insulin-dependent diabetes mellitus.[7] Second, MSAFP levels are approximately 20% lower in patients with insulin-dependent diabetes mellitus compared with the general population.[8] Although recent publications have suggested that this adjustment factor may no longer be necessary,[9] guidelines still suggest including an adjustment.[10]

In cases of open spina bifida and anencephaly, openings in the spine or skull result in leakage of AFP into the amniotic fluid, which then diffuses into the maternal blood

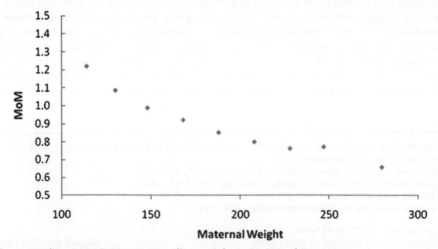

Fig. 1. Median AFP MoM versus median weight in 21,972 white patients.

causing significant increases in MSAFP levels. The median MoM value in open spina bifida at 16 weeks of gestation is 3.8 MoM, whereas the median MoM value for anencephaly is 6.5 MoM.[11] The typical cutoff for MSAFP screening is 2.0 to 2.5 MoM. Using a cutoff of 2 MoM can increase detection of open spina bifida by approximately 10%. Using this 2-MoM cutoff, the detection rate for open spina bifida is 90% and virtually all cases of anencephaly are detected unless gestational age dating is significantly incorrect.[12]

Twin pregnancies can be evaluated for open neural tube defects. However, the discrimination between the distribution of AFP levels in neural tube defect and unaffected pregnancy is much less than in singleton pregnancy. In an affected twin pregnancy, the median MoM is 4.4 in open spina bifida and 7.5 in anencephaly.[13] Compared with the unaffected twin median (1.9 MoM), this represents a 2.3- and 3.9-fold increase in affected cases for open spina bifida and anencephaly, respectively, compared with a 3.8- and 6.5-fold increase in a singleton pregnancy. The reason for the smaller discrimination is that the AFP level in affected twin pregnancy represents a mixture of AFP levels from both the unaffected and affected fetus. Thus, whereas the median MoM in unaffected twin pregnancy is approximately double that of a singleton pregnancy, the median MoM in an affected twin pregnancy is not twice as great as that in an affected singleton pregnancy.

Using a cutoff of 4 multiples of the singleton median, the detection rate in twins is 93% for anencephaly and 58% for open spina bifida with a 7.8% false-positive rate. Using a 5-MoM cutoff, the detection rate is 83.0% for anencephaly and 39.0% for open spina bifida with a 3.3% false-positive rate.[13] Laboratories may report the results in twins based on the singleton median, in which case the cutoff is 4 or 5 MoM, or they may adjust the MoM for twins, in which case the cutoff is identical to the cutoff used in singleton pregnancy (2.0–2.5 MoM).

Laboratories usually provide a patient-specific risk for open spina bifida, anencephaly, and ventral wall defect on patient reports. Risks are determined by factoring in the distribution of AFP MoM values and the prior incidence of these disorders. The incidence of open neural tube defects is approximately 1 to 2 per 1000 in the United States; however, these incidence rates vary from region to region. Incidence rates are highest in the southeastern United States and are lowest in the northwest. In addition, incidence rates vary by ethnic group with African Americans having a lower incidence than whites.[14] In addition, the incidence of neural tube defects is increased in patients who previously have had a child with open neural tube defect and to a lesser extent if there is family history of open neural tube defect.[15] There is a 1% risk of open spina bifida in patients taking valproic acid or carbamazepine medication.[16,17]

Although patient-specific risk information is desirable as a way of providing understandable information to patients, the risk calculations are based in part on reference data that may no longer be applicable. For example, the precision of AFP assays has significantly improved over the last 30 years. The standard deviation of log MoM in unaffected pregnancies was estimated to be 0.216 in 1982.[10] More recently, the standard deviation of log MoM in unaffected pregnancies was estimated to be 0.1468.[18] This improved precision not only leads to better screening performance but results in three- to seven-fold higher risk estimates for MoM values between 2.5 and 3 than previously estimated.

In addition, since the early 1990s, the American College of Obstetricians and Gynecologists have recommended that pregnant women ingest 400 mg of folic acid daily to prevent neural tube defects, thus lowering the incidence of open neural tube defects.[19] Also, because a large number of affected pregnancies are terminated, incidence rates at birth are less accurate. As a result, it is difficult to quantify the incidence rates compared with historically observed data. Thus risk figures provided by laboratories that rely on historical incidence rates may not be as precise as they were in the past. Furthermore, it is now possible to detect anencephaly during the nuchal translucency examination that is undertaken as part of first trimester Down syndrome screening.[20] Indeed, if nuchal translucency is performed, the risk of anencephaly quantitated based on MSAFP levels is not relevant. However, if cell-free DNA screening is performed and the first trimester ultrasound is not performed then anencephaly risk information is relevant.

Specimens with results between 2.0 and 2.5 MoM may be considered to be borderline elevated. In such cases, a repeat maternal serum blood specimen can better differentiate between false-positives and affected pregnancies. A second blood test result tends to have regression to the mean such that this second specimen lies closer to the mean than an initial specimen. In the case of open neural tube defects, the regression to the mean phenomenon has a significant advantage because the MSAFP levels in open spina bifida and anencephaly are significantly greater than 2.5 MoM. As a result, a second maternal serum blood specimen tends to regress toward these higher MoM values, whereas a second maternal serum blood specimen from an unaffected pregnancy tends to regress toward 1.0 MoM. Therefore, in open spina bifida and anencephaly pregnancies, a second blood specimen tends to be higher, whereas in unaffected pregnancy, a second blood specimen tends to be lower, thus improving screening performance.

For patients with MSAFP results greater than 2.5 MoM or those with two results greater than 2.0 MoM, follow-up testing should be offered. For those who opt to have amniocentesis, elevated amniotic fluid AFP with confirmation by acetylcholinesterase is an effective diagnostic test for neural tube defects. However, follow-up assessment with ultrasound to visualize the defect should be performed before any decision is made regarding continuation of the pregnancy. In recent years, it has been argued that it may be preferable to perform the detailed ultrasound before amniocentesis and offer amniocentesis only to confirm neural tube defects visualized on ultrasound.

In normal pregnancy, amniotic fluid AFP decreases by approximately 20% per week from a level of 15 mg/mL at 15 weeks of gestation to 4.4 mg/mL at 21 weeks of gestation. In cases of neural tube defect, AFP leaks into the amniotic fluid through openings in either the skull or spine, causing an increase in measured amniotic fluid AFP. Elevated amniotic fluid AFP may be associated with conditions other than neural tube defects. As a result, confirmation should be performed using acetylcholinesterase.

In cases where open neural tube defect has been ruled out, elevated MSAFP still imparts increased risk of adverse pregnancy outcome. Approximately 25% of patients with elevated MSAFP have an adverse pregnancy outcome.[5,12] **Table 1** shows the increase in risk attributable to elevated MSAFP for specific disorders.[12,21–23] In addition, elevated AFP (>2.5 MoM) concurrent with elevated free β-human chorionic gonadotropin (>2.5 moM) is associated with a 32.2-fold increase in the risk of placenta accreta,[21] whereas elevated AFP (>2.0 MoM) concurrent with elevated inhibin (>2.0 MoM) is associated with a 20-fold for preterm birth (<32 weeks), 18-fold for early fetal loss (<24 weeks), nine-fold for late fetal loss (>24 weeks), and 4.3-fold for preeclampsia.[24]

As an alternative to maternal serum screening, ultrasound may be used to identify neural tube defects.[25,26] Although such screening performs well in high-risk pregnancies, its performance in low-risk pregnancies in a decentralized health system, such as

Table 1
Incidence of adverse outcomes associated with elevated maternal serum AFP

Outcome	Relative Risk	Reference
Major nonchromosomal congenital defect	4.7	12
Fetal death	8.1	12
Neonatal death	4.7	12
Newborn complications	3.6	12
Oligohydramnios	3.4	12
Abruption	3	12
Preeclampsia	2.4	21
Placenta accreta	9.7	22
Preterm birth (<37 wk)	4.8	23
Low birth weight (<10th percentile)	2.8	23

Data from Refs.[12,21–23]

the United States, may not be as strong.[27] In addition, by forgoing the opportunity to assess MSAFP levels in the second trimester, the chance to identify pregnancies at high risk for adverse outcome is lost. As a result, it is likely that MSAFP screening for open neural tube defects will continue to play a significant role in prenatal care.

REFERENCES

1. Brock DJ, Bolton AE, Monaghan JM. Prenatal diagnosis of anencephaly through maternal serum-alphafetoprotein measurement. Lancet 1973;2(7835):923–4.

2. Macri JN, Weiss RR, Schell NB, et al. Progress in screening for neural tube defects. JAMA 1977;237:2187.

3. Merkatz IR, Nitowsky HM, Macri JN, et al. An association between low maternal serum alpha-fetoprotein and fetal chromosomal abnormalities. Am J Obstet Gynecol 1984;148:886–94.

4. Committee Opinion No. 640: cell-free DNA screening for fetal aneuploidy. Obstet Gynecol 2015;126(3):e31–7.

5. Macri JN, Anderson RW, Krantz DA, et al. Prenatal maternal dried blood screening with alpha-fetoprotein and free beta-human chorionic gonadotropin for open neural tube defect and Down syndrome. Am J Obstet Gynecol 1996; 174:566–72.

6. Wald N, Cuckle H, Boreham J, et al. The effect of maternal weight on maternal serum alpha-fetoprotein levels. Br J Obstet Gynaecol 1981;88:1094–6.

7. Mills JL, Knopp RH, Simpson JL, et al. Lack of relation of increased malformation rates in infants of diabetic mothers to glycemic control during organogenesis. N Engl J Med 1988;318:671–6.

8. Henriques CU, Damm P, Tabor A, et al. Decreased alpha-fetoprotein in amniotic fluid and maternal serum in diabetic pregnancy. Obstet Gynecol 1993;82:960–4.

9. Sancken U, Bartels I. Biochemical screening for chromosomal disorders and neural tube defects (NTD): is adjustment of maternal alpha-fetoprotein (AFP) still appropriate in insulin-dependent diabetes mellitus (IDDM)? Prenat Diagn 2001; 21:383–6.

10. Bradley LA, Palomaki GE, McDowell GA, ONTD Working Group, ACMG Laboratory Quality Assurance Committee. Technical standards and guidelines: prenatal screening for open neural tube defects. Genet Med 2005;7:355–69.
11. Fourth report of the UK collaborative study on alpha-fetoprotein in relation to neural tube defects. Estimating an individual's risk of having a fetus with open spina bifida and the value of repeat alpha-fetoprotein testing. J Epidemiol Community Health 1982;36(2):87–95.
12. Milunsky A, Jick SS, Bruell CL, et al. Predictive values, relative risks, and overall benefits of high and low maternal serum alpha-fetoprotein screening in singleton pregnancies: new epidemiologic data. Am J Obstet Gynecol 1989;161:291–7.
13. Cuckle H, Wald N, Stevenson JD, et al. Maternal serum alpha-fetoprotein screening for open neural tube defects in twin pregnancies. Prenat Diagn 1990;10(2):71–7.
14. Greenberg F, James LM, Oakley GP Jr. Estimates of birth prevalence rates of spina bifida in the United States from computer-generated maps. Am J Obstet Gynecol 1983;145:570–3.
15. Main DM, Mennuti MT. Neural tube defects: issues in prenatal diagnosis and counseling. Obstet Gynecol 1986;1:67.
16. Robert E, Guibaud P. Maternal valproic acid and congenital neural tube defects. Lancet 1982;320:937.
17. Rosa FW. Spina bifida in infants of women treated with carbamazepine during pregnancy. N Engl J Med 1991;324:675–7.
18. Wald NJ, Hackshaw AK, George LM. Assay precision of serum alpha fetoprotein in antenatal screening for neural tube defects and Down's syndrome. J Med Screen 2000;7:74–7.
19. Centers for Disease Control (CDC). Use of folic acid for prevention of spina bifida and other neural tube defects—1983–1991. MMWR Morb Mortal Wkly Rep 1991; 40:513–6.
20. Johnson SP, Sebire NJ, Snijders RJ, et al. Ultrasound screening for anencephaly at 10–14 weeks of gestation. Ultrasound Obstet Gynecol 1997;9:14–6.
21. Morris RK, Cnossen JS, Langejans M, et al. Serum screening with Down's syndrome markers to predict pre-eclampsia and small for gestational age: systematic review and meta-analysis. BMC Pregnancy Childbirth 2008;8:33.
22. Dreux S, Salomon LJ, Muller F, et al, ABA Study Group. Second-trimester maternal serum markers and placenta accreta. Prenat Diagn 2012;32:1010–2.
23. Krause TG, Christens P, Wohlfahrt J, et al. Second-trimester maternal serum alpha-fetoprotein and risk of adverse pregnancy outcome. Obstet Gynecol 2001;97:277–82.
24. Dugoff L, Hobbins JC, Malone FD, et al, FASTER Trial Research Consortium. Quad screen as a predictor of adverse pregnancy outcome. Obstet Gynecol 2005;106:260–7.
25. Lennon CA, Gray DL. Sensitivity and specificity of ultrasound for the detection of neural tube and ventral wall defects in a high risk population. Obstet Gynecol 1999;94:562–6.
26. Boyd PA, Wellesley DG, De Walle HE, et al. Evaluation of prenatal diagnosis of neural tube defects by fetal ultrasonographic examination in different centres across Europe. J Med Screen 2000;7:169–74.
27. Jenkins TM, Wapner RJ. Prenatal diagnosis of congenital disorders. In: Creasy RK, Resnick R, Iams JD, editors. Maternal-fetal medicine principals and practice. 5th edition. Philadelphia: WB Saunders; 2004. p. 235–80.

Toxoplasmosis, Parvovirus, and Cytomegalovirus in Pregnancy

Deborah M. Feldman, MD[a],*, Rebecca Keller, MD[b],
Adam F. Borgida, MD[a]

KEYWORDS

- Toxoplasmosis • Parvovirus • Cytomegalovirus • Diagnosis • Management

KEY POINTS

- There are several infections in adults that warrant special consideration in pregnant women given the potential fetal consequences.
- Among these are toxoplasmosis, parvovirus B19, and cytomegalovirus; these infections have an important impact on the developing fetus, depending on the timing of infection.
- Most fetal outcomes are favorable, even for those with documented infection during pregnancy.

TOXOPLASMOSIS

Toxoplasmosis is caused by the *Toxoplasma gondii* protozoan, an obligate intracellular parasite. The organism can infect any warm-blooded animal and may be found in soil, but its definitive hosts are in the cat family. The organism completes its sexual cycle in feline intestinal epithelial cells and oocysts are shed in the feces for several weeks after the reproductive cycle is completed.[1] Three routes of infection have been identified. Oocysts may be ingested from contaminated cat feces, water, or fruits and vegetables, as well as by gardening in contaminated soil. Tissue cysts are ingested in infected raw or undercooked meat. In a study of 148 patients, including 76 pregnant women with recently acquired infection, aged greater than or equal to 50 years, male sex, Midwest region, working with meat, having 3 or more kittens, and eating locally produced cured, dried, or smoked meat, rare lamb, raw ground

This article is an update of an article previously published in *Clinics in Laboratory Medicine*, Volume 30, Issue 3, September 2010.

[a] Division of Maternal Fetal Medicine, Prenatal Testing Center, Hartford Hospital, University of Connecticut School of Medicine, 85 Jefferson Street, #625, Farmington, CT 06102, USA; [b] Maternal Fetal Medicine, Obstetrics and Gynecology, UConn Health Center, University of Connecticut School of Medicine, 263 Farmington Avenue, Farmington, CT 06030, USA
* Corresponding author.
E-mail address: Deborah.feldman@hhchealth.org

beef, and unpasteurized goat's milk were associated with infection.[2] A third route of infection is via vertical transmission. Vertical transmission from a pregnant woman to her fetus can cause congenital toxoplasmosis, with consequences including still-birth, chorioretinitis, deafness, microcephaly, and developmental delay.[3,4]

The true prevalence of toxoplasmosis is unknown because it is not a reportable dis-ease in the United States; however, it was estimated by the fourth National Health and Nutrition Examination Survey performed from 1999 to 2000.[1] In 4234 people tested for immunoglobulin (Ig) G antibodies to *Toxoplasma*, 15.8% were positive. Of 2221 women aged 12 to 49 years, 14.9% were seropositive, leaving 85% of women of child-bearing age susceptible to infection. In a more recent study of 635,000 infants in the New England Regional Newborn Screening Program, the rate was 1 per 10,000 live births.[3] With approximately 4 million live births in the United States annually, it can be estimated that between 400 and 4000 infants will be born with congenital toxoplasmosis.

Vertical transmission of infection to the fetus is most likely to occur with a primary infection during the pregnancy. However, immunocompromised women with chronic infection may also transmit the disease.[5] More than 90% of pregnant women who ac-quire a primary infection are asymptomatic, as are 85% of neonates born with congen-ital toxoplasmosis.[6] Transmission is rare in early pregnancy and increases with duration of pregnancy. Transmission frequency is approximately 15% in the first trimester, 30% in the second trimester, and 60% in the third trimester.[6] Exposure to infection acquired in the first trimester causes more severe congenital toxoplasmosis, with fetuses exposed in the third trimester most likely to be asymptomatic. However, although most infected infants are asymptomatic at birth, some studies have shown that up to 90% of affected infants show symptoms later in life, including visual impair-ment, hearing loss, and developmental delays.[7] These infants require treatment to prevent manifestations later in life. Transmission can be decreased by antenatal treat-ment, and appropriate therapy should be initiated for suspected fetal infection.

DIAGNOSIS

Diagnosis can be made by testing maternal serum for antibodies. Initial testing should measure IgG and IgM antibodies. If both are negative, infection has not occurred. A negative IgM result with a positive IgG result during the first or second trimester often indicates an infection that predated the pregnancy; this is also likely in the third trimester but the infection could have occurred early in pregnancy with the IgM level decreased to undetectable levels.[8] A positive IgM result with or without IgG to *Toxo-plasma* requires further testing to determine the status of the infection. IgM antibodies may represent false-positive results or chronic or past infection, because they can persist for 1 year or more.[9] Serum antibody screening for toxoplasmosis can have high false-positive and false-negative rates with inconsistent standardization across facilities.[10,11]

Up to 60% of patients positive for IgM in the community have results inconsistent with recent infection on confirmatory testing at the reference laboratory.[12] Therefore, confirmation is important before consideration of elective termination of pregnancy. In one study, confirmatory testing decreased the rate of abortion from 17.2% to 0.4%.[12]

Confirmatory testing consists of the *Toxoplasma* serologic profile, performed at reference laboratories such as the Toxoplasma Serology Laboratory of the Palo Alto Medical Foundation. The panel of tests available includes the Sabin-Feldman test, the differential agglutination test, IgG avidity, and enzyme-linked immunosorbent assay (ELISA) for IgM, IgE, and IgA.

ELISA is used to qualitatively determine the presence or absence of antibodies by adding serum to a well containing *T gondii* antigen bound to an enzyme. A fluorescent substrate is then added that fluoresces if antigen-antibody linking has occurred.[13,14] The presence of IgA and IgE on ELISA implies recent infection.

The IgG avidity test measures the strength of antigen-antibody binding, which increases with duration of infection. Avidity is determined by diluting the substrates in an immunoassay with urea and comparing the ratio of antibody titer in an untreated well with that of the urea-treated well.[11] High avidity requires at least 3 months to develop, and so helps to rule out acute infection.

Ultrasonography can be used to detect certain fetal manifestations of infection. Findings suggestive of congenital toxoplasmosis include unilateral or bilateral ventriculomegaly, ascites, intracranial or intrahepatic calcifications, hepatomegaly, splenomegaly, and intrauterine growth restriction.[8,15] In the absence of abnormalities, monthly ultrasonographic monitoring should continue throughout the pregnancy.

Amniocentesis should be offered for polymerase chain reaction (PCR) testing of the amniotic fluid to assist in the diagnosis of congenital toxoplasmosis. The procedure should be performed after 18 weeks' gestation and 4 or more weeks after the estimated date of infection. Amplification of the B1 gene of the parasite is used to assess for the presence of infection. In a study performed at 3 centers in France, overall sensitivity was 64% with a negative predictive value of 98.8%. There were no false-positives, yielding a specificity of 100%, as well as a positive predictive value of 100%.[16] The sensitivity of PCR diagnosis was highest when maternal infection occurred between 17 and 21 weeks. Although other studies have suggested a higher sensitivity,[17,18] a negative PCR result does not rule out congenital disease and adequate treatment and follow-up are still indicated for these patients.

TREATMENT

Vertical transmission of newly acquired infection during early pregnancy at less than or equal to 18 weeks can be reduced by administration of oral spiramycin, 1 g every 8 hours; however, spiramycin does not definitively prevent fetal infection.[6,19] This macrolide antibiotic does not cross the placenta, so is not appropriate for fetal treatment of congenital infection. In the absence of signs of fetal infection, spiramycin should be continued until delivery. The drug is not commercially available in the United States, but can be obtained at no cost from the Food and Drug Administration or the reference laboratories that perform confirmatory testing.[6] Spiramycin does not seem to have any fetal effects, although a small percentage of women develop gastrointestinal side effects.[6,20]

If seroconversion occurs after 18 weeks or fetal infection is confirmed by PCR or ultrasonography findings, treatment should be initiated. Pyrimethamine 50 mg twice daily for 2 days followed by 50 mg per day, sulfadiazine 75 mg/kg per day in 2 divided doses for 2 days followed by 50 mg twice daily, and folinic acid 10 to 20 mg per day may reduce the severity of congenital infection at later gestational ages and also treat the fetus.[6] Pyrimethamine is a folic acid antagonist that is teratogenic early in pregnancy, therefore its use in the first trimester should be avoided. It is not associated with hyperbilirubinemia, but may cause bone marrow depression.[21] Folinic acid may help prevent hematologic toxicity.

Immunocompromised women with chronic infection may, rarely, transmit the parasite to the fetus, resulting in congenital infection. This possibility includes women with acquired immunodeficiency syndrome as well as those on immunosuppressive treatment. Vertical transmission occurs in up to 4% of cases, particularly when the CD4 count is less than 100/mm^3.[3,22] The risk of transmission is low when the CD4 count is greater than 200/mm^3. Screening is recommended for all immunosuppressed women or human immunodeficiency virus (HIV)–positive women, for evidence of a history of infection to establish an early diagnosis of reactivation. Seropositive women with low CD4 counts should receive trimethoprim-sulfamethoxazole to prevent reactivation of *Toxoplasma*. Because of reports of congenital toxoplasmosis in mild or moderately immunosuppressed women, it is recommended that women infected with HIV with CD4 counts less than 200/mm^3 or immunocompromised women not infected with HIV be treated with spiramycin for the duration of pregnancy.[6]

PREVENTION

In a recent survey of pregnant women in the United States, only 48% of respondents had heard of toxoplasmosis but 60% were aware that *Toxoplasma* is shed in the feces of cats and can be contracted by changing cat litter. Only 30% knew of the association with raw or undercooked meat.[23] A 2009 survey of obstetricians practicing in the United States showed that 87.7% counsel patients about how and why to prevent toxoplasmosis, with 78% of counseling occurring only at the first prenatal visit.[24] The rate of primary infection may be decreased by as much as 63% to 92% by counseling pregnant woman on how to avoid infection.[25]

Secondary prevention strategies to prevent fetal infection in women who contract the disease are in place in many countries with a higher incidence of toxoplasmosis than the United States, including France and Austria. In these countries, all women are screened for antibodies to *Toxoplasma* on initiation of prenatal care. Seronegative women are rechecked monthly to allow for intervention if a new infection is detected. In the United States, several states have instituted newborn serologic screening for *Toxoplasma* IgM. However, this does not allow for prenatal intervention, and may miss neonates infected early in gestation or late in the third trimester.[5] At present, routine prenatal screening for toxoplasmosis in the United States, in the absence of risk factors, is not recommended.

PARVOVIRUS

Parvovirus B19 is a small, single-stranded DNA virus that infects only humans. It most commonly presents as erythema infectiosum, or fifth disease, a common viral exanthem in children. Typically, the disease is characterized by fever and an erythematous rash on the cheeks. It is self-limited, and symptoms resolve within 7 to 10 days. Immunity after the disease is lifelong, and at least 50% of adults are immune from exposure to the virus during childhood. Clinical manifestations for those adults who are susceptible to the virus include malaise, a reticular rash, joint pain/swelling that may last from days to months, and transient aplastic crisis in patients with preexisting hemoglobinopathy.[26] Approximately 20% to 30% of patients have no symptoms.[27]

Transmission of parvovirus B19 occurs most commonly through spread of respiratory droplets. The incubation period is 5 to 10 days after exposure and before any symptoms. By the time a rash is present, respiratory secretions and serum are usually free of the virus and the patient is no longer contagious.[28]

Because parvovirus B19 preferentially infects rapidly dividing cells and is cytotoxic for erythroid progenitor cells, there is concern about the effect of fetal transmission from an infected mother. Among the first reported associations between parvovirus B19 and fetal nonimmune hydrops was a case series published in the mid to late 1980s after an outbreak of the virus in a Connecticut community in 1986.[29] Since then, several hundred publications have reported the potential risks and outcomes, and management plans for parvovirus in pregnancy have been outlined.

DIAGNOSIS OF MATERNAL INFECTION

Maternal serology using ELISA, Western blot, or radioimmunoassay is the most common method of detecting the presence of IgG and IgM immunoglobulins, which are both produced in response to infection with parvovirus B19. The sensitivity of these assays to detect IgG and IgM is generally around 70% to 80%.[30] The IgM-specific antibody is usually present by the third to the fifth day after symptoms present, and may persist for several weeks to months. Positive IgM antibody indicates acute infection. The presence of IgG antibodies is noted approximately 7 days after the onset of symptoms and lasts indefinitely. In the absence of IgM antibodies, a positive IgG test indicates an old infection and therefore immunity. Cases of recurrent or persistent parvovirus are extremely rare. The prevalence of IgG antibodies to the virus increases with age, from 2% to 10% rates of seropositivity in preschool-aged children to 60% of adolescents and adults.[31]

DIAGNOSIS OF FETAL INFECTION

Diagnosis of fetal infection is mainly done by qualitative PCR of amniotic fluid. In addition, ultrasonography can be used to identify evidence of fetal anemia resulting from congenital parvovirus B19 infection, which should prompt amniotic fluid testing for fetal parvovirus.[32] Because of the affinity of the virus for erythroid stem cells, infected fetuses may become profoundly anemic. In addition, the virus can attack the myocardium, causing a cardiomyopathy, as well as direct hepatic injury, which may impair protein synthesis and decrease colloid oncotic pressure. All of these effects may lead to hydrops fetalis, which is readily diagnosed with ultrasonography (**Fig. 1**). Hydrops occurs in up to 10% of pregnancies in which parvovirus infection is documented before 20 weeks. Of note, when infection occurs before 20 weeks, this is the time period were infection leads to more severe fetal disease.[33-35] The risk for hydrops decreases significantly if infection occurs in the late second or third trimester. Infection early in the first trimester is associated with a higher risk for spontaneous abortion than in noninfected pregnancies.[26,27]

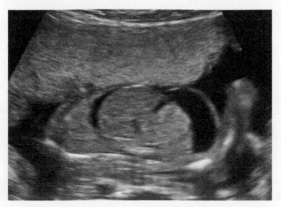

Fig. 1. Fetal hydrops diagnosed by ascites and pleural effusions in a fetus with known parvovirus B19 infection.

MANAGEMENT OF PARVOVIRUS B19 INFECTION DURING PREGNANCY

Following an exposure to parvovirus B19, pregnant patients should be tested for the presence of IgG and IgM antibodies. If immunity is documented by the presence of IgG and the absence of IgM antibodies, the patient can be reassured that her fetus is not at risk for prenatal infection. If both IgG and IgM antibodies are undetectable, this indicates that the patient is susceptible to infection and titers should be repeated in 3 to 4 weeks. If they remain negative, the patient remains susceptible to the disease without evidence of infection. Continued hand washing and avoidance of possible sources of infection are recommended. There is no vaccine or known medical treatment of the virus. At present, routine screening for parvovirus in pregnancy or targeted screening in low-risk pregnancies is not recommended. In addition, exclusion of pregnant women from their working environments, particularly in endemic periods or locations, is also not recommended. Instead, testing should be completed for symptomatic patients or patients with known or suspected exposure to parvovirus B19.[36]

If the patient has evidence of seroconversion with positive titers of both IgG and IgM antibodies, ultrasonography surveillance of the fetus should be initiated. Transmission rates from mother to fetus can be as high as 33%.[8] Also, although some cases of fetal infection have spontaneous resolution, other outcomes, including risk of hydrops, stillbirth, and spontaneous miscarriage, warrant increased surveillance.[37] Attention should be focused on the presence of ascites, pleural or pericardial effusions, or scalp edema. In addition, middle cerebral artery (MCA) Doppler should be used to evaluate for fetal anemia (**Fig. 2**), because this may be detected before fetal hydrops.[38,39] The

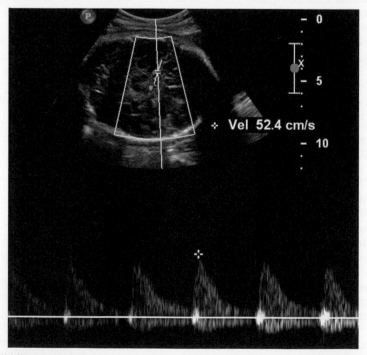

Fig. 2. Middle cerebral artery-peak systolic velocity (vel) to screen for fetal anemia after acute parvovirus B19 infection.

incubation period for congenital infection may be longer than in adults, and reports of fetal hydrops have been made as long as 8 to 10 weeks after exposure. Therefore, the authors recommend weekly ultrasonography scans for approximately 10 weeks after exposure to the virus. If no hydrops or evidence of anemia has been shown by then, the likelihood of its development is very small.[40] Very few cases of fetal death in the absence of hydrops have been attributed to parvovirus B19.

If there is evidence of fetal hydrops or anemia from an increased peak systolic velocity through the MCA, a cordocentesis should be performed when technically possible. Although the disease is often self-limited and there have been cases of spontaneous resolution of hydrops reported,[13] an in-utero blood transfusion is indicated in cases of severe anemia, and is best performed intravascularly through the umbilical vein using ultrasonography guidance.[41,42]

NEONATAL OUTCOMES AFTER PARVOVIRUS INFECTION

There have been few data published on the long-term outcomes of fetuses requiring in-utero blood transfusion because of parvovirus B19 infection. Barring any complications related to the procedure itself, most fetuses do well after intravascular transfusion even if they are profoundly anemic before the procedure. However, results regarding the neurodevelopment of these infants after birth are conflicting. Most studies suggest normal neurologic outcomes after appropriate therapy. One small, retrospective study reported a higher rate of delayed psychomotor development in children aged 6 to 8 years who had undergone intrauterine transfusion for parvovirus B19 infection, suggesting a potential effect of the virus on the central nervous system.[43] A larger, controlled study suggested a similar rate of developmental delay among infants born to mothers with acute parvovirus infection during pregnancy compared with controls.[44]

CYTOMEGALOVIRUS

Human cytomegalovirus (CMV) is an enveloped DNA herpes virus. It has numerous characteristics of a herpes virus, including mode of transmission (sexual contact; contact with infected blood, urine, and saliva), and also the ability to cause congenital infection. The seroprevalence of CMV is approximately 50% in adults in industrialized countries. Based on an epidemiologic study, seroprevalence of cytomegalovirus infection in the United States was 58% in reproductive-aged women.[45] Approximately 0.6% to 0.7% of infants born in the United States are congenitally infected, making it the most common cause of infection-related congenital disorder.[46] Vertical transmission of CMV depends on numerous factors, including type and timing of infection. Treatment of congenital CMV infection is an active area of research, and the Institute of Medicine has rated the development of a CMV vaccine a highest priority.[47]

CMV infection is typically asymptomatic in immunocompetent adults. Less than 5% of pregnant women with a primary CMV infection are symptomatic, making the diagnosis of infection in pregnancy difficult.[48] CMV infection is known to cause neurologic sequelae in newborns; however, prediction of vertical transmission can be difficult. Neurologic handicap is possible after either primary or recurrent infection. However, after primary infections with CMV, about one-third of newborns acquire a CMV infection but only approximately 1% to 2% of newborns acquire CMV after a recurrent infection.[46,49] Up to 90% of infants who are symptomatic at birth have serious long-term handicaps, including hearing loss, visual impairment, mental retardation, and/or mild cognitive impairment.[50] In contrast, asymptomatic newborns are at much less risk for serious long-term impairment, in the range of 5% to 15%.[49,51] The timing in gestation has also been described as an important risk factor for vertical transmission. Third-trimester infection seems to have a higher rate of vertical transmission, but the incidence of symptomatic newborns with these late infections is much less than that of first-trimester vertical transmission.[52] In contrast, the rate of vertical transmission after maternal infection early in pregnancy is low, but, in cases of congenital infection, the rate of severe disease is much higher.[53,54]

MATERNAL INFECTION

Diagnosis for CMV in adults is typically done by serologic testing. Acute maternal infection to CMV can be considered if a woman has seroconversion of CMV IgG during her pregnancy. In this situation, her nonimmune status would have to have previously been established, usually by collecting samples 3 to 4 weeks apart and testing for seroconversion from negative to positive IgG, or an increase in IgG titers greater than 4-fold. Another possible indicator of acute maternal infection is CMV IgG and/ or IgM antibodies. However, CMV IgM antibodies can persist for more than 6 months, making it difficult to determine the precise timing of infection.[55] In addition, there has been concern over the accuracy of commercially available CMV antibody test kits.[56] CMV IgM may also be present, and reinfection and false-positive results have been reported from other viral infections.[56,57]

When there is a question of acute maternal CMV infection, IgG avidity testing may be the most reliable way to confirm the diagnosis. Low-avidity IgG antibodies are present in acute or recent primary CMV infections.[58] If testing is performed at 16 to 18 weeks' gestation, anti-CMV IgG avidity testing has been reported to have a 100% sensitivity for newborn infection.[59] If high-avidity CMV IgG is detected by 16 weeks, a recent infection can be ruled out.

FETAL INFECTION

If acute maternal infection is suspected in pregnancy, fetal infection can then be investigated. Historically, fetal blood sampling was performed by cordocentesis to determine fetal immune status. Because the fetus may not be immunocompetent in early gestation, fetal immune status may not be helpful until late in pregnancy. There is also concern over the safety and availability of cordocentesis, and as such this technique is no longer recommended for fetal testing.[60] Amniocentesis, which is much safer than cordocentesis, can obtain amniotic fluid for CMV detection by PCR or culture. PCR of amniotic fluid has a reported sensitivity and specificity of more than 90% for vertical transmission of CMV.[61,62] Viral culture or CMV early antigen testing has also been performed to confirm vertical transmission, but the speed and accuracy of PCR have made it the standard diagnostic test for fetal infection with CMV.

Fetal infection may be suspected during pregnancy because of ultrasonography findings suspicious for CMV infection. These findings include early-onset intrauterine growth restriction, microcephaly, ventriculomegaly, hepatosplenomegaly, ascites, liver calcifications, echogenic bowel, and fetal hydrops (**Fig. 3**). However, only about 5% to 25% of infected newborns have ultrasonography evidence of congenital infection.[63] However, if fetal anomalies are detected, it implies a more severely affected newborn.[64] Any ultrasonography findings suspicious for congenital CMV infection should prompt a serologic and/or invasive diagnostic evaluation to determine whether an acute infection is present. Amniocentesis with CMV PCR has been reported to be most accurate for diagnosing fetal infection when performed after 20 weeks' gestation, making this the ideal time for the procedure.[65,66]

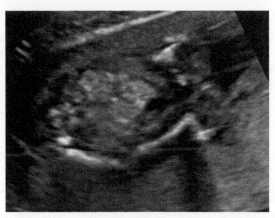

Fig. 3. Echogenic bowel noted in the abdomen of a fetus with early CMV infection.

TREATMENT

Once fetal CMV infection has been confirmed, no standard therapy for in-utero treatment has been established. A recent nonrandomized trial of CMV hyperimmune globulin was promising for treatment of acute fetal CMV infection. Women who received CMV hyperimmune globulin during pregnancy had only a 3% incidence of a symptomatic newborn at birth and 2 years of age, whereas untreated women had a 50% incidence. However, use of this treatment modality is not recommended outside of a research protocol.[67] There are no specific antiviral regimens for fetal treatment of CMV infection but postnatal treatment of severely affected newborns has been reported with ganciclovir and valganciclovir with varying degrees of efficacy.[58,68] In cases of known maternal CMV infection, additional surveillance with serial ultrasonography scans for growth following fetal anatomic assessment is warranted in addition to referral to a maternal fetal medicine and/or infectious diseases specialist. Pregnancy termination remains an option for pregnancies with CMV infection, but this should be reserved for cases with documented acute fetal infection after a thorough diagnostic evaluation and extensive counseling.

Routine screening for CMV infection in pregnancy is not recommended. At present, an efficacious treatment of acute fetal infection is not available. A recent study evaluated 3 screening strategies and showed that universal screening could be cost-effective if treatment of CMV in pregnancy could achieve at least a 47% reduction in disease.[69] Until then, education on prevention with good hygiene is best for women known to be at risk for primary CMV infection.

SUMMARY

There are many infections that may be asymptomatic or cause only mild clinical symptoms in an immunocompetent adult, but that cause more significant consequences in a developing fetus. Depending on the gestational age of infection, there is wide variation in the pregnancy outcomes of women who acquire toxoplasmosis, parvovirus, or CMV during pregnancy. Most fetal outcomes are favorable even for those with documented infection during pregnancy. However, there remains much anxiety among patients who develop these infections. With proper screening, maternal and fetal testing, and treatment where appropriate, clinicians can provide these patients with the best possible pregnancy outcomes.

REFERENCES

1. Jones J, Kruszon-Moran D, Wilson M. *Toxoplasma gondii* infection in the United States, 1999–2000. Emerg Infect Dis 2003;9(11):1371–4. Available at: http://www.cdc.gov/ncidod/EID/vol9no11/03-0098.htm. Accessed October 22, 2009.
2. Jones J, Dargelas V, Roberts J, et al. Risk factors for *Toxoplasma gondii* infection in the United States. Clin Infect Dis 2009;49:878–84.
3. Guerina NG, Hsu H-W, Meissner H, et al. Neonatal serologic screening and early treatment for congenital *Toxoplasma gondii* infection. N Engl J Med 1994;330:1858–63.
4. McClure E, Goldenberg R. Infection and stillbirth. Semin Fetal Neonatal Med 2009;14:182–9.
5. Centers for Disease Control and Prevention. Preventing congenital toxoplasmosis. MMWR Recomm Rep 2000;49:57–75.
6. Montoya J, Remington J. Management of *Toxoplasma gondii* infection during pregnancy. Clin Infect Dis 2008;47:554–66.
7. Wilson CB, Remington JS, Stagno S, et al. Development of adverse sequelae in children born with subclinical congenital Toxoplasma infection. Pediatrics 1980;66:767–74.
8. Montoya J, Rosso F. Diagnosis and management of toxoplasmosis. Clin Perinatol 2005;32:705–26.
9. Del Bono V, Canessa A, Bruzzi P, et al. Significance of specific immunoglobulin M in the chronological diagnosis of 38 cases of toxoplasmic lymphadenopathy. J Clin Microbiol 1989;27:2133–5.
10. Ashburn D, Evans R, Skinner LJ, et al. Comparison of relative uses of commercial assays for *Toxoplasma gondii* IgM antibodies. J Clin Pathol 1992;45(6):483–6.
11. Liesenfeld O, Press C, Montoya JG, et al. False-positive results in immunoglobulin M (IgM) toxoplasma antibody tests and importance of confirmatory testing: the Platelia Toxo IgM test. J Clin Microbiol 1997;35(1):174–8.
12. Liesenfeld O, Montoya J, Tathineni N, et al. Confirmatory serologic testing for acute toxoplasmosis and the rate of induced abortions among women reported to have positive *Toxoplasma* immunoglobulin M antibody titers. Am J Obstet Gynecol 2001;184:140–5.
13. Lequin RM. Enzyme immunoassay (EIA)/enzyme-linked immunosorbent assay (ELISA). Clin Chem 2005;51:2415–8.
14. Lefevre-Pettrazzoni M, Le Cam S, Wallon M. Delayed maturation of immunoglobulin G avidity: implication for the diagnosis of toxoplasmosis in pregnant women. Eur J Clin Microbiol Infect Dis 2006;25:687–93.
15. Byrne JL. Toxoplasmosis. In: Woodward PJ, Kennedy A, Sohaey R, et al, editors. Diagnostic imaging obstetrics. 2nd edition. Manitoba, Canada: Amirsys Publishing; 2011. p. 14–8, 14–9.
16. Romand S, Wallon M, Franck F, et al. Prenatal diagnosis using polymerase chain reaction on amniotic fluid for congenital toxoplasmosis. Obstet Gynecol 2001;97:296–300.
17. Foulon W, Pinon J, Stray-Pederson B, et al. Prenatal diagnosis of congenital toxoplasmosis: a multicenter evaluation of different diagnostic parameters. Am J Obstet Gynecol 1999;181:843–7.
18. Bessieres M, Berrebi A, Cassaing S, et al. Diagnosis of congenital toxoplasmosis: prenatal and neonatal evaluation of methods used in Toulouse University Hospital and incidence of congenital toxoplasmosis. Mem Inst Oswaldo Cruz 2009;104:389–92.

19. Peyron F, Wallon M, Liou C, et al. Treatments for toxoplasmosis in pregnancy. Cochrane Database Syst Rev 1999;(3):CD001684.

20. Cook G. Use of antiprotozoan and anthelmintic drugs during pregnancy: side effects and contra-indications. J Infect 1992;25:1–9.

21. Peters PJ, Thigpen MC, Parise ME, et al. Safety and toxicity of sulfadoxine/pyrimethamine: implications for malaria prevention in pregnancy using intermittent preventive treatment. Drug Saf 2007;30:481–501.

22. Bachmeyer C, Mouchnino G, Thulliez P, et al. Congenital toxoplasmosis from an HIV-infected woman as a result of reactivation. J Infect 2006;52:e55–7.

23. Jones J, Ogunmodede G, Scheftel J, et al. Toxoplasmosis-related knowledge and practices among pregnant women in the United States. Infect Dis Obstet Gynecol 2003;11:139–45.

24. Ross D, Rasmussen S, Cannon M, et al. Obstetrician/gynecologists' knowledge, attitudes, and practices regarding prevention of infections in pregnancy. J Womens Health 2009;18:1187–93.

25. Breugelmans M, Naessens A, Foulon W. Prevention of toxoplasmosis during pregnancy–an epidemiologic survey over 22 consecutive years. J Perinat Med 2004;32:211–4.

26. Brown KE. Parvovirus infections. In: Longo DL, Fauci AS, Kasper DL, et al, editors. Harrison's principles of internal medicine. 18th edition. New York: McGraw-Hill; 2012. p. 1478–9.

27. Chorba T, Coccia P, Holman RC, et al. The role of parvovirus B19 in anaplastic crisis and erythema infectiosum (fifth disease). J Infect Dis 1986;154:383–93.

28. Thurn J. Human parvovirus B19: historical and clinical review. Rev Infect Dis 1988;10:1005–11.

29. Rodis JF, Hodick TJ, Quinn DL, et al. Human parvovirus in pregnancy. Obstet Gynecol 1988;72(5):733–8.

30. Anderson LJ, Tsou C, Parker RA, et al. Detection antibodies and antigens of human parvovirus B19 by enzyme-linked immunosorbent assay. J Clin Microbiol 1986;24:522–6.

31. Hall SM, Cohen BJ, Mortimer PP, et al. Prospective study of human parvovirus (B19) infection in pregnancy. Public health laboratory service working party on fifth disease. BMJ 1990;300(6733):1166–70.

32. Lamont RF, Sobel JD, Vaisbuch E, et al. Parvovirus B19 infection in human pregnancy. BJOG 2011;118:175–86.

33. Rodis JF, Quinn DL, Gary GW Jr, et al. Management and outcomes of pregnancies complicated by human B19 parvovirus infection: a prospective study. Am J Obstet Gynecol 1990;163(4 Pt 1):1168–71.

34. Riipinen A, Vaisanen E, Nuutila M, et al. Parvovirus B19 infection in fetal deaths. Clin Infect Dis 2008;47(12):1519–25.

35. Kovacs BW, Carlson DE, Shahbahrami B, et al. Prenatal diagnosis of human parvovirus B19 in nonimmune hydrops fetalis by polymerase chain reaction. Am J Obstet Gynecol 1992;167:461–6.

36. Crane J, Mundle W, Boucoiran I, et al, Maternal Fetal Medicine Committee. Parvovirus B19 infection in pregnancy. J Obstet Gynaecol Can 2014;36(12):1107–16.

37. Levy R, Weissman A, Blomberg G, et al. Infection by parvovirus B 19 during pregnancy: a review. Obstet Gynecol Surv 1997;52:254–9.

38. Moise KJ Jr. The usefulness of middle cerebral artery Doppler assessment in the treatment of the fetus at risk for anemia. Am J Obstet Gynecol 2008;198(2):161.e1–4.

39. Borna S, Mirzaie F, Hanthoush-Zadeh S, et al. Middle cerebral artery peak systolic velocity and ductus venosus velocity in the investigation of nonimmune hydrops. J Clin Ultrasound 2009;37(7):385–8.

40. Rodis JF, Borgida AF, Wilson M, et al. Management of parvovirus infection in pregnancy and outcomes of hydrops: a survey of members of the society of perinatal obstetricians. Am J Obstet Gynecol 1998;79(4):985–8.

41. Schild RL, Bald R, Plath H, et al. Intrauterine management of fetal parvovirus B19 infection. Ultrasound Obstet Gynecol 1999;13(3):161–6.

42. Odibo AO, Campbell WA, Feldman DM, et al. Resolution of human parvovirus B19-induced nonimmune hydrops after intrauterine transfusion. J Ultrasound Med 1998;17(9):547–50.

43. Nagel HT, de Haan TR, Vandenbussche FP, et al. Long-term outcome after fetal transfusion for hydrops associated with parvovirus B19 infection. Obstet Gynecol 2007;109(1):42–7.

44. Rodis JF, Rodner C, Hansen AA, et al. Long-term outcome of children following maternal human parvovirus B19 infection. Obstet Gynecol 1998;91(1):125–8.

45. Staras SA, Dollard SC, Radford KW, et al. Seroprevalence of cytomegalovirus infection in the United States, 1988-1994. Clin Infect Dis 2006;43(9):1143–51.

46. Kenneson A, Cannon MJ. Review and meta-analysis of the epidemiology of congenital cytomegalovirus (CMV) infection. Rev Med Virol 2007;17:253–76.

47. Institute of Medicine Committee to Study Priorities for Vaccine Development. Vaccines for the 21st Century: a tool for decision making. In: Stratton KR, Durch JS, Lawrence RS, editors. Vaccines for the 21st Century: a tool for decision making. Washington, DC: National Academy Press; 2000. p. 460.

48. Pass RF. Cytomegalovirus. In: Jeffries DJ, Hudson CN, editors. Viral infections in obstetrics and gynecology. New York: Arnold; 1999. p. 35–6.

49. Fowler FB, Stagno S, Pass RF, et al. The outcome of congenital cytomegalovirus in relation to maternal antibody status. N Engl J Med 1992;326:663–7.

50. Boppana SB, Pass RF, Britt WJ, et al. Symptomatic congenital cytomegalovirus infection: neonatal morbidity and mortality. Pediatr Infect Dis J 1992;11:93–9.

51. Fowler KB, Dahle AJ, Boppana SB, et al. Newborn hearing screening: will children with hearing loss caused by congenital cytomegalovirus infection be missed? J Pediatr 1999;135:60–4.

52. Gindes L, Teperberg-Oikawa M, Sherman D, et al. Congenital cytomegalovirus infection following primary maternal infection in the third trimester. BJOG 2008; 115:830–5.

53. Daiminger GJ, Bader U, Enders G. Pre- and periconceptional primary cytomegalovirus infection: risk of vertical transmission and congenital disease. Br J Obstet Gynaecol 2005;112:166–72.

54. Leisnard C, Donner C, Brancart F, et al. Prenatal diagnosis of congenital cytomegalovirus infection: prospective study of 237 pregnancies at risk. Obstet Gynecol 2000;95:881–8.

55. Stagno S, Pass RF, Cloud G, et al. Primary cytomegalovirus infection in pregnancy: incidence, transmission to fetus and clinical outcome. JAMA 1986;256: 1904–8.

56. Lazzarotto T, Brojanac S, Maine GT, et al. Search for cytomegalovirus-specific immunoglobulin M: comparison between a new western blot, conventional Western blot and nine commercially available assays. Clin Diagn Lab Immunol 1997;4: 483–6.

57. Lazzarotto T, Gabrielli L, Lanari M, et al. Congenital cytomegalovirus infection: recent advances in the diagnosis of maternal infection. Hum Immunol 2004;65: 410–5.

58. Lazzarotto T, Spezzacatena P, Pradelli P, et al. Avidity of immunoglobulin G directed against human cytomegalovirus during primary and secondary infections in immunocompetent and immunocompromised subjects. Clin Diagn Lab Immunol 1997;4:469–73.

59. Lazzarotto T, Varani S, Spezzacatena P, et al. Maternal IgG avidity and IgM detected by blot as diagnostic tools to identify pregnancy women at risk of transmitting cytomegalovirus. Viral Immunol 2000;13:137–41.

60. Weiner CP. Cordocentesis. Obstet Gynecol Clin North Am 1988;15:283–301.

61. Lipitz S, Yagel S, Shalev E, et al. Prenatal diagnosis of fetal primary cytomegalovirus infection. Obstet Gynecol 1997;89:763–7.

62. Guerra B, Lazzarotto T, Quarta S, et al. Prenatal diagnosis of symptomatic congenital cytomegalovirus infection. Am J Obstet Gynecol 2000;183:476–82.

63. Ville Y. The megalovirus. Ultrasound Obstet Gynecol 1998;12:151–3.

64. Guerra B, Simonazzi G, Puccetti C, et al. Ultrasound prediction of symptomatic congenital cytomegalovirus infection. Am J Obstet Gynecol 2008;198(380):e1–7.

65. Pass RF, Fowler KB, Boppana SB, et al. Congenital cytomegalovirus infection following first trimester maternal infection: symptoms at birth and outcome. J Clin Virol 2006;35:216–20.

66. Reullan-Eugene G, Barjot P, Campet M, et al. Evaluation of virological procedures to detect fetal human cytomegalovirus infection: avidity of IgG antibodies, virus detection in amniotic fluid and maternal serum. J Med Virol 1996;50:9–15.

67. Nigro G, Adler SP, La Torre R, et al. Passive immunization during pregnancy for congenital cytomegalovirus infection. N Engl J Med 2005;353:1350–62.

68. Muller A, Eis-Hubinger AM, Brandhorts G, et al. Oral valganciclovir for symptomatic congenital cytomegalovirus infection in an extremely low birth weight infant. J Perinatol 2008;25:74–6.

69. Cahill AG, Odibo AO, Stamillo DM, et al. Screening and treating for primary cytomegalovirus infection in pregnancy: where do we stand? A decision-analytic and economic analysis. Am J Obstet Gynecol 2009;201(466):e1–7.

Prenatal Screening for Thrombophilias

Indications and Controversies, an Update

Adetola F. Louis-Jacques, MD*, Lindsay Maggio, MD, MPH,
Stephanie T. Romero, MD

KEYWORDS

- Thrombophilia • Adverse pregnancy outcomes • Venous thromboembolism
- Inherited thrombophilias • Acquired thrombophilias • Pregnancy

KEY POINTS

- Thrombophilias are disorders of hemostasis that predispose a person to a thrombotic event.
- Acquired and inherited thrombophilias lead to an increased risk of venous thromboembolism (VTE) during pregnancy and in the postpartum period.
- Acquired thrombophilias are associated with adverse pregnancy outcomes.
- Universal screening of pregnant women is not cost-effective or indicated because of the low incidence of VTE during pregnancy.

INTRODUCTION

There are numerous procoagulant physiologic changes in pregnancy. There is an increase in levels of fibrinogen; von Willebrand factor; and clotting factors II, VII, VIII, IX, X[1,2]; there is a decrease in levels of physiologic anticoagulants such as protein S (PS), and an increase in protein C (PC) resistance. Pregnancy is associated with increased clotting potential, decreased anticoagulant activity, and decreased fibrinolysis.[3,4]

A thrombophilia is defined as a disorder of hemostasis that predisposes a person to a thrombotic event.[5] Data suggest that at least 50% of cases of venous thromboembolism[6] (VTE) in pregnant women are associated with thrombophilias.[7,8] Inherited

This article is an update to the article, "Prenatal Screening for Thrombophilias: Indications and Controversies," previously published in *Clinics in Laboratory Medicine*, Volume 30, Issue 3, September 2010.
Disclosure: The authors have nothing to disclose.
Division of Maternal Fetal Medicine, Department of Obstetrics and Gynecology, University of South Florida Morsani College of Medicine, 2 Tampa General Circle, 6th Floor, Tampa, FL 33606, USA
* Corresponding author.
E-mail address: alouisjacques@health.usf.edu

and/or acquired thrombophilias have been associated with an increased risk of maternal thromboembolism and adverse pregnancy outcomes such as recurrent pregnancy loss, intrauterine fetal demise, preterm preeclampsia, and fetal growth restriction (FGR), although there is controversy regarding these associations. It is important to be able to identify which patients have indications for thrombophilia testing, and, in those who do, what laboratory testing should be performed.

INHERITED THROMBOPHILIAS

There are several types of inherited thrombophilias, including factor V Leiden (FVL) mutation, prothrombin (PT) gene (G20210A) mutation, PC deficiency, PS deficiency, and antithrombin III (ARIII) deficiency.[9–11]

Factor V Leiden

FVL mutation is present in approximately 5% to 9% of the white European population and is the most common heritable thrombophilia among this ethnic group. It is rare in populations of African and Asian ancestry.[9] In most cases, it is a result of a point mutation in the factor V gene located at nucleotide position 1691. This mutation leads to substitution of glutamine (Q) for arginine (R) at amino acid position 506 (FVR506Q or FV:Q506). This substitution impairs the proteolysis of factor V by activated PC (aPC), producing a hypercoagulable state.[10] This point mutation, first described in 1994, is the leading cause of aPC resistance and has an autosomal dominant inheritance pattern.[12,13]

Forty-four percent of patients presenting with VTE during pregnancy or postpartum are found to carry the FVL mutation, and most are heterozygotes.[14] In pregnant women who are heterozygotes for FVL and have never had a VTE or a first-degree relative with a VTE, there is a thrombotic risk of 0.5% to 1.2%. In women who are homozygous for FVL without a history or first-degree family history of VTE, the risk of VTE is 4%.[14,15] The thrombotic risk per pregnancy increases in women with a personal history of VTE, with a 10% probability in FVL heterozygotes and 17% in FVL homozygotes (**Table 1**).[11,14,16–20]

Screening can be performed by assessing aPC resistance using a second-generation coagulation assay followed by genotyping for the FVL mutation or simply gene analysis for the factor V exon to detect FVL.[10] DNA analysis for FVL is accurate during pregnancy, acute thrombotic events, and while on anticoagulation (**Table 2**).

Prothrombin Gene (G20210A)

The PT gene (G20210A) point mutation, discovered in 1996, leads to a substitution of guanine to adenine at nucleotide position 20210 in the factor II gene, causing hyperprothrombinemia.[21]

PT gene mutation is present in 3% of the white European population and is associated with 17% of the VTE in pregnancy (see **Table 1**).[14] The probability of VTE in patients without a history of a thrombotic event is 0.37% for PT heterozygotes, and 2% to 4% for homozygotes.[11,16] Individuals who are compound heterozygotes for FVL and PT mutations are characterized by further hypercoagulability. The incidence of compound heterozygosity is 1 in 10,000 people. The risk of VTE per pregnancy in this population is 4.7% without a personal or family history of VTE and is more than 20% with a positive history.[16]

Gene analysis using polymerase chain reaction is used to detect the PT gene mutation.[21] Increased plasma levels of PT should not be used for screening. Similar to

Table 1
Risk of VTE with different thrombophilias

	Prevalence in General Population (%)	VTE Risk per Pregnancy; No History (%)	VTE Risk per Pregnancy; Previous VTE (%)	Percentage of all VTE	References
Factor V Leiden heterozygote	1–15	0.5–1.2	10	40	10,14,16,17
Factor V Leiden homozygote	<1	4	17	2	10,14,16,17
PT gene heterozygote	2–5	<0.5	>10	17	10,14,16,17
PT gene homozygote	<1	2–4	>17	0.5	10,14,16,17
Factor V Leiden/PT double heterozygote	0.01	4–5	>20	1–3	10,14,16,17
ATIII activity (<60%)	0.02	3–7	40	1	10,18,19
PC activity (<50%)	0.2–0.4	0.1–0.8	4–17	14	10,18,20
PS free antigen (<55%)	0.03–0.13	0.1	0–22	3	10,27,30,31

From American College of Obstetricians and Gynecologists Women's Health Care Physicians. ACOG practice bulletin no. 138: inherited thrombophilias in pregnancy. Obstet Gynecol 2013;122(3):706–17; with permission.

Table 2
How to test for thrombophilias

Thrombophilia	Testing Method	Is Testing Reliable During Pregnancy?	Is Testing Reliable During Acute Thrombosis?	Is Testing Reliable with Anticoagulation?
Factor V Leiden mutation	Activated PC resistance assay (second generation)	Yes	Yes	No
	If abnormal DNA analysis	Yes	Yes	Yes
PT G20210A mutation	DNA analysis	Yes	Yes	Yes
PC deficiency	PC activity (<60%)	Yes	No	No
PS deficiency	Functional assay (<55%)	No[a]	No	No
Antithrombin deficiency	Antithrombin activity (<60%)	Yes	No	No

[a] If screening in pregnancy is necessary, cutoff values for free PS antigen levels in the second and third trimesters have been identified at less than 30% and less than 24%, respectively.

From American College of Obstetricians and Gynecologists Women's Health Care Physicians. ACOG practice bulletin no. 138: inherited thrombophilias in pregnancy. Obstet Gynecol 2013;122(3):706–17; with permission.

FVL DNA testing, PT gene mutation testing is reliable during pregnancy, acute VTE, and while on anticoagulation (see **Table 2**).

Protein C

PC is a vitamin K–dependent protein synthesized in the liver. PC is activated once thrombin binds to thrombomodulin, an endothelial receptor. aPC inhibits thrombin formation by inactivating coagulation factors V_a and VIII_a.[10] The inhibitory effect of aPC is significantly enhanced by cofactor PS. The gene for PC is located on chromosome 2q13-14, spans approximately 10 kb, and contains 9 exons.[22,23] Heterogeneous mutations in the PC gene cause a loss in function, which results in low plasma levels of PC. One-hundred and sixty-one mutations have been identified[10] and PC deficiency is inherited in an autosomal dominant pattern.[9]

PC deficiency is present in up to 1 in 500 of the general population (see **Table 1**).[24] The risk of thrombosis with PC deficiency per pregnancy ranges from 0.1% to 0.8%.[11,16] Most affected patients are heterozygous; homozygous forms result in severe neonatal disease called purpura fulminans.[11]

Diagnosis is established by the measurement of the plasma PC activity using immunologic and functional assays.[10] PC activity is affected by active thrombosis and anticoagulation (see **Table 2**).

Protein S

PS deficiency is typically inherited in an autosomal dominant pattern. There are 2 PS genes (PROS1 and PROS2) mapped to chromosome 3. PROS1 produces PS; PROS2 is a pseudogene.[10,25] There are more than 130 mutations that result in PS deficiency. PS deficiency may be quantitative with reduced total and/or free PS antigen levels, or qualitative causing decreased PS activity.[10] PS is a vitamin K–dependent glycoprotein and is a cofactor to PC. In the presence of PS, aPC inactivates factors Va and VIIIa, resulting in reduced thrombin generation.[26]

PS deficiency is present in 0.03% to 0.13% of the general population.[27] Seligsohn and Lubetsky[28] reported that VTE occurred during pregnancy and postpartum in up to 20% of women with a deficiency of either PC or PS. Similar to PC, most of the affected patients are heterozygous; purpura fulminans is noted in homozygous neonates.[11] Diagnosis is established by measuring free plasma PS antigen and activity levels using immunologic and functional assays.[10,29,30] PS deficiency should not be tested during pregnancy. There is significant variation in the levels of PS because of the fluctuating levels of PS binding protein in pregnancy.[30] Nevertheless, if screening is performed during pregnancy, cutoff values for free PS antigen levels in the second and third trimesters are less than 30% and less than 24%, respectively.[31]

Antithrombin III Deficiency

ATIII deficiency was the first inherited thrombophilia identified (in 1965) and is part of the serine proteinase inhibitor superfamily of proteins.[32] ATIII is the main inhibitor of thrombin, and it also inhibits factors IX_a, X_a, XI_a, and XII.[10] It is the most thrombogenic of the inherited thrombophilias.[9] The ATIII gene is localized on chromosome 1q23-25. There are more than 250 mutations that cause deficiency in ATIII and these are usually inherited in an autosomal dominant fashion. These mutations decrease gene transcription, resulting in a reduction of antigen level and activity. Mutations can also modify structure and function, causing decreased activity but normal antigen levels.[10]

ATIII deficiency is rare, present in 0.2 per 1000 to 11 per 1000 of the population, and the prevalence of ATIII deficiency in thrombotic patients ranges from 1% to 8%.[10] However, up to 60% of pregnant women with this thrombophilia experience VTE.[28]

ATIII deficiency is diagnosed by measuring ATIII activity. Screening for ATIII deficiency should not occur in the setting of acute thrombosis or anticoagulation.

THROMBOPHILIA TESTING

Although VTE is one of the leading causes of pregnancy-related deaths,[33] the incidence of VTE is low at approximately 1 to 2 per 1000 pregnancies.[34,35] Because of the low incidence of VTE in pregnancy, universal screening of pregnant women is not cost-effective or indicated.[36]

Screening for inherited thrombophilias should be considered in women with a personal history of nonprovoked VTE or a first-degree relative with a known thrombophilia. Those with a personal history of thrombosis associated with a nonrecurrent risk factor such as fractures, surgery, or prolonged immobilization should not be routinely screened.[37] In patients for whom screening is appropriate, testing should include the following heritable thrombophilias: FVL, PT gene mutation, ATIII, PC, and PS. Testing should occur at least 6 weeks after the thrombotic event, after the completion of anticoagulation therapy, and ideally not during pregnancy or while on hormone therapy except for FVL and PT gene mutation analyses, which can be performed at any time.

ACQUIRED THROMBOPHILIAS
Antiphospholipid Antibody Syndrome

Phospholipids are molecules composed of 2 fatty acid tails attached to a glycerol head and are the basic structural component of cell membranes. The antiphospholipid antibody syndrome (APS) is the predominant acquired thrombophilia; it can be diagnosed in any patient, but is more common in those with a coexisting autoimmune disease such as lupus. The international consensus statement for APS states that a patient must have 1 clinical criterion and 1 laboratory criterion (positive on 2 occasions 12 weeks apart) to make the diagnosis.[38]

The clinical criteria for APS testing are separated into 2 categories: obstetric outcomes and thrombosis. The obstetric criteria are (1) 3 or more consecutive euploid spontaneous abortions before the 10th week of gestation, (2) unexplained fetal deaths in 1 or more morphologically normal fetuses at greater than or equal to 10 weeks' gestation, or (3) preterm delivery at less than or equal to 34 weeks' gestation resulting from severe preeclampsia or placental insufficiency.[12] Encompassed in the category of placental insufficiency are multiple findings including nonreassuring fetal testing suggestive of fetal hypoxemia, abnormal umbilical Doppler flow velocimetry, oligohydramnios (AFI [amniotic fluid index] ≤ 5 cm), or estimated fetal weight less than the 10th percentile (FGR) requiring delivery at less than or equal to 34 weeks' gestation. However, as that consensus statement acknowledges, placental insufficiency is not well defined, nor are there any characteristic placental abnormalities seen on pathology and therefore this criterion is left to the discretion of the provider. The thrombotic criteria are clearer: 1 or more clinical episodes of arterial, venous, or small-vessel thrombosis, in any tissue or organ.[38] There are other clinical findings associated with APS (thrombocytopenia, livedo reticularis) but these are not included in the diagnostic criteria.[39]

Once clinical criteria are met, antiphospholipid antibody testing should be performed to establish laboratory criteria. Patients should be tested for the presence of 3 factors: (1) lupus anticoagulant, (2) anticardiolipin immunoglobulin (Ig) G and IgM antibody, and (3) anti–β_2-glycoprotein-1 IgG and IgM antibody. If any of these laboratory criteria are positive, a confirmatory test must be performed in 12 weeks.[38] Other factors have been proposed, including anticardiolipin IgA, anti–β_2-glycoprotein-1 IgA, or antibodies against other phospholipids, such as phosphatidylserine; however, these are not part of the diagnostic criteria and should not be included in testing for APS.

Antiphospholipid Antibodies

The lupus anticoagulant is a prothrombotic immunoglobulin. It blocks phospholipid-dependent clotting assays by interfering with the assembly of the PT complex. Because there are other inhibitors and analytical variables that can cause abnormal test results, several different tests are used to confirm the presence of a lupus anticoagulant. Typically, these include activated partial thromboplastin time, PT, dilute or modified Russell viper venom screen, and a hexagonal (II) phase phospholipid assay (Staclot-LA test) or kaolin clotting time. Regardless of the assay used, the result is reported as present or absent.

Anticardiolipin antibodies react to the complex of negatively charged phospholipids. These antibodies are detected using conventional immunoassays using purified cardiolipin as the phospholipid matrix. Anticardiolipin IgG or IgM antibodies must be present in medium to high titers greater than 40 GPL (IgG phospholipid units)/MPL (IgM phospholipid units).

Anti-B2-glycoprotein-1 is a phospholipid-dependent inhibitor of coagulation. These antibodies are measured by standardized enzyme-linked immunosorbent assay. Antibodies IgG and IgM must have titers greater than the 99th percentile for a positive result. Antiphospholipid antibodies can be accurately tested during pregnancy.[37]

ADVERSE PREGNANCY OUTCOMES

Although it is clear that screening women with a personal history of VTE for both inherited and acquired thrombophilias is prudent, there is controversy in screening women for thrombophilias after adverse pregnancy outcomes. There are insufficient data to suggest causality between inherited thrombophilias and adverse pregnancy outcomes, and treatment of thrombophilias has not been shown to improve outcomes in most circumstances.[37]

PREGNANCY LOSS
Acquired Thrombophilia

APS is associated with both early pregnancy loss at less than 10 weeks and fetal loss[40]; however, the greatest proportion of losses caused by APS are fetal death (>10 weeks).[39] Several randomized trials have been performed comparing treatment of women with APS and the results indicate that treatment can improve pregnancy outcomes; however, many did not use the currently accepted definition of APS as their inclusion criterion. The 2 studies that included women with APS by strict criteria found higher rates of live births (71%–80%) with use of heparin and aspirin than with aspirin alone (42%–44%).[41,42] One study included women with persistent antibodies only after 8 weeks, rather than the recommended 12 weeks.[41] In a different study, treatment did not improve outcomes; however, the patients in this study also did not meet laboratory criteria for the diagnosis for APS.[43] Similarly, in a randomized controlled trial of low-molecular-weight heparin and aspirin compared with aspirin alone, there was no difference in the rates of live birth.[44]

Inherited Thrombophilia

Older meta-analysis data suggested an association between inherited thrombophilias and pregnancy loss. One systematic review found that stillbirth was associated with heterozygous FVL, PC, and PS deficiency.[45] The included studies were either very small in size, retrospective, or case control in design, limiting their interpretation. Similarly, a meta-analysis of case-control, cohort, and cross-sectional studies found that FVL, PT gene mutation, and PS deficiency were associated with recurrent early pregnancy loss and late fetal loss.[46]

In a secondary analysis of a multicenter, prospective, observational cohort study, there was no association between PT gene mutation and pregnancy loss.[47] In another prospective study, there was no association between women with FVL mutations and pregnancy loss.[48] Other investigators found that the presence of 1 thrombophilia or more than 1 thrombophilia seemed to be protective against fetal loss before 10 weeks (1 thrombophilia: OR, 0.55; 95% CI, 0.33–0.92. >1 thrombophilia: OR, 0.48; 95% CI, 0.29–0.78).[49] Although robust randomized data are lacking in this topic, the strongest quality of evidence suggests that there is no relationship between inherited thrombophilias and pregnancy loss, early or late. In addition, the associations that are shown may be caused purely by the high frequency of these mutations in the population, and may not reflect causality.

PREECLAMPSIA
Acquired Thrombophilia

Several studies have established the association of early onset severe preeclampsia and APS. One large observational study showed that 50% of women with APS developed preeclampsia.[50] The association of APS and preeclampsia seems to be strongest with preeclampsia before 34 weeks. In one study, 16% of women with severe preeclampsia before 34 weeks had antiphospholipid antibodies.[51] In another study, the presence of anticardiolipin antibody was associated with an 11-fold increase in developing hypertension in pregnancy and a 20-fold increase in developing severe preeclampsia.[52] Similarly, in one meta-analysis there was an 11-fold increased risk of severe preeclampsia in women with anticardiolipin antibodies.[53] In another meta-analysis the relationship of lupus anticoagulant and anticardiolipin antibodies to preeclampsia was not consistent among case-control studies and cohort studies. This study showed a relationship of both antibodies to preeclampsia in case-control studies, but did not in cohort studies.[54]

Inherited Thrombophilia

The association of preeclampsia with inherited thrombophilias is more controversial. In a prospective study of mothers with preeclampsia, there was no difference in the detection of FVL mutation.[55] In another prospective study, there were similar rates of PT gene mutation and FVL mutation in women with preeclampsia compared with the general population.[56] Several studies have failed to find an association between preeclampsia and inherited thrombophilias.[47,57–60] In addition, earlier meta-analyses and systematic reviews of some different studies do not show an association.[59,61] One meta-analysis showed that women with preeclampsia were more likely to be FVL mutation heterozygotes, PT gene mutation heterozygotes, MTHFR (methylenetetrahydrofolate reductase) mutation homozygotes, have PC deficiency, PS deficiency, or aPC resistance compared with controls; however, the published studies included are too small to adequately assess the size of the association.[45] Another meta-analysis showed that the risk of preeclampsia was significantly associated with FVL heterozygosity (OR, 2.19; 95% CI, 1.46–3.27), PT gene mutation heterozygosity (OR, 2.54; 95% CI, 1.52–4.23), MTHFR homozygosity (OR, 1.37; 95% CI, 1.07–1.76), and anticardiolipin antibodies (OR, 2.73; 95% CI, 1.65–4.51).[62] Other investigators showed an increased risk of preeclampsia (OR, 3.21; 95% CI, 1.20–8.58) in patients with acquired and inherited thrombophilias.[49]

FETAL GROWTH RESTRICTION
Acquired Thrombophilia

FGR is most commonly defined as an estimated fetal weight less than the 10th percentile for gestational age.[31] FGR is associated with an increase in fetal and neonatal mortality and morbidity.[63–69] FGR occurs in up to 30% of patients diagnosed with APS.[50,70,71] Some retrospective studies suggest an increased risk of FGR in women with antiphospholipid antibodies in isolation (without the clinical criteria for APS). One study showed a statistically significant 8-fold increased risk in women with lupus anticoagulant.[52] These investigators also found a 6-fold increased rate of FGR[72] when anticardiolipin antibodies were present in the first trimester, which was confirmed by other investigators.[73] In a prospective study, there was no association between increased antiphospholipid antibody levels and FGR.[74]

Inherited Thrombophilia

The association between inherited thrombophilias and FGR has not been well shown. Several investigators have not found that the risk of FGR is higher in women with a thrombophilia.[47,48,75,76] In contrast, some case-control studies have found an association. For example, one study found a significant relationship between FVL as well as PT gene mutation and FGR.[77] One meta-analysis examining the relationship between FGR and FVL and PT gene mutation showed that the associations seen were only in case-control studies and were most likely caused by publication bias.[78] In another meta-analysis and systematic review of case-control studies, there was a significant association between FVL and FGR (OR, 2.7; 95% CI, 1.3–5.5) and PT gene mutation and FGR (OR, 2.5; 95% CI, 1.3–5.0).[79] Although the data are conflicting, there are no well-developed studies that have determined definitive causality.

PLACENTAL ABRUPTION

Some studies have shown a possible association between abruption and thrombophilias. One study found a significant 3-fold increase in the rate of abruption[49]; other investigators reported a 4.7-fold increase in the association of FVL and abruption and a 7.7-fold increase with PT gene mutation.[62] Similarly, it has been reported that placental abruption was more often associated with FVL, heterozygous PT gene mutation, homocysteinemia, PC deficiency, and anticardiolipin IgG antibodies.[45] Prospective studies have failed to show this association.[47,48]

SUMMARY

Thrombophilias, both acquired and inherited, lead to an increased risk of thrombosis during pregnancy and in the postpartum period. The relationship between these disorders and adverse pregnancy outcomes remains controversial. All patients with a personal history of a thrombotic event should be tested for inherited and acquired thrombophilias, noting whether testing can be performed during pregnancy, an acute thrombus, or while on anticoagulation. Given the high incidence of thrombophilia in the population and the low incidence of VTE, universal screening is not cost-effective. Women with acquired thrombophilias seem to be at an increased risk for adverse pregnancy outcomes, but the relationship with inherited thrombophilia is much less certain. With the exception of recurrent pregnancy loss in the setting of APS, there is no clear evidence that thromboprophylaxis during pregnancy improves perinatal outcomes. Until it is definitively shown that thromboprophylaxis prevents recurrent adverse pregnancy outcomes, universal screening should not become standard of care.

REFERENCES

1. Brenner B. Thrombophilia and adverse pregnancy outcome. Obstet Gynecol Clin North Am 2006;33(3):443–56, ix.
2. ACOG educational bulletin. Thromboembolism in pregnancy. Number 234, March 1997. American College of Obstetricians and Gynecologists. Int J Gynaecol Obstet 1997;57(2):209–18.
3. Creasky R, Resnik R, Iams J. Creasy and Resnik's maternal-fetal medicine: principles and practice. 6th edition. Philadelphia: Saunders/Elsevier; 2009.
4. Hellgren M. Hemostasis during normal pregnancy and puerperium. Semin Thromb Hemost 2003;29(2):125–30.
5. Haemostasis and Thrombosis Task Force, British Committee for Standards in Haematology. Investigation and management of heritable thrombophilia. Br J Haematol 2001;114(3):512–28.
6. Marik PE, Plante LA. Venous thromboembolic disease and pregnancy. N Engl J Med 2008;359(19):2025–33.
7. Greer IA. Thrombosis in pregnancy: maternal and fetal issues. Lancet 1999; 353(9160):1258–65.
8. Rosendaal FR. Venous thrombosis: a multicausal disease. Lancet 1999; 353(9159):1167–73.
9. Lockwood CJ. Inherited thrombophilias in pregnant patients: detection and treatment paradigm. Obstet Gynecol 2002;99(2):333–41.
10. Franco RF, Reitsma PH. Genetic risk factors of venous thrombosis. Hum Genet 2001;109(4):369–84.
11. Marlar RA, Neumann A. Neonatal purpura fulminans due to homozygous protein C or protein S deficiencies. Semin Thromb Hemost 1990;16(4):299–309.
12. Zöller B, Dahlbäck B. Linkage between inherited resistance to activated protein C and factor V gene mutation in venous thrombosis. Lancet 1994;343(8912): 1536–8.
13. Voorberg J, Roelse J, Koopman R, et al. Association of idiopathic venous thromboembolism with single point-mutation at Arg506 of factor V. Lancet 1994; 343(8912):1535–6.
14. Gerhardt A, Scharf RE, Beckmann MW, et al. Prothrombin and factor V mutations in women with a history of thrombosis during pregnancy and the puerperium. N Engl J Med 2000;342(6):374–80.
15. Bates SM, Greer IA, Middeldorp S, et al. VTE, thrombophilia, antithrombotic therapy, and pregnancy: antithrombotic therapy and prevention of thrombosis, 9th ed: American College of Chest Physicians evidence-based clinical practice guidelines. Chest 2012;141(2 Suppl):e691S–736.
16. Zotz RB, Gerhardt A, Scharf RE. Inherited thrombophilia and gestational venous thromboembolism. Best Pract Res Clin Haematol 2003;16(2):243–59.
17. Haverkate F, Samama M. Familial dysfibrinogenaemia and thrombophilia. Report on a study of the SSC Subcommittee on fibrinogen. Thromb Haemost 1995;73: 151–61.
18. Carraro P, European Communities Confederation of Clinical Chemistry and Laboratory Medicine, Working Group on Guidelines for Investigation of Disease. Guidelines for the laboratory investigation of inherited thrombophilias. Recommendations for the first level clinical laboratories. Clin Chem Lab Med 2003;41: 382–91.
19. Friederich PW, Sanson BJ, Simioni P, et al. Frequency of pregnancy-related venous thromboembolism in anticoagulant factor-deficient women: implications

for prophylaxis. Ann Intern Med 1996;125:955–60 [Erratum appears in Ann Intern Med 1997;127:1138; 1997;126:835].

20. Vossen CY, Preston FE, Conard J, et al. Hereditary thrombophilia and fetal loss: a prospective follow-up study. J Thromb Haemost 2004;2:592–6.

21. Poort SR, Rosendaal FR, Reitsma PH, et al. A common genetic variation in the 3′-untranslated region of the prothrombin gene is associated with elevated plasma prothrombin levels and an increase in venous thrombosis. Blood 1996; 88(10):3698–703.

22. Foster DC, Yoshitake S, Davie EW. The nucleotide sequence of the gene for human protein C. Proc Natl Acad Sci U S A 1985;82(14):4673–7.

23. Plutzky J, Hoskins JA, Long GL, et al. Evolution and organization of the human protein C gene. Proc Natl Acad Sci U S A 1986;83(3):546–50.

24. Tait RC, Walker ID, Reitsma PH, et al. Prevalence of protein C deficiency in the healthy population. Thromb Haemost 1995;73(1):87–93.

25. Ploos van Amstel JK, van der Zanden AL, Bakker E, et al. Two genes homologous with human protein S cDNA are located on chromosome 3. Thromb Haemost 1987;58(4):982–7.

26. Esmon CT. The protein C anticoagulant pathway. Arterioscler Thromb Vasc Biol 1992;12(2):135–45.

27. Dykes AC, Walker ID, McMahon AD, et al. A study of Protein S antigen levels in 3788 healthy volunteers: influence of age, sex and hormone use, and estimate for prevalence of deficiency state. Br J Haematol 2001;113(3):636–41.

28. Seligsohn U, Lubetsky A. Genetic susceptibility to venous thrombosis. N Engl J Med 2001;344(16):1222–31.

29. MacCallum PK, Cooper JA, Martin J, et al. Associations of protein C and protein S with serum lipid concentrations. Br J Haematol 1998;102(2):609–15.

30. Goodwin AJ, Rosendaal FR, Kottke-Marchant K, et al. A review of the technical, diagnostic, and epidemiologic considerations for protein S assays. Arch Pathol Lab Med 2002;126(11):1349–66.

31. Paidas MJ, Ku DH, Lee M-J, et al. Protein Z, protein S levels are lower in patients with thrombophilia and subsequent pregnancy complications. J Thromb Haemost 2005;3(3):497–501.

32. Egeberg O. Thrombophilia caused by inheritable deficiency of blood antithrombin. Scand J Clin Lab Invest 1965;17:92.

33. Creanga AA, Berg CJ, Syverson C, et al. Pregnancy-related mortality in the United States, 2006-2010. Obstet Gynecol 2015;125(1):5–12.

34. James AH, Jamison MG, Brancazio LR, et al. Venous thromboembolism during pregnancy and the postpartum period: incidence, risk factors, and mortality. Am J Obstet Gynecol 2006;194(5):1311–5.

35. Heit JA, Kobbervig CE, James AH, et al. Trends in the incidence of venous thromboembolism during pregnancy or postpartum: a 30-year population-based study. Ann Intern Med 2005;143(10):697–706.

36. Wu O, Robertson L, Twaddle S, et al. Screening for thrombophilia in high-risk situations: systematic review and cost-effectiveness analysis. The Thrombosis: Risk and Economic Assessment of Thrombophilia Screening (TREATS) study. Health Technol Assess 2006;10(11):1–110.

37. American College of Obstetricians and Gynecologists Women's Health Care Physicians. ACOG practice bulletin no. 138: inherited thrombophilias in pregnancy. Obstet Gynecol 2013;122(3):706–17.

38. Miyakis S, Lockshin MD, Atsumi T, et al. International consensus statement on an update of the classification criteria for definite antiphospholipid syndrome (APS). J Thromb Haemost 2006;4(2):295–306.

39. Oshiro BT, Silver RM, Scott JR, et al. Antiphospholipid antibodies and fetal death. Obstet Gynecol 1996;87(4):489–93.

40. Levine JS, Branch DW, Rauch J. The antiphospholipid syndrome. N Engl J Med 2002;346(10):752–63.

41. Rai P, Rajaram S, Goel N, et al. Oral micronized progesterone for prevention of preterm birth. Int J Gynaecol Obstet 2009;104(1):40–3.

42. Kutteh WH. Antiphospholipid antibody-associated recurrent pregnancy loss: treatment with heparin and low-dose aspirin is superior to low-dose aspirin alone. Am J Obstet Gynecol 1996;174(5):1584–9.

43. Farquharson RG, Quenby S, Greaves M. Antiphospholipid syndrome in pregnancy: a randomized, controlled trial of treatment. Obstet Gynecol 2002;100(3):408–13.

44. Laskin CA, Spitzer KA, Clark CA, et al. Low molecular weight heparin and aspirin for recurrent pregnancy loss: results from the randomized, controlled HepASA trial. J Rheumatol 2009;36(2):279–87.

45. Alfirevic Z, Roberts D, Martlew V. How strong is the association between maternal thrombophilia and adverse pregnancy outcome? A systematic review. Eur J Obstet Gynecol Reprod Biol 2002;101(1):6–14.

46. Rey E, Kahn SR, David M, et al. Thrombophilic disorders and fetal loss: a meta-analysis. Lancet 2003;361(9361):901–8.

47. Silver RM, Zhao Y, Spong CY, et al. Prothrombin gene G20210A mutation and obstetric complications. Obstet Gynecol 2010;115(1):14–20.

48. Dizon-Townson D, Miller C, Sibai B, et al. The relationship of the factor V Leiden mutation and pregnancy outcomes for mother and fetus. Obstet Gynecol 2005;106(3):517–24.

49. Roqué H, Paidas MJ, Funai EF, et al. Maternal thrombophilias are not associated with early pregnancy loss. Thromb Haemost 2004;91(2):290–5.

50. Branch DW, Silver RM, Blackwell JL, et al. Outcome of treated pregnancies in women with antiphospholipid syndrome: an update of the Utah experience. Obstet Gynecol 1992;80(4):614–20.

51. Branch DW, Andres R, Digre KB, et al. The association of antiphospholipid antibodies with severe preeclampsia. Obstet Gynecol 1989;73(4):541–5.

52. Yamada H, Atsumi T, Kobashi G, et al. Antiphospholipid antibodies increase the risk of pregnancy-induced hypertension and adverse pregnancy outcomes. J Reprod Immunol 2009;79(2):188–95.

53. Do Prado AD, Piovesan DM, Staub HL, et al. Association of anticardiolipin antibodies with preeclampsia: a systematic review and meta-analysis. Obstet Gynecol 2010;116(6):1433–43.

54. Abou-Nassar K, Carrier M, Ramsay T, et al. The association between antiphospholipid antibodies and placenta mediated complications: a systematic review and meta-analysis. Thromb Res 2011;128(1):77–85.

55. Currie L, Peek M, McNiven M, et al. Is there an increased maternal-infant prevalence of factor V Leiden in association with severe pre-eclampsia? BJOG 2002;109(2):191–6.

56. Van Pampus MG, Wolf H, Koopman MM, et al. Prothrombin 20210 G: a mutation and factor V Leiden mutation in women with a history of severe preeclampsia and (H)ELLP syndrome. Hypertens Pregnancy 2001;20(3):291–8.

57. Kahn SR, Platt R, McNamara H, et al. Inherited thrombophilia and preeclampsia within a multicenter cohort: The Montreal Preeclampsia Study. Am J Obstet Gynecol 2009;200(2):151.e1–9 [discussion: e1-5].

58. D'Elia AV, Driul L, Giacomello R, et al. Frequency of factor V, prothrombin and methylenetetrahydrofolate reductase gene variants in preeclampsia. Gynecol Obstet Invest 2002;53(2):84–7.

59. Morrison ER, Miedzybrodzka ZH, Campbell DM, et al. Prothrombotic genotypes are not associated with pre-eclampsia and gestational hypertension: results from a large population-based study and systematic review. Thromb Haemost 2002; 87(5):779–85.

60. Livingston JC, Barton JR, Park V, et al. Maternal and fetal inherited thrombophilias are not related to the development of severe preeclampsia. Am J Obstet Gynecol 2001;185(1):153–7.

61. Lin J, August P. Genetic thrombophilias and preeclampsia: a meta-analysis. Obstet Gynecol 2005;105(1):182–92.

62. Robertson L, Wu O, Langhorne P, et al. Thrombophilia in pregnancy: a systematic review. Br J Haematol 2006;132(2):171–96.

63. Kramer MS, Olivier M, McLean FH, et al. Impact of intrauterine growth retardation and body proportionality on fetal and neonatal outcome. Pediatrics 1990;86(5): 707–13.

64. McIntire DD, Bloom SL, Casey BM, et al. Birth weight in relation to morbidity and mortality among newborn infants. N Engl J Med 1999;340(16):1234–8.

65. Barker DJP. Adult consequences of fetal growth restriction. Clin Obstet Gynecol 2006;49(2):270–83.

66. Henriksen T. Foetal nutrition, foetal growth restriction and health later in life. Acta Paediatr Suppl 1999;88(429):4–8.

67. Clausson B, Cnattingius S, Axelsson O. Outcomes of post-term births: the role of fetal growth restriction and malformations. Obstet Gynecol 1999;94(5 Pt 1): 758–62.

68. Pallotto EK, Kilbride HW. Perinatal outcome and later implications of intrauterine growth restriction. Clin Obstet Gynecol 2006;49(2):257–69.

69. Resnik R. Intrauterine growth restriction. Obstet Gynecol 2002;99(3):490–6.

70. Lima F, Khamashta MA, Buchanan NM, et al. A study of sixty pregnancies in patients with the antiphospholipid syndrome. Clin Exp Rheumatol 1996;14(2):131–6.

71. Committee on Practice Bulletins—Obstetrics, American College of Obstetricians and Gynecologists. Practice bulletin no. 132: antiphospholipid syndrome. Obstet Gynecol 2012;120(6):1514–21.

72. Yasuda M, Takakuwa K, Tokunaga A, et al. Prospective studies of the association between anticardiolipin antibody and outcome of pregnancy. Obstet Gynecol 1995;86(4 Pt 1):555–9.

73. Polzin WJ, Kopelman JN, Robinson RD, et al. The association of antiphospholipid antibodies with pregnancies complicated by fetal growth restriction. Obstet Gynecol 1991;78(6):1108–11.

74. Lynch A, Marlar R, Murphy J, et al. Antiphospholipid antibodies in predicting adverse pregnancy outcome. A prospective study. Ann Intern Med 1994; 120(6):470–5.

75. Infante-Rivard C, Rivard G-E, Yotov WV, et al. Absence of association of thrombophilia polymorphisms with intrauterine growth restriction. N Engl J Med 2002; 347(1):19–25.

76. Franchi F, Cetin I, Todros T, et al. Intrauterine growth restriction and genetic predisposition to thrombophilia. Haematologica 2004;89(4):444–9.

77. Verspyck E, Borg JY, Le Cam-Duchez V, et al. Thrombophilia and fetal growth restriction. Eur J Obstet Gynecol Reprod Biol 2004;113(1):36–40.
78. Facco F, You W, Grobman W. Genetic thrombophilias and intrauterine growth restriction: a meta-analysis. Obstet Gynecol 2009;113(6):1206–16.
79. Howley HEA, Walker M, Rodger MA. A systematic review of the association between factor V Leiden or prothrombin gene variant and intrauterine growth restriction. Am J Obstet Gynecol 2005;192(3):694–708.

Sleep Disordered Breathing and Adverse Pregnancy Outcomes

Mary Ashley Cain, MD[a],*, Judette M. Louis, MD, MPH[a,b]

KEYWORDS

- Obstructive sleep apnea • Pregnancy • Preeclampsia • Obesity

KEY POINTS

- Sleep disordered breathing is likely underdiagnosed among women of reproductive age.
- Current guidelines for screening and diagnosis of obstructive sleep apnea follow those of the nonpregnant population.
- Sleep disordered breathing in pregnancy is associated with gestational diabetes, hypertension, and fetal growth abnormalities.
- Limited research exits regarding treatment of sleep disordered breathing in pregnancy.

INTRODUCTION

Sleep disordered breathing (SDB) encompasses a group of disorders characterized by abnormalities in respiration and ventilation occurring during sleep. These disorders range from snoring to the most severe form, obstructive sleep apnea (OSA). A substantial body of evidence shows an association between OSA and SDB and morbidities, including diabetes mellitus, heart disease, and stroke, in the nonpregnant population.[1,2] This article reviews the prevalence, risk factors, diagnosis, associated pregnancy morbidities, and treatment options for SDB among pregnant women.

EPIDEMIOLOGY

An estimated 40 million American have a sleep disorder; of these, 18 million have OSA.[3] Although OSA occurs most often in elderly men, 0.6% to 15% of

Disclosure: The authors have nothing to disclose.
[a] Division of Maternal Fetal Medicine, Department of Obstetrics and Gynecology, University of South Florida Morsani College of Medicine, 2 Tampa General Circle, 6th Floor, Tampa, FL 33606, USA; [b] Department of Community and Family Health, College of Public Health, University of South Florida, 2 Tampa General Circle, 6th Floor, Tampa, FL 33606, USA
* Corresponding author.
E-mail address: mcain@health.usf.edu

Clin Lab Med 36 (2016) 435–446
http://dx.doi.org/10.1016/j.cll.2016.01.001   **labmed.theclinics.com**

reproductive-aged women have OSA.[4,5] Approximately 90% of women with OSA may be undiagnosed.[6] Causes for underdiagnosis in women include a lack of identification by the physician, attribution of symptoms to alternative causes, and a tendency to present with unconventional symptoms of depression and anxiety.[7,8] Several studies show a similar prevalence among pregnant populations. Olivarez and colleagues[9] performed sleep studies on 100 pregnant women at a mean gestational age of 32 weeks, hospitalized for a variety of obstetric and nonobstetric medical complications. The investigators noted a 20% incidence of SDB (apnea hypopnea index [AHI] $\geq$5); mean AHI was 12.2.[9] Louis and colleagues[10] noted an OSA prevalence of 15.4% in a study assessing SDB with ambulatory sleep assessments in 175 obese pregnant women with an average gestational age of 21 weeks. In addition, the prevalence seems to increase with advancing gestational age.[11,12] Pien and colleagues[12] studied 105 subjects with in-laboratory polysomnography (PSG). SDB was present in 10.5% of women in the first trimester (median, 12.1 weeks). By the third trimester (median, 33.6 weeks), the prevalence increased to 26.7%.

RISK FACTORS

Pregnancy-specific risk factors for SDB are ill defined. Prior studies showed an association between obesity and increasing maternal age, which are known risk factors for SDB outside of pregnancy, with SDB in early pregnancy.[11,12] In theory, gestational weight gain may affect the development of SDB in later gestation. Limited studies of SDB across pregnancy did not note any association between gestational weight gain and the development of SDB in the third trimester.[12] At present, because of limited data, providers may use the risk factors noted in the general populations as indicators for screening and testing.

Risk factors for SDB in the general population include[3]:

- Male gender
- Obesity
- Increased neck circumference
- Older age
- African American and Asian race
- Craniofacial abnormalities[3,13]

Differences in craniofacial structure lead to increased risk among specific racial backgrounds. In addition, risk increases as body mass index (BMI), neck circumference, and waist/hip ratio increase.[4]

SCREENING IN PREGNANCY

Recognition and diagnosis of OSA in pregnancy can be difficult. Typical OSA symptoms, including excessive daytime sleepiness, fatigue, and frequent nocturnal wakening, overlap with normal changes of pregnancy. Outside of pregnancy, providers use screening tools such as the Berlin Questionnaire and the Epworth Sleepiness Scale to identify patients at risk for OSA, who require further testing. Because of the high prevalence of excessive daytime sleepiness in pregnancy, these validated questionnaires have not been predictive of SDB in the pregnant population.[14–18] A study using PSG to assess for SDB in the first and third trimesters found maternal weight before pregnancy and maternal age to be the major predictors of SDB risk.[12] Among nonpregnant patients, habitual snoring has good correlation with PSG and may be an important symptom to elicit.[19,20] Despite these studies, no predominant screening strategy for pregnant women exists. In the absence of strong recommendations, risk factors to consider among pregnant patients include:

- Habitual snoring
- Chronic hypertension
- Maternal baseline BMI greater than 25 to 30 kg/m^2
- Advanced maternal age

Despite these challenges, increasing recognition of the disease among reproductive-aged women may lead to improvement in screening and diagnosis. Because of alterations in anatomy and physiology in pregnancy, women at risk for OSA may experience a worsening of symptoms across gestation, which can improve postpartum. A prospective cohort of women undergoing PSG in the first and third trimesters found a significant increase in the mean AHI from the first to the third trimester (2.07 first trimester vs 3.74 third trimester; $P = .009$).[12] The prevalence of OSA also increased from 10.5% in the first trimester to 26.7% in the third trimester.[12] A case control study noted a postpartum improvement in AHI among 10 women who underwent PSG in the late third trimester and again 3 months after delivery.[21]

Physiologic changes during pregnancy that increase risk of OSA:

- Gestational weight gain
- Pharyngeal edema
- Progesterone effect on pharyngeal dilator muscles
- Tracheal shortening
- Abdominal mass loading
- Decreased lung volume
- Nasal congestion

DIAGNOSIS IN PREGNANCY

At present, no specific guidelines for OSA diagnosis among pregnant women exist and providers must use standard guidelines created for the general population. Women suspected of having sleep apnea should be evaluated by a sleep specialist and undergo a sleep-directed history and physical examination and sleep testing.[22] Patients deemed at risk for OSA following a screening history and physical then undergo an overnight sleep study. The gold standard for diagnosis is in-laboratory PSG.[12] In the general population, home monitoring has also been used but there are limitations caused by the poor negative predictive value. The American Academy of Sleep Medicine recommends portable monitoring in only those patients with a high pretest probability of moderate to severe OSA and no comorbid medical conditions.[22] These conditions include cardiac, pulmonary, psychiatric, or neurologic disease and apply to the pregnant patient population.[23] Compared with portable monitors with only 3 channels (**Fig. 1**), in-laboratory PSG records an electroencephalogram, electrooculogram, chin electromyogram, airflow, oxygen saturation, respiratory effort, and electrocardiogram.[24,25] In-laboratory PSG studies are attended by trained specialists who monitor the patient and recordings throughout the study. The patient's AHI is determined using the number of apneas and hypopneas per hour of sleep. An apnea episode occurs when the patient has complete cessation of airflow for greater than 10 seconds; hypopnea occurs with a 50% or more decrease in airflow with a 3% or more decrease in oxygen saturation. Patients with an AHI greater than 15 or greater than 5 in the presence of nonrestorative sleep, excessive daytime sleepiness, snoring, breath holding during sleep, or unintentional sleep during the daytime are given the diagnosis of OSA (**Table 1**).[22]

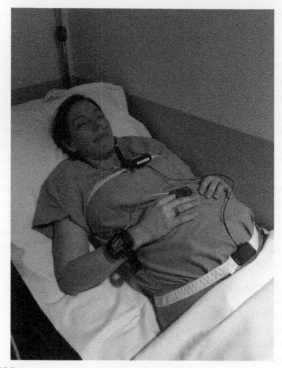

Fig. 1. Portable PSG.

OBSTRUCTIVE SLEEP APNEA AND PREGNANCY MORBIDITY
Potential Mechanisms for Adverse Pregnancy Outcomes

The underlying mechanistic pathways linking sleep disturbances and adverse pregnancy outcomes are likely multifactorial. Notable overlap exists between the biological pathways in SDB and adverse pregnancy outcomes.[26] Recurrent episodes of partial or complete pharyngeal collapse during sleep results in intermittent hypoxia, reoxygenation, sleep fragmentation secondary to repetitive arousals, and a decrease in the total sleep duration.[27] These events result in physiologic consequences that include inducing oxidative stress, sympathetic activity, hypothalamic-pituitary axis activation, inflammation, and alterations in appetite-regulating hormones, which in turn contribute to endothelial and metabolic dysfunction.[28–30] Furthermore, increased oxidative stress is a physiologic trigger for inflammation, insulin resistance, glucose intolerance, and dyslipidemia.[31–33] Sympathetic nervous system and hypothalamic-pituitary axis activation caused by sleep fragmentation, intermittent hypoxia, and intrathoracic pressure changes linked to SDB lead to increased release of the

Table 1 OSA severity	
OSA Severity	**AHI**
Mild	≥5
Moderate	≥15
Severe	≥30

glucocorticoid cortisol.[34–40] Disproportionate sympathetic activation persists into the daytime, leading to increased peripheral vascular reactivity and catecholamine production, blunted baroreflex sensitivity, hindered pancreatic insulin secretion, and altered hepatic glucose release.[33] All of these downstream effects of SDB are linked to the development of hypertension, endothelial dysfunction, impaired glucose metabolism, and pathophysiologic derangements often observed in preeclampsia.[33,41–43] Chronic cortisol secretion also increases susceptibility to insulin resistance and predisposes to the development of gestational diabetes[36,37,44] **(Fig. 2)**.

The role of inflammation is a little more complex. SDB tracks with obesity, a proinflammatory state. SDB-related events are strongly linked with increased systemic inflammation, including increased interleukin-6, tumor necrosis factor, and C-reactive protein levels.[45–51] Increased expression of proinflammatory cytokines may contribute to endothelial dysfunction and metabolic dysregulation.[40,52–54] These mechanistic pathways are also linked to adverse pregnancy outcomes, particularly preeclampsia and fetal growth restriction.[40,52,53,55–57]

Hypertensive Disorders of Pregnancy

The traditional risk factors for hypertensive disease include obesity and increased maternal age, which overlap with some of the risk factors for SDB. However, a substantial body of evidence suggests a link between SDB and pregnancy-related hypertension, with most studies showing a 2-fold increase in the odds of gestational

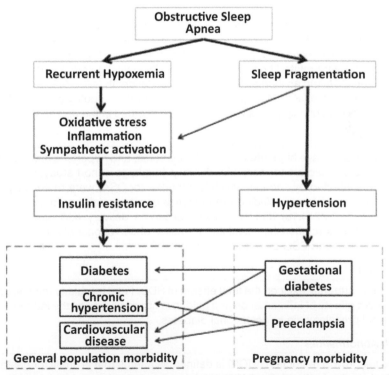

Fig. 2. Mechanisms for the adverse effects of OSA and the implications for future health. (*From* Cain MA, Ricciuti J, Louis JM. Sleep-disordered breathing and future cardiovascular disease risk. Semin Perinatol 2015;39(4):306; with permission.)

hypertension and preeclampsia.[7,10,58,59] In 2 of the largest epidemiologic studies to date, after adjusting for confounding variables, a diagnosis of OSA was associated with preeclampsia with an adjusted odds ratio (aOR) 1.60 (2.16–11.26) and 1.89 (1.67–2.14).[58,60] Although these 2 large studies showed limitations in the quality of data and quantification of SDB exposure and pregnancy outcome assessment, smaller studies using symptoms-based or PSG-diagnosed SDB reported similar findings with a magnitude of 2-fold increased odds of preeclampsia among pregnancies complicated by SDB.[61,62]

Diabetes in Pregnancy

In the general population a well-established relationship exists between SDB and diabetes. Despite the lack of a proven causal link, SDB has been noted to precede the onset of diabetes. In addition, the initiation of continuous positive airway pressure (CPAP) among nonpregnant patients with OSA leads to improved glucose control.[63,64] Prior studies evaluated SDB and diabetes as both outcome and predictor variables. Recent evidence identifies a similar relationship among SDB and gestational diabetes. A systematic review of 5 observational studies showed an increased risk of gestational diabetes among pregnant women with SDB, identified through questionnaires or PSG (aOR, 1.86; 95% confidence interval [CI], 1.30–2.42).[62] A prospective study using longitudinal, objective assessment of SDB noted a dose-response relationship between SDB and gestational diabetes. The rates of gestational diabetes with no SDB, mild SDB, and moderate/severe SDB were 25%, 43%, and 63% respectively.[65]

Severe Maternal Morbidity

An increase in maternal mortality in recent years increased interest in decreasing severe maternal morbidities.[66] Although most studies were underpowered to detect severe morbidity, one examined a large database of hospital discharge data, including 55,781,965 delivery-related hospital discharges. The investigators noted an association between OSA and an increased risk of in-hospital death (aOR, 5.28 [2.42–11.53]), pulmonary embolism (aOR, 4.47 [2.25–8.88]), and cardiomyopathy (aOR, 9.01 [7.47–10.87]).[58] This relationship persisted and was exacerbated in the presence of obesity.

Cesarean Delivery

Women with SDB have high rates of obesity, diabetes, and hypertension. These conditions are all risk factors for cesarean delivery. In a large cohort study, women with pregnancies affected by snoring, which is a marker for OSA, were more likely to undergo cesarean delivery, including both elective cesarean delivery (odds ratio [OR], 2.25; 95% CI, 1.22–4.18) and emergency cesarean delivery (OR, 1.68; 95% CI, 1.22–2.30).[67] This relationship persists in smaller observational studies using both symptom-based and PSG-based diagnosis of SDB.[7,10,18]

Fetal Effects

Limited data currently exist on the fetal effects of SDB. Fetal morbidity may be caused by the direct effects of inflammation and oxidative stress as well as the indirect effects of maternal preeclampsia or gestational diabetes.

Growth Abnormalities

Intrauterine growth restriction (IUGR) is defined as a fetus that is small for gestational age. Most studies further define IUGR as a fetus measuring less than the tenth percentile for gestational age.[68] Prior research links IUGR with increased perinatal morbidity and mortality.[69] The findings of recent retrospective and observational studies are mixed, with some failing to show an association between SDB and poor fetal growth. However, a cumulative assessment of the existing studies of growth restriction suggested that pregnant women with moderate to severe SDB had higher odds of developing fetal growth restriction (OR, 1.44; 95% CI, 1.22–1.71).[70]

A large percentage of research involving growth abnormalities and SDB focuses on growth restriction. In contrast, SDB in pregnancy may also be associated with large-for-gestational-age (LGA) neonates. LGA neonates have higher rates of birth trauma, respiratory morbidity, and short-term and long-term morbidity.[68] One study found more LGA among women with SDB compared with obese and normal-weight controls (17% vs 8% and 2.6%, respectively).[7]

Low birthweight is defined as birthweight less than 2500 g. Both preterm delivery and intrauterine growth restriction can lead to low birthweights. Regardless of the cause, low birthweight is associated with increased short-term and long-term morbidity, and increased health care costs.[68] Among the pooled studies, SDB was associated with low birthweight (unadjusted OR, 1.39; 95% CI, 1.14–1.65).[62] Most studies have not been able to report a difference in birthweight, as a continuous number, among women with and without SDB.[62] Two studies found a statistically significant difference between mean birthweights among women with and without SDB. The SDB-exposed neonates weighed 100 g less than unexposed neonates, which may be of little clinical relevance.[7,17]

Preterm Delivery

Preterm births, occurring before 37 weeks of completed gestation, account for 11.6% of births. These births are responsible for a significant amount of neonatal morbidity and mortality. Preterm birth may be classified as spontaneous in occurrence or medically indicated. Medically indicated preterm births are precipitated by obstetric intervention, usually for maternal or fetal benefit.[68] Large cross-sectional studies of SDB in pregnancy reported an increased risk of preterm delivery.[58,60] Because of the nature of the data, these studies did not differentiate between spontaneous and medically indicated preterm birth. One smaller retrospective study noted an increase in medically indicated preterm delivery associated with preeclampsia among women with SDB.[7] In this study the rate of preterm birth among pregnant women with SDB compared with normal-weight controls was 29.8% versus 12.3% (aOR, 2.6; 95% CI, 1.02–6.6). Most cases of preterm birth were related to preeclampsia.

Miscarriages and Stillbirth

Miscarriage, or spontaneous abortion, involves the loss of a pregnancy, usually within the first 3 months of conception. Risk factors for miscarriage include extremes of age, smoking history, increased BMI, previous miscarriage, hypertension, and diabetes. All of these risk factors overlap with the risk factors for SDB. Limited data exist linking SDB and miscarriage. One retrospective review of 147 premenopausal women, referred to a sleep disorders clinic, noted an association between SDB and number of miscarriages. The investigators noted higher rates of miscarriage among overweight/obese women with SDB, especially those with moderate-severe SDB, compared with women without SDB.[71]

The term stillbirth identifies any fetal death at or beyond 20 weeks of gestation.[68] Recognized risk factors for stillbirth overlap with SDB risk factors and include advancing age, African American race, smoking, maternal medical conditions such as diabetes and hypertension, obesity, growth restriction, and previous adverse pregnancy outcomes.[72] Although this overlap lends biological plausibility, there are no large-scale studies examining an association between SDB and stillbirth. This lack of data may be caused by the infrequent occurrence of stillbirth and the large number that would be needed to examine the association.

TREATMENT

Among the nonpregnant population with OSA, first-line treatment involves the use of a CPAP device worn while sleeping. The use of CPAP decreases the number of apneic events and improves the recurrent hypoxia and sleep fragmentation. Prospective studies note a decrease in hypertension and neurocognitive performance among patients with OSA treated with CPAP compared with placebo.[73–75] Although effective, patient CPAP compliance remains low. Hypertension and OSA severity are patient factors associated with improved compliance.[76,77] Alternative treatments, including surgery or lifestyle modification for obesity, oral appliances, and in limited cases upper airway reconstructive surgery, have not proved as effective as CPAP.[78]

Limited information exists on the utility of CPAP in preventing pregnancy morbidity among patients with OSA. A small randomized controlled trial including 16 hypertensive pregnant patients with excessive snoring treated with CPAP versus placebo noted a decrease in blood pressure among patients in the treatment group.[79] As data regarding pregnancy morbidity and OSA increase, the need for research into effective treatment strategies grows.

SUMMARY

OSA in reproductive-aged women may be difficult to recognize and diagnose. Increasing evidence notes a relationship between OSA and pregnancy morbidities. Consistent evidence indicates an increase in hypertensive disorders of pregnancy among women who have OSA. These findings persist even after controlling for obesity. Future studies are needed to evaluate effective treatment strategies designed to decrease pregnancy morbidities.

REFERENCES

1. Alam I, Lewis K, Stephens JW, et al. Obesity, metabolic syndrome and sleep apnoea: all pro-inflammatory states. Obes Rev 2007;8(2):119–27.

2. Jordan AS, McSharry DG, Malhotra A. Adult obstructive sleep apnoea. Lancet 2014;383(9918):736–47.

3. Young T, Peppard PE, Gottlieb DJ. Epidemiology of obstructive sleep apnea: a population health perspective. Am J Respir Crit Care Med 2002;165(9):1217–39.

4. Young T, Skatrud J, Peppard PE. Risk factors for obstructive sleep apnea in adults. JAMA 2004;291(16):2013–6.

5. Young T, Palta M, Dempsey J, et al. The occurrence of sleep-disordered breathing among middle-aged adults. N Engl J Med 1993;328(17):1230–5.

6. Young T, Evans L, Finn L, et al. Estimation of the clinically diagnosed proportion of sleep apnea syndrome in middle-aged men and women. Sleep 1997;20(9): 705–6.

7. Louis JM, Auckley D, Sokol RJ, et al. Maternal and neonatal morbidities associated with obstructive sleep apnea complicating pregnancy. Am J Obstet Gynecol 2010;202(3):261.e1–5.

8. Pillar G, Lavie P. Psychiatric symptoms in sleep apnea syndrome: effects of gender and respiratory disturbance index. Chest 1998;114(3):697–703.

9. Olivarez SA, Maheshwari B, McCarthy M, et al. Prospective trial on obstructive sleep apnea in pregnancy and fetal heart rate monitoring. Am J Obstet Gynecol 2010;202(6):552.e1–7.

10. Louis J, Auckley D, Miladinovic B, et al. Perinatal outcomes associated with obstructive sleep apnea in obese pregnant women. Obstet Gynecol 2012; 120(5):1085–92.

11. Facco FL, Ouyang DW, Zee PC, et al. Sleep disordered breathing in a high-risk cohort prevalence and severity across pregnancy. Am J Perinatol 2014;31(10): 899–904.

12. Pien GW, Pack AI, Jackson N, et al. Risk factors for sleep-disordered breathing in pregnancy. Thorax 2014;69(4):371–7.

13. Redline S, Tishler PV, Hans MG, et al. Racial differences in sleep-disordered breathing in African-Americans and Caucasians. Am J Respir Crit Care Med 1997;155(1):186–92.

14. Antony KM, Agrawal A, Arndt ME, et al. Obstructive sleep apnea in pregnancy: reliability of prevalence and prediction estimates. J Perinatol 2014;34(8):587–93.

15. Facco FL, Ouyang DW, Zee PC, et al. Development of a pregnancy-specific screening tool for sleep apnea. J Clin Sleep Med 2012;8(4):389–94.

16. Netzer NC, Stoohs RA, Netzer CM, et al. Using the Berlin Questionnaire to identify patients at risk for the sleep apnea syndrome. Ann Intern Med 1999;131(7): 485–91.

17. Higgins N, Leong E, Park CS, et al. The Berlin Questionnaire for assessment of sleep disordered breathing risk in parturients and non-pregnant women. Int J Obstet Anesth 2011;20(1):22–5.

18. Bourjeily G, Raker CA, Chalhoub M, et al. Pregnancy and fetal outcomes of symptoms of sleep-disordered breathing. Eur Respir J 2010;36(4):849–55.

19. Bliwise DL, Nekich JC, Dement WC. Relative validity of self-reported snoring as a symptom of sleep apnea in a sleep clinic population. Chest 1991;99(3):600–8.

20. Nieto FJ, Young TB, Lind BK, et al. Association of sleep-disordered breathing, sleep apnea, and hypertension in a large community-based study. Sleep Heart Health Study. JAMA 2000;283(14):1829–36.

21. Edwards N, Blyton DM, Hennessy A, et al. Severity of sleep-disordered breathing improves following parturition. Sleep 2005;28(6):737–41.

22. Epstein LJ, Kristo D, Strollo PJ Jr, et al. Clinical guideline for the evaluation, management and long-term care of obstructive sleep apnea in adults. J Clin Sleep Med 2009;5(3):263–76.

23. Collop N, Anderson WM, Boehlecke B, et al. Clinical guidelines for the use of unattended portable monitors in the diagnosis of obstructive sleep apnea in adult patients. J Clin Sleep Med 2007;3(7):737–47.

24. Whittle AT, Finch SP, Mortimore IL, et al. Use of home sleep studies for diagnosis of the sleep apnoea/hypopnoea syndrome. Thorax 1997;52(12):1068–73.

25. Boyer S, Kapur V. Role of portable sleep studies for diagnosis of obstructive sleep apnea. Curr Opin Pulm Med 2003;9(6):465–70.

26. Dempsey JA, Veasey SC, Morgan BJ, et al. Pathophysiology of sleep apnea. Physiol Rev 2010;90(1):47–112.

27. Polotsky VY, Rubin AE, Balbir A, et al. Intermittent hypoxia causes REM sleep deficits and decreases EEG delta power in NREM sleep in the C57BL/6J mouse. Sleep Med 2006;7(1):7–16.

28. Ryan S, Taylor CT, McNicholas WT. Selective activation of inflammatory pathways by intermittent hypoxia in obstructive sleep apnea syndrome. Circulation 2005; 112(17):2660–7.

29. Narkiewicz K, Somers VK. Sympathetic nerve activity in obstructive sleep apnoea. Acta Physiol Scand 2003;177(3):385–90.

30. Cho JG, Witting PK, Verma M, et al. Tissue vibration induces carotid artery endothelial dysfunction: a mechanism linking snoring and carotid atherosclerosis? Sleep 2011;34(6):751–7.

31. Xu J, Long YS, Gozal D, et al. Beta-cell death and proliferation after intermittent hypoxia: role of oxidative stress. Free Radic Biol Med 2009;46:783–90.

32. Gozal D, Reeves SR, Row BW, et al. Respiratory effects of gestational intermittent hypoxia in the developing rat. Am J Respir Crit Care Med 2003;167(11):1540–7.

33. Levy P, Ryan S, Oldenburg O, et al. Sleep apnoea and the heart. Eur Respir Rev 2013;22:333–52.

34. Qiu C, Enquobahrie D, Frederick IO, et al. Glucose intolerance and gestational diabetes risk in relation to sleep duration and snoring during pregnancy: a pilot study. BMC Womens Health 2010;10(17):2–9.

35. Tamisier R, Pepin JL, Remy J, et al. 14 nights of intermittent hypoxia elevate daytime blood pressure and sympathetic activity in healthy humans. Eur Respir J 2011;37(1):119–28.

36. Szelenyi J, Vizi ES. The catecholamine cytokine balance: interaction between the brain and the immune system. Ann N Y Acad Sci 2007;1113:311–24.

37. Stamatakis KA, Punjabi NM. Effects of sleep fragmentation on glucose metabolism in normal subjects. Chest 2010;137(1):95–101.

38. Steiger A. Sleep and the hypothalamo-pituitary-adrenocortical system. Sleep Med Rev 2002;6(2):125–38.

39. Gozal D, Kheirandish-Gozal L. Cardiovascular morbidity in obstructive sleep apnea: oxidative stress, inflammation, and much more. Am J Respir Crit Care Med 2008;177(4):369–75.

40. Reutrakul S, van Cauter E. Interactions between sleep, circadian function, and glucose metabolism: implications for risk and severity of diabetes. Ann N Y Acad Sci 2014;1311:1–23.

41. Blyton DM, Sullivan CE, Edwards N. Reduced nocturnal cardiac output associated with preeclampsia is minimized with the use of nocturnal nasal CPAP. Sleep 2004;27(1):79–84.

42. Edwards N, Blyton DM, Kirjavainen T, et al. Nasal continuous positive airway pressure reduces sleep-induced blood pressure increments in preeclampsia. Am J Respir Crit Care Med 2000;162(1):252–7.

43. Edwards N, Blyton DM, Kirjavainen TT, et al. Hemodynamic responses to obstructive respiratory events during sleep are augmented in women with preeclampsia. Am J Hypertens 2001;14(11 Pt 1):1090–5.

44. Venihaki M, Dikkes P, Carrigan A, et al. Corticotropin-releasing hormone regulates IL-6 expression during inflammation. J Clin Invest 2001;108(8):1159–66.

45. Okun ML, Coussons-Read ME. Sleep disruption during pregnancy: how does it influence serum cytokines? J Reprod Immunol 2007;73(2):158–65.

46. Prather AA, Epel ES, Cohen BE, et al. Gender differences in the prospective associations of self-reported sleep quality with biomarkers of systemic inflammation and coagulation: findings from the Heart and Soul Study. J Psychiatr Res 2013; 47(9):1228–35.

47. Kaushal N, Ramesh V, Gozal D. TNF-alpha and temporal changes in sleep architecture in mice exposed to sleep fragmentation. PLoS One 2012;7(9):e45610.

48. Rosa Neto JC, Lira FS, Venancio DP, et al. Sleep deprivation affects inflammatory marker expression in adipose tissue. Lipids Health Dis 2010;9:125.

49. Irwin MR, Carrillo C, Olmstead R. Sleep loss activates cellular markers of inflammation: sex differences. Brain Behav Immun 2010;24(1):54–7.
50. Thomas KS, Motivala S, Olmstead R, et al. Sleep depth and fatigue: role of cellular inflammatory activation. Brain Behav Immun 2011;25(1):53–8.
51. Altman NG, Izci-Balserak B, Schopfer E, et al. Sleep duration versus sleep insufficiency as predictors of cardiometabolic health outcomes. Sleep Med 2012; 13(10):1261–70.
52. Facco FL, Lappen J, Lim C, et al. Preeclampsia and sleep-disordered breathing: a case-control study. Pregnancy Hypertens 2013;3(2):133–9.
53. Izci-Balserak B, Pien GW. Sleep-disordered breathing and pregnancy: potential mechanisms and evidence for maternal and fetal morbidity. Curr Opin Pulm Med 2010;16(6):574–82.
54. Izci-Balserak B, Pien GW. The relationship and potential mechanistic pathways between sleep disturbances and maternal Hyperglycemia. Curr Diab Rep 2014;14:459.
55. Okun ML, Schetter CD, Glynn LM. Poor sleep quality is associated with preterm birth. Sleep 2011;34(11):1493–8.
56. Jelic S, Padeletti M, Kawut SM, et al. Inflammation, oxidative stress, and repair capacity of the vascular endothelium in obstructive sleep apnea. Circulation 2008;117(17):2270–8.
57. Bourjeily G, Barbara N, Larson L, et al. Clinical manifestations of obstructive sleep apnoea in pregnancy: more than snoring and witnessed apnoeas. J Obstet Gynaecol 2012;32:434–8.
58. Louis JM, Mogos MF, Salemi JL, et al. Obstructive sleep apnea and severe maternal-infant morbidity/mortality in the United States, 1998-2009. Sleep 2014; 37(5):843–9.
59. O'Brien LM, Bullough AS, Owusu JT, et al. Pregnancy-onset habitual snoring, gestational hypertension, and preeclampsia: prospective cohort study. Am J Obstet Gynecol 2012;207(6):487.e1–9.
60. Chen Y-H, Kang J-H, Lin C-C, et al. Obstructive sleep apnea and the risk of adverse pregnancy outcomes. Am J Obstet Gynecol 2012;206(2):136.e1–5.
61. Venkata C, Venkateshiah SB. Sleep-disordered breathing during pregnancy. J Am Board Fam Med 2009;22(2):158–68.
62. Pamidi S, Pinto LM, Marc I, et al. Maternal sleep-disordered breathing and adverse pregnancy outcomes: a systematic review and metaanalysis. Am J Obstet Gynecol 2014;210(1):52.e1–14.
63. Lévy P, Bonsignore MR, Eckel J. Sleep, sleep-disordered breathing and metabolic consequences. Eur Respir J 2009;34(1):243–60.
64. Steiropoulos P, Papanas N, Nena E, et al. Continuous positive airway pressure treatment in patients with sleep apnoea: does it really improve glucose metabolism? Curr Diabetes Rev 2010;6(3):156–66.
65. Facco FL, Ouyang DW, Zee PC, et al. Implications of sleep-disordered breathing in pregnancy. Am J Obstet Gynecol 2013;210(6):559.e1–6.
66. Berg CJ, Callaghan WM, Syverson C, et al. Pregnancy-related mortality in the United States, 1998 to 2005. Obstet Gynecol 2010;116(6):1302–9.
67. O'Brien LM, Bullough AS, Owusu JT, et al. Snoring during pregnancy and delivery outcomes: a cohort study. Sleep 2012;36(11):1625–32.
68. Dashe JS. Williams Obstetrics. New York: McGraw-Hill Education; 2014.
69. American College of Obstetricians and Gynecologists. ACOG practice bulletin no. 134: fetal growth restriction. Obstet Gynecol 2013;121(5):1122–33.

70. Ding X-X, Wu Y-L, Xu S-J, et al. A systematic review and quantitative assessment of sleep-disordered breathing during pregnancy and perinatal outcomes. Sleep Breath 2014;18:1–11.
71. Lee EK, Gutcher ST, Douglass AB. Is sleep-disordered breathing associated with miscarriages? An emerging hypothesis. Med Hypotheses 2014;82(4):481–5.
72. Aune D, Saugstad O, Henriksen T, et al. Maternal body mass index and the risk of fetal death, stillbirth, and infant death: a systematic review and meta-analysis. JAMA 2014;311(15):1536–46.
73. Hack M, Davies RJ, Mullins R, et al. Randomised prospective parallel trial of therapeutic versus subtherapeutic nasal continuous positive airway pressure on simulated steering performance in patients with obstructive sleep apnoea. Thorax 2000;55(3):224–31.
74. Faccenda JF, Mackay TW, Boon NA, et al. Randomized placebo-controlled trial of continuous positive airway pressure on blood pressure in the sleep apnea-hypopnea syndrome. Am J Respir Crit Care Med 2001;163(2):344–8.
75. Haentjens P, Van Meerhaeghe A, Moscariello A, et al. The impact of continuous positive airway pressure on blood pressure in patients with obstructive sleep apnea syndrome: evidence from a meta-analysis of placebo-controlled randomized trials. Arch Intern Med 2007;167(8):757–64.
76. Campos-Rodriguez F, Martinez-Alonso M, Sanchez-de-la-Torre M, et al. Long-term adherence to continuous positive airway pressure therapy in non-sleepy sleep apnea patients. Sleep Med 2016;17:1–6.
77. Hoy CJ, Vennelle M, Kingshott RN, et al. Can intensive support improve continuous positive airway pressure use in patients with the sleep apnea/hypopnea syndrome? Am J Respir Crit Care Med 1999;159(4 Pt 1):1096–100.
78. Malhotra A, White DP. Obstructive sleep apnoea. Lancet 2002;360(9328):237–45.
79. Poyares D, Guilleminault C, Hachul H, et al. Pre-eclampsia and nasal CPAP: part 2. Hypertension during pregnancy, chronic snoring, and early nasal CPAP intervention. Sleep Med 2007;9(1):15–21.

Printed and bound by CPI Group (UK) Ltd, Croydon, CR0 4YY

07/10/2024

01040506-0004